Emerging Trends in Complications Associated with SARS-CoV-2 Infection

Emerging Trends in Complications Associated with SARS-CoV-2 Infection

Editors

Elena Cecilia Rosca
Amalia Cornea

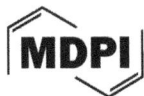

Basel • Beijing • Wuhan • Barcelona • Belgrade • Novi Sad • Cluj • Manchester

Editors

Elena Cecilia Rosca
Department of Neurology
Victor Babes University of
Medicine and Pharmacy
Timisoara
Romania

Amalia Cornea
Department of Neurology
Victor Babes University of
Medicine and Pharmacy
Timisoara
Romania

Editorial Office
MDPI
St. Alban-Anlage 66
4052 Basel, Switzerland

This is a reprint of articles from the Special Issue published online in the open access journal *Biomedicines* (ISSN 2227-9059) (available at: www.mdpi.com/journal/biomedicines/special_issues/ GAW108L704).

For citation purposes, cite each article independently as indicated on the article page online and as indicated below:

Lastname, A.A.; Lastname, B.B. Article Title. *Journal Name* **Year**, *Volume Number*, Page Range.

ISBN 978-3-7258-0118-3 (Hbk)
ISBN 978-3-7258-0117-6 (PDF)
doi.org/10.3390/books978-3-7258-0117-6

© 2024 by the authors. Articles in this book are Open Access and distributed under the Creative Commons Attribution (CC BY) license. The book as a whole is distributed by MDPI under the terms and conditions of the Creative Commons Attribution-NonCommercial-NoDerivs (CC BY-NC-ND) license.

Contents

Preface vii

Elena Cecilia Rosca, Amalia Cornea and Mihaela Simu
Emerging Trends in Complications Associated with SARS-CoV-2 Infection
Reprinted from: *Biomedicines* 2023, 12, 4, doi:10.3390/biomedicines12010004 1

Vladimir Zdravković, ore Stevanović, Neda Ćićarić, Nemanja Zdravković, Ivan Čekerevac and Mina Poskurica et al.
Anthropometric Measurements and Admission Parameters as Predictors of Acute Respiratory Distress Syndrome in Hospitalized COVID-19 Patients
Reprinted from: *Biomedicines* 2023, 11, 1199, doi:10.3390/biomedicines11041199 6

Luana Orlando, Gianluca Bagnato, Carmelo Ioppolo, Maria Stella Franzè, Maria Perticone and Antonio Giovanni Versace et al.
Natural Course of COVID-19 and Independent Predictors of Mortality
Reprinted from: *Biomedicines* 2023, 11, 939, doi:10.3390/biomedicines11030939 19

Jose Iglesias, Andrew Vassallo, Justin Ilagan, Song Peng Ang, Ndausung Udongwo and Anton Mararenko et al.
Acute Kidney Injury Associated with Severe SARS-CoV-2 Infection: Risk Factors for Morbidity and Mortality and a Potential Benefit of Combined Therapy with Tocilizumab and Corticosteroids
Reprinted from: *Biomedicines* 2023, 11, 845, doi:10.3390/biomedicines11030845 28

Thomas McDonnell, Henry H. L. Wu, Philip A. Kalra and Rajkumar Chinnadurai
COVID-19 in Elderly Patients Receiving Haemodialysis: A Current Review
Reprinted from: *Biomedicines* 2023, 11, 926, doi:10.3390/biomedicines11030926 48

Giuseppe Regolisti, Paola Rebora, Giuseppe Occhino, Giulia Lieti, Giulio Molon and Alessandro Maloberti et al.
Elevated Serum Urea-to-Creatinine Ratio and In-Hospital Death in Patients with Hyponatremia Hospitalized for COVID-19
Reprinted from: *Biomedicines* 2023, 11, 1555, doi:10.3390/biomedicines11061555 65

Francesco Cei, Ludia Chiarugi, Simona Brancati, Silvia Dolenti, Maria Silvia Montini and Matteo Rosselli et al.
Clinical and Personal Predictors of Helmet-CPAP Use and Failure in Patients Firstly Admitted to Regular Medical Wards with COVID-19-Related Acute Respiratory Distress Syndrome (hCPAP-f Study)
Reprinted from: *Biomedicines* 2023, 11, 207, doi:10.3390/biomedicines11010207 79

Daniel Duda-Seiman, Nilima Rajpal Kundnani, Daniela Dugaci, Dana Emilia Man, Dana Velimirovici and Simona Ruxanda Dragan
COVID-19 Related Myocarditis and Myositis in a Patient with Undiagnosed Antisynthetase Syndrome
Reprinted from: *Biomedicines* 2022, 11, 95, doi:10.3390/biomedicines11010095 95

Arianna Di Stadio, Elena Cantone, Pietro De Luca, Claudio Di Nola, Eva A. Massimilla and Giovanni Motta et al.
Parosmia COVID-19 Related Treated by a Combination of Olfactory Training and Ultramicronized PEA-LUT: A Prospective Randomized Controlled Trial
Reprinted from: *Biomedicines* 2023, 11, 1109, doi:10.3390/biomedicines11041109 102

Amalia Cornea, Irina Lata, Mihaela Simu and Elena Cecilia Rosca
Parsonage-Turner Syndrome Following SARS-CoV-2 Infection: A Systematic Review
Reprinted from: *Biomedicines* **2023**, *11*, 837, doi:10.3390/biomedicines11030837 . . . . **112**

Chiara Lauri, Giuseppe Campagna, Andor W. J. M. Glaudemans, Riemer H. J. A. Slart, Bram van Leer and Janesh Pillay et al.
SARS-CoV-2 Affects Thyroid and Adrenal Glands: An ^{18}F-FDG PET/CT Study
Reprinted from: *Biomedicines* **2023**, *11*, 2899, doi:10.3390/biomedicines11112899 . . . . **129**

Célia Regina Malveste Ito, André Luís Elias Moreira, Paulo Alex Neves da Silva, Mônica de Oliveira Santos, Adailton Pereira dos Santos and Geovana Sôffa Rézio et al.
Viral Coinfection of Children Hospitalized with Severe Acute Respiratory Infections during COVID-19 Pandemic
Reprinted from: *Biomedicines* **2023**, *11*, 1402, doi:10.3390/biomedicines11051402 . . . . **143**

Ionela Maniu, George Constantin Maniu, Elisabeta Antonescu, Lavinia Duica, Nicolae Grigore and Maria Totan
SARS-CoV-2 Antibody Responses in Pediatric Patients: A Bibliometric Analysis
Reprinted from: *Biomedicines* **2023**, *11*, 1455, doi:10.3390/biomedicines11051455 . . . . **158**

Preface

Coronavirus disease 2019 (COVID-19) is a serious respiratory disease that results from infection with severe acute respiratory syndrome coronavirus 2 (SARS-COV-2). Although several vaccines have been developed and programs implemented globally, patients may present various complications, including some that are life-threatening.

Different studies have shown several potential acute and chronic complications in patients with COVID-19. The spectrum of acute complications ranges from respiratory failure to cardiac and cardiovascular injury, liver and renal disorders, neurologic manifestations, secondary infections, and coinfections, as well as disseminated intravascular coagulation.

Unfortunately, COVID-19 is not only a short-term infection; patients may also present with long-term complications. Post-COVID-19 conditions are found more often after severe illness, but any patient may experience long COVID-19, even those who have mild illness or no symptoms.

Also, due to the intrinsic characteristics of SARS-CoV-2 infection, the elderly and patients with certain medical conditions have been demonstrated to be particularly at risk for various complications.

At present, our research critically analyzes and discusses current knowledge on the clinical characteristics of SARS-CoV-2 infection, focusing on acute and long-term complications.

Elena Cecilia Rosca and Amalia Cornea
Editors

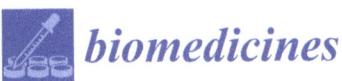

Editorial

Emerging Trends in Complications Associated with SARS-CoV-2 Infection

Elena Cecilia Rosca [1,2,*], Amalia Cornea [1,2] and Mihaela Simu [1,2]

1 Department of Neurology, Victor Babes University of Medicine and Pharmacy Timisoara, Eftimie Murgu Sq. no. 2, 300041 Timisoara, Romania; amalia.cornea@yahoo.com (A.C.); mihaelasimu6713@gmail.com (M.S.)
2 Department of Neurology, Clinical Emergency County Hospital Timisoara, Bd. Iosif Bulbuca no. 10, 300736 Timisoara, Romania
* Correspondence: roscacecilia@yahoo.com; Tel.: +40-746-173-794

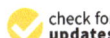

Citation: Rosca, E.C.; Cornea, A.; Simu, M. Emerging Trends in Complications Associated with SARS-CoV-2 Infection. *Biomedicines* **2024**, *12*, 4. https://doi.org/10.3390/biomedicines12010004

Received: 5 December 2023
Accepted: 14 December 2023
Published: 19 December 2023

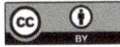

Copyright: © 2023 by the authors. Licensee MDPI, Basel, Switzerland. This article is an open access article distributed under the terms and conditions of the Creative Commons Attribution (CC BY) license (https:// creativecommons.org/licenses/by/ 4.0/).

The coronavirus disease 2019 (COVID-19) pandemic has presented a remarkable challenge to global health, sparking a surge in research aimed at understanding the multifaceted impacts of the virus. COVID-19 is a severe respiratory disease caused by severe acute respiratory syndrome coronavirus 2 (SARS-CoV-2). Despite the development of various vaccines and global programs, some patients may experience life-threatening complications. The acute complications can range from respiratory failure to cardiac and cardiovascular injury, liver and renal disorders, neurologic manifestations, secondary infections, coinfections, and disseminated intravascular coagulation. However, COVID-19 is not only a short-term infection, but can also present long-term complications. Post-COVID-19 conditions are more common after severe illness, but any patient can experience long COVID, even those with mild or no symptoms.

Recent studies have delved into diverse aspects of the impact of the virus, shedding light on its metabolic, cardiovascular, pediatric, and neurological dimensions.

Acute respiratory distress syndrome (ARDS) is more common than initially thought, with 10% of intensive care units patients and 23% of mechanically ventilated patients meeting the criteria [1]. Hospital mortality rates range from 35 to 45%, with a 31% mortality rate even in rapidly resolved cases [2]. The COVID-19 pandemic has highlighted this critical care condition [3]. Among ARDS predictors in hospitalized COVID-19 patients, body mass index (BMI), body fat percentage (BF%), and visceral fat (VF) are significant characteristics, with obesity emerging as a crucial risk factor for ARDS. Additionally, admission predictors of ARDS have been delineated: having a very high BMI, $SaO_2 < 87.5$, $IL\text{-}6 > 59.75$, a low lymphocyte count, being of female sex, and aged <68.5. Obesity was found to be a significant risk factor for ARDS clinical deterioration. These findings support the need for targeted interventions in obese patients to mitigate the risk of ARDS [4].

Prognostic markers also include the evaluation of N-terminal pro-brain natriuretic peptide (NT-pro-BNP) [5]. Studies have revealed that NT-pro-BNP levels and other clinical parameters are independently associated with in-hospital mortality [6,7]. Furthermore, mortality has been reported to be increased in patients of older age, with a lower GCS and PaO_2/FiO_2 ratio, elevated D-dimer values, INR, creatinine values, and shorter PT. They showed an increased frequency of heart failure and higher NT-pro-BNP values. Multivariable logistic regression analysis demonstrated that higher NT-pro-BNP values and lower PT and PaO_2/FiO_2 at admission were independent predictors of mortality during hospitalization. Although further longitudinal studies are needed in order to confirm these findings, the authors underscore the significance of monitoring NT-pro-BNP levels in COVID-19 pneumonia patients to identify those at highest risk [7].

A common complication in COVID-19 patients is acute kidney injury (AKI) [8], with older age, higher admission serum creatinine, an elevated Sequential Organ Failure Assessment (SOFA) score, elevated D-dimer, elevated C-reactive protein (CRP) on day 2, mechanical ventilation, vasopressor requirement, and azithromycin usage being significant risk factors [9]. However, the combined use of Tocilizumab and corticosteroids has been independently associated with reduced AKI risk. Therefore, the early administration of anti-inflammatory agents may improve clinical outcomes, and anti-inflammatory agents should be considered when managing COVID-19-associated AKI. Nonetheless, the association of AKI with the usage of common anti-COVID-19 drugs (e.g., remdesivir, tocilizumab, and lopinavir/ritonavir) should be further investigated [10], and further research is required to assess the risks and benefits of Tocilizumab treatment in critically ill COVID-19 patients with renal impairment [11].

The COVID-19 pandemic has highlighted high-risk groups for poor COVID-19 outcomes [12], including elderly patients receiving hemodialysis, with factors such as age, immunosenescence, and increased exposure to infection sources influencing COVID-19 incidence, severity, and mortality. Preventative measures such as regular screening and vaccination programs have been reported to be crucial to reducing COVID-19 cases and complications, especially for elderly hemodialysis patients. The pandemic has led to the development of medications for treating viral and inflammatory diseases, but elderly hemodialysis patients have been underrepresented in many trials. Nonetheless, contemporary treatments for COVID-19 in this population, with an up-to-date guide, are now available [13].

Shifting the focus to another critical aspect, the elevated serum urea-to-creatinine ratio (UCR) emerges as a potential proxy for hypovolemia, with a 5-unit increase linked to an 8% rise in all-cause mortality. Notably, patients with a baseline UCR > 40 face higher odds of in-hospital death when experiencing > 10 mmol/L increases in serum sodium within the first week [14]. These findings underscore the importance of monitoring sodium levels and implementing targeted interventions for at-risk patients [15].

The COVID-19 pandemic has led to various levels of prevalence and geographical areas of ARDS in hospitalized patients, with unclear optimal respiratory support and high mortality rates due to early intubation experiences and the lack of international guidelines for noninvasive modalities. Numerous studies have attempted to compare supplemental high-flow nasal cannula (HFNC) oxygen and normal oxygen therapy (NIV) in COVID-19 patients, with inconclusive results [16,17]. However, other researchers have evaluated the use and success rate of helmet continuous positive airway pressure (hCPAP) in regular medical wards, offering a tailored approach for COVID-19-associated ARDS, with a computed hCPAP-f Score emerging as a valuable tool for predicting hCPAP failure, offering a nuanced approach to patient management. Factors associated with hCPAP use include a PaO_2/FiO_2 ratio < 270, IL-6 serum levels over 46 pg/mL, AST > 33 U/L, LDH > 570 U/L, age > 78 years, and neuropsychiatric conditions. The failure of hCPAP was associated with being of male sex, polypharmacotherapy, a platelet count < 180 × 109/L, and a PaO2/FiO2 ratio < 240 [18].

The clinical presentation of SARS-CoV-2 varies [19], with respiratory tract infections and multi-organ damage being common findings. Proper investigation is crucial due to the high risk of systemic inflammation, such as myositis and myocarditis, which can lead to fatal outcomes. Among the atypical presentations of COVID-19, myocarditis, mimicking autoimmune disease, necessitates further exploration into the autoimmune aspects of COVID-19 [20].

Although parosmia was a previously known disorder with limited clinical interventions, it is only since the COVID-19 epidemic that researchers have had to deal with an ever-increasing number of patients [21], contributing to an expansion of knowledge and innovative techniques [22]. For example, researchers have confirmed the efficacy of combining ultramicronized palmitoylethanolamide and Luteolin (umPEA-LUT) with olfactory training as a therapy for COVID-19-related quantitative smell alteration, emphasizing the importance of addressing both the central and peripheral aspects of olfactory dysfunction [23].

Recently, at least 74 different clinical manifestations were demonstrated to be associated with COVID-19 [19]. Parsonage–Turner syndrome (PTS), an inflammatory disorder of the brachial plexus with immune-mediated causes, was also reported following SARS-CoV-2 infection. A systematic review revealed 26 cases of PTS in patients who had previously contracted COVID-19 [24]. The spectrum was heterogeneous, with 93.8% experiencing severe pain, 80.8% suffering motor deficit, and 53.8% undergoing muscle wasting. Paresthesia was noted in 46.2% of PTS individuals, and sensory loss in 34.6%. This review emphasizes the need for a high index of suspicion for PTS and underscores the necessity for standardized investigation and reporting protocols [24].

SARS-CoV-2 does not show selective tropism to the respiratory system; it has widespread effects on many tissues, including endocrine gland impairment [25,26]. Recent research has examined the activity of the thyroid and adrenal glands through 18F-FDG PET/CT scans, revealing a persistent low 18F-FDG uptake in adrenal glands, suggesting chronic hypofunction. Conversely, the thyroid's metabolic activity, initially comparable to normal subjects, exhibited an intriguing shift post recovery, hinting at the onset of inflammatory thyroiditis. These observations advocate for heightened vigilance regarding the pituitary–adrenal axis and thyroid functionality in COVID-19 patients during infection and recovery [27].

Regarding pediatric cases, researchers have also investigated the prevalence of respiratory viruses and their coinfections in children with severe respiratory infections (SARIs) [28]. The five most frequent coinfections identified were human rhinovirus (hRV)/SARS-CoV-2 (17.91%), hRV/respiratory syncytial virus (RSV) (14.18%), RSV/SARS-CoV-2 (12.69%), hRV/human bocavirus (BoV) (10.45%), and hRV/adenovirus (AdV) (8.21%) [29]. These findings offer valuable insights into the complexity of pediatric respiratory infections and the need for tailored interventions.

Bibliometric analysis is an approach that uses a set of quantitative methods to measure, track, and analyze the scholarly literature [30], providing an overview of a field of research. It has been used in SARS-CoV-2-infection-related research. For example, a bibliometric review exploring studies that assessed SARS-CoV-2 antibody responses in the pediatric population highlighted collaborative networks, international interactions, and key findings regarding antibody titers and correlations with immune markers. This study offers insights into future research directions in pediatric SARS-CoV-2 antibody responses [31].

Together, these papers provide a wealth of information, revealing the many facets of COVID-19's effects on various physiological systems. Each study adds a piece to the puzzle, including topics such as neurological symptoms, pediatric responses, metabolic abnormalities, and cardiovascular and metabolic consequences. As we examine these findings, the importance of standardized approaches, vigilant monitoring, and tailored interventions becomes clear. The multidisciplinary nature of these studies underscores the need for collaborative efforts and for pushing the boundaries of knowledge to better understand not only the SARS-CoV-2 infection but also any new pathogens.

Author Contributions: Conceptualization, A.C., M.S. and E.C.R.; methodology, A.C. and E.C.R.; software, A.C. and E.C.R.; investigation, A.C., M.S. and E.C.R.; resources, A.C. and E.C.R.; writing—original draft preparation, A.C.; writing—review and editing, M.S. and E.C.R.; supervision, M.S. and E.C.R.; project administration, E.C.R. All authors have read and agreed to the published version of the manuscript.

Funding: This research received no external funding.

Conflicts of Interest: The authors declare no conflict of interest.

References

1. Bellani, G.; Laffey, J.G.; Pham, T.; Fan, E.; Brochard, L.; Esteban, A.; Gattinoni, L.; van Haren, F.; Larsson, A.; McAuley, D.F.; et al. Epidemiology, Patterns of Care, and Mortality for Patients With Acute Respiratory Distress Syndrome in Intensive Care Units in 50 Countries. *JAMA* **2016**, *315*, 788–800. [CrossRef] [PubMed]
2. Madotto, F.; Pham, T.; Bellani, G.; Bos, L.D.; Simonis, F.D.; Fan, E.; Artigas, A.; Brochard, L.; Schultz, M.J.; Laffey, J.G. Resolved versus confirmed ARDS after 24 h: Insights from the LUNG SAFE study. *Intensive Care Med.* **2018**, *44*, 564–577. [CrossRef] [PubMed]
3. Meyer, N.J.; Gattinoni, L.; Calfee, C.S. Acute respiratory distress syndrome. *Lancet* **2021**, *398*, 622–637. [CrossRef] [PubMed]
4. Zdravković, V.; Stevanović, Đ.; Ćićarić, N.; Zdravković, N.; Čekerevac, I.; Poskurica, M.; Simić, I.; Stojić, V.; Nikolić, T.; Marković, M.; et al. Anthropometric Measurements and Admission Parameters as Predictors of Acute Respiratory Distress Syndrome in Hospitalized COVID-19 Patients. *Biomedicines* **2023**, *11*, 1199. [CrossRef] [PubMed]
5. Smadja, D.M.; Fellous, B.A.; Bonnet, G.; Hauw-Berlemont, C.; Sutter, W.; Beauvais, A.; Fauvel, C.; Philippe, A.; Weizman, O.; Mika, D.; et al. D-dimer, BNP/NT-pro-BNP, and creatinine are reliable decision-making biomarkers in life-sustaining therapies withholding and withdrawing during COVID-19 outbreak. *Front. Cardiovasc. Med.* **2022**, *9*, 935333. [CrossRef] [PubMed]
6. Gao, L.; Jiang, D.; Wen, X.S.; Cheng, X.C.; Sun, M.; He, B.; You, L.N.; Lei, P.; Tan, X.W.; Qin, S.; et al. Prognostic value of NT-proBNP in patients with severe COVID-19. *Respir. Res.* **2020**, *21*, 83. [CrossRef]
7. Orlando, L.; Bagnato, G.; Ioppolo, C.; Franzè, M.S.; Perticone, M.; Versace, A.G.; Sciacqua, A.; Russo, V.; Cicero, A.F.G.; De Gaetano, A.; et al. Natural Course of COVID-19 and Independent Predictors of Mortality. *Biomedicines* **2023**, *11*, 939. [CrossRef]
8. Hilton, J.; Boyer, N.; Nadim, M.K.; Forni, L.G.; Kellum, J.A. COVID-19 and Acute Kidney Injury. *Crit. Care Clin.* **2022**, *38*, 473–489. [CrossRef]
9. Iglesias, J.; Vassallo, A.; Ilagan, J.; Ang, S.P.; Udongwo, N.; Mararenko, A.; Alshami, A.; Patel, D.; Elbaga, Y.; Levine, J.S. Acute Kidney Injury Associated with Severe SARS-CoV-2 Infection: Risk Factors for Morbidity and Mortality and a Potential Benefit of Combined Therapy with Tocilizumab and Corticosteroids. *Biomedicines* **2023**, *11*, 845. [CrossRef]
10. Zhou, Y.; Li, J.; Wang, L.; Zhu, X.; Zhang, M.; Zheng, J. Acute Kidney Injury and Drugs Prescribed for COVID-19 in Diabetes Patients: A Real-World Disproportionality Analysis. *Front. Pharmacol.* **2022**, *13*, 833679. [CrossRef]
11. Aljuhani, O.; Al Sulaiman, K.; Korayem, B.G.; Alharbi, A.; Altebainawi, A.F.; Aldkheel, S.A.; Alotaibi, S.G.; Vishwakarma, R.; Alshareef, H.; Alsohimi, S.; et al. The use of Tocilizumab in COVID-19 critically ill patients with renal impairment: A multicenter, cohort study. *Ren. Fail.* **2023**, *45*, 2268213. [CrossRef] [PubMed]
12. Alfano, G.; Ferrari, A.; Magistroni, R.; Fontana, F.; Cappelli, G.; Basile, C. The frail world of haemodialysis patients in the COVID-19 pandemic era: A systematic scoping review. *J. Nephrol.* **2021**, *34*, 1387–1403. [CrossRef] [PubMed]
13. McDonnell, T.; Wu, H.H.L.; Kalra, P.A.; Chinnadurai, R. COVID-19 in Elderly Patients Receiving Haemodialysis: A Current Review. *Biomedicines* **2023**, *11*, 926. [CrossRef] [PubMed]
14. Regolisti, G.; Rebora, P.; Occhino, G.; Lieti, G.; Molon, G.; Maloberti, A.; Algeri, M.; Giannattasio, C.; Valsecchi, M.G.; Genovesi, S. Elevated Serum Urea-to-Creatinine Ratio and In-Hospital Death in Patients with Hyponatremia Hospitalized for COVID-19. *Biomedicines* **2023**, *11*, 1555. [CrossRef]
15. Hata, T.; Goto, T.; Yamanaka, S.; Matsumoto, T.; Yamamura, O.; Hayashi, H. Prognostic value of initial serum sodium level in predicting disease severity in patients with COVID-19: A multicenter retrospective study. *J. Infect. Chemother.* **2023**. [CrossRef]
16. Grieco, D.L.; Menga, L.S.; Cesarano, M.; Rosà, T.; Spadaro, S.; Bitondo, M.M.; Montomoli, J.; Falò, G.; Tonetti, T.; Cutuli, S.L.; et al. Effect of Helmet Noninvasive Ventilation vs High-Flow Nasal Oxygen on Days Free of Respiratory Support in Patients With COVID-19 and Moderate to Severe Hypoxemic Respiratory Failure: The HENIVOT Randomized Clinical Trial. *JAMA* **2021**, *325*, 1731–1743. [CrossRef] [PubMed]
17. Arabi, Y.M.; Aldekhyl, S.; Al Qahtani, S.; Al-Dorzi, H.M.; Abdukahil, S.A.; Al Harbi, M.K.; Al Qasim, E.; Kharaba, A.; Albrahim, T.; Alshahrani, M.S.; et al. Effect of Helmet Noninvasive Ventilation vs Usual Respiratory Support on Mortality Among Patients With Acute Hypoxemic Respiratory Failure Due to COVID-19: The HELMET-COVID Randomized Clinical Trial. *JAMA* **2022**, *328*, 1063–1072. [CrossRef]
18. Cei, F.; Chiarugi, L.; Brancati, S.; Dolenti, S.; Montini, M.S.; Rosselli, M.; Filippelli, M.; Ciacci, C.; Sellerio, I.; Gucci, M.M.; et al. Clinical and Personal Predictors of Helmet-CPAP Use and Failure in Patients Firstly Admitted to Regular Medical Wards with COVID-19-Related Acute Respiratory Distress Syndrome (hCPAP-f Study). *Biomedicines* **2023**, *11*, 207. [CrossRef]
19. Luo, X.; Lv, M.; Zhang, X.; Estill, J.; Yang, B.; Lei, R.; Ren, M.; Liu, Y.; Wang, L.; Liu, X.; et al. Clinical manifestations of COVID-19: An overview of 102 systematic reviews with evidence mapping. *J. Evid.-Based Med.* **2022**, *15*, 201–215. [CrossRef]
20. Duda-Seiman, D.; Kundnani, N.R.; Dugaci, D.; Man, D.E.; Velimirovici, D.; Dragan, S.R. COVID-19 Related Myocarditis and Myositis in a Patient with Undiagnosed Antisynthetase Syndrome. *Biomedicines* **2022**, *11*, 95. [CrossRef]
21. Walker, A.; Kelly, C.; Pottinger, G.; Hopkins, C. Parosmia—A common consequence of COVID-19. *BMJ* **2022**, *377*, e069860. [CrossRef] [PubMed]
22. Capra, A.P.; Ardizzone, A.; Crupi, L.; Calapai, F.; Campolo, M.; Cuzzocrea, S.; Esposito, E. Efficacy of Palmitoylethanolamide and Luteolin Association on Post-COVID Olfactory Dysfunction: A Systematic Review and Meta-Analysis of Clinical Studies. *Biomedicines* **2023**, *11*, 2189. [CrossRef] [PubMed]

23. Di Stadio, A.; Cantone, E.; De Luca, P.; Di Nola, C.; Massimilla, E.A.; Motta, G.; La Mantia, I.; Motta, G. Parosmia COVID-19 Related Treated by a Combination of Olfactory Training and Ultramicronized PEA-LUT: A Prospective Randomized Controlled Trial. *Biomedicines* **2023**, *11*, 1109. [CrossRef] [PubMed]
24. Cornea, A.; Lata, I.; Simu, M.; Rosca, E.C. Parsonage-Turner Syndrome Following SARS-CoV-2 Infection: A Systematic Review. *Biomedicines* **2023**, *11*, 837. [CrossRef] [PubMed]
25. Khan, S.; Karim, M.; Gupta, V.; Goel, H.; Jain, R. A Comprehensive Review of COVID-19-Associated Endocrine Manifestations. *South Med. J.* **2023**, *116*, 350–354. [CrossRef] [PubMed]
26. Durcan, E.; Hacioglu, A.; Karaca, Z.; Unluhizarci, K.; Gonen, M.S.; Kelestimur, F. Hypothalamic-pituitary axis function and adrenal insufficiency in COVID-19 patients. *Neuroimmunomodulation* **2023**, *30*, 215–225. [CrossRef]
27. Lauri, C.; Campagna, G.; Glaudemans, A.; Slart, R.; van Leer, B.; Pillay, J.; Colandrea, M.; Grana, C.M.; Stigliano, A.; Signore, A. SARS-CoV-2 Affects Thyroid and Adrenal Glands: An (18)F-FDG PET/CT Study. *Biomedicines* **2023**, *11*, 2899. [CrossRef]
28. Westbrook, A.; Wang, T.; Bhakta, K.; Sullivan, J.; Gonzalez, M.D.; Lam, W.; Rostad, C.A. Respiratory Coinfections in Children With SARS-CoV-2. *Pediatr. Infect. Dis. J.* **2023**, *42*, 774–780. [CrossRef]
29. Malveste Ito, C.R.; Moreira, A.L.E.; Silva, P.; Santos, M.O.; Santos, A.P.D.; Rézio, G.S.; Brito, P.N.; Rezende, A.P.C.; Fonseca, J.G.; Peixoto, F.A.O.; et al. Viral Coinfection of Children Hospitalized with Severe Acute Respiratory Infections during COVID-19 Pandemic. *Biomedicines* **2023**, *11*, 1402. [CrossRef]
30. Donthu, N.; Kumar, S.; Mukherjee, D.; Pandey, N.; Lim, W.M. How to conduct a bibliometric analysis: An overview and guidelines. *J. Bus. Res.* **2021**, *133*, 285–296. [CrossRef]
31. Maniu, I.; Maniu, G.C.; Antonescu, E.; Duica, L.; Grigore, N.; Totan, M. SARS-CoV-2 Antibody Responses in Pediatric Patients: A Bibliometric Analysis. *Biomedicines* **2023**, *11*, 1455. [CrossRef] [PubMed]

Disclaimer/Publisher's Note: The statements, opinions and data contained in all publications are solely those of the individual author(s) and contributor(s) and not of MDPI and/or the editor(s). MDPI and/or the editor(s) disclaim responsibility for any injury to people or property resulting from any ideas, methods, instructions or products referred to in the content.

Anthropometric Measurements and Admission Parameters as Predictors of Acute Respiratory Distress Syndrome in Hospitalized COVID-19 Patients

Vladimir Zdravković [1,2], Đorđe Stevanović [1,2,*], Neda Ćićarić [1], Nemanja Zdravković [3], Ivan Čekerevac [2,4], Mina Poskurica [1], Ivan Simić [1,2], Vladislava Stojić [5], Tomislav Nikolić [2,6], Marina Marković [2,7], Marija Popović [1], Ana Divjak [8,9], Dušan Todorović [10,11] and Marina Petrović [2,3]

1. Department of Interventional Cardiology, Cardiology Clinic, University Clinical Center Kragujevac, 34000 Kragujevac, Serbia
2. Department of Internal Medicine, Faculty of Medical Sciences, University of Kragujevac, 34000 Kragujevac, Serbia
3. Department of Pathophysiology, Faculty of Medical Sciences, University of Kragujevac, 34000 Kragujevac, Serbia
4. Pulmonology Clinic, University Clinical Center Kragujevac, 34000 Kragujevac, Serbia
5. Department of Medical Statistics and Informatics, Faculty of Medical Sciences, University of Kragujevac, 34000 Kragujevac, Serbia
6. Urology and Nephrology Clinic, University Clinical Center Kragujevac, 34000 Kragujevac, Serbia
7. Center of Medical Oncology, University Clinical Center Kragujevac, 34000 Kragujevac, Serbia
8. Department of Physical Medicine and Rehabilitation, University Clinical Center Kragujevac, 34000 Kragujevac, Serbia
9. Department of Physical Medicine and Rehabilitation, Faculty of Medical Sciences, University of Kragujevac, 34000 Kragujevac, Serbia
10. Department of Ophtamology, Faculty of Medical Sciences, University of Kragujevac, 34000 Kragujevac, Serbia
11. Ophtalmology Clinic, University Clinical Center Kragujevac, 34000 Kragujevac, Serbia
* Correspondence: djordje.stevanovic.kg@gmail.com; Tel.: +381-6069-69077 or +381-3450-5088

Abstract: Aim: We aimed to single out admission predictors of acute respiratory distress syndrome (ARDS) in hospitalized COVID-19 patients and investigate the role of bioelectrical impedance (BIA) measurements in ARDS development. **Method**: An observational, prospective cohort study was conducted on 407 consecutive COVID-19 patients hospitalized at the University Clinical Center Kragujevac between September 2021 and March 2022. Patients were followed during the hospitalization, and ARDS was observed as a primary endpoint. Body composition was assessed using the BMI, body fat percentage (BF%), and visceral fat (VF) via BIA. Within 24 h of admission, patients were sampled for blood gas and laboratory analysis. **Results**: Patients with BMI above 30 kg/m^2, very high BF%, and/or very high VF levels were at a significantly higher risk of developing ARDS compared to nonobese patients (OR: 4.568, 8.892, and 2.448, respectively). In addition, after performing multiple regression analysis, six admission predictors of ARDS were singled out: (1) very high BF (aOR 8.059), (2) SaO_2 < 87.5 (aOR 5.120), (3) IL-6 > 59.75 (aOR 4.089), (4) low lymphocyte count (aOR 2.880), (5) female sex (aOR 2.290), and (6) age < 68.5 (aOR 1.976). **Conclusion**: Obesity is an important risk factor for the clinical deterioration of hospitalized COVID-19 patients. BF%, assessed through BIA measuring, was the strongest independent predictor of ARDS in hospitalized COVID-19 patients.

Keywords: ARDS; bioelectrical impedance analysis; body fat percentage; COVID-19; obesity

1. Introduction

Severe acute respiratory syndrome coronavirus 2 (SARS-CoV-2) is responsible for a significant number of deaths and health impairments worldwide [1]. The illness is characterized mostly by respiratory clinical manifestations ranging from mild to severe clinical forms [2]. However, in 10–20% of patients, the disease is complicated by respiratory failure, acute respiratory distress syndrome (ARDS), and multisystem organ failure [3,4].

Despite continuous research efforts, the exact mechanisms of clinical deterioration are not fully elucidated. In a practical manner, it would be beneficial to single out conditions and clinical characteristics associated with ARDS development in order to construct prediction models and promptly single out patients at risk of clinical deterioration. According to the available literature, many parameters are associated with COVID-19 ARDS, such as older age, male sex, certain comorbidities, smoking, impaired gas exchange, elevated biomarkers of inflammation, and impaired coagulation [5–11]. However, the exact selection of predictors and their impact on ARDS development in hospitalized COVID-19 patients are not uniform across the literature, mostly due to the significant heterogeneity of cohort characteristics and methodological approach.

Obesity, according to body mass index (BMI), is associated with disease severity and the need for ICU treatment (OR 1.2–5.5) [12–15]. However, BMI is a basic anthropometric measurement that neglects body composition and the presence of adipose tissue. Given that most of the pathophysiological mechanisms through which obesity possibly affects the COVID-19 course are the effect of adipose tissue, assessing body composition solely using the BMI could be suboptimal [16–18].

Therefore, we aimed to single out admission predictors of ARDS in hospitalized COVID-19 patients, based on sociodemographic and medical history data, as well as blood gas and laboratory analysis on admission. Additionally, we aimed to examine the impact of obesity on COVID-19 ARDS, as well as compare BMI with anthropometric measurements given by BIA method, such as total body and visceral fat. To the best of the authors' knowledge, this is the first registry regarding BIA measurements and COVID-19 outcomes.

2. Materials and Methods

2.1. Study Population

An observational, prospective cohort study included 407 consecutive COVID-19 patients hospitalized at the University Clinical Center Kragujevac between September 2021 and March 2022. The study was granted approval by the University Clinical Center Kragujevac (Serbia) Ethical committee.

Our COVID-19 center consisted of standard, semi-intensive, and intensive care units focused on severe to critically ill patients [19]. Patients were followed during the hospitalization, and ARDS development was observed as a primary endpoint. The ARDS is an acute onset clinical syndrome characterized by diffuse, bilateral alveolar damage, inflammation, and edema, resulting in respiratory failure [20]. ARDS was defined using the Berlin criteria [21]: (1) timing within 1 week of clinical insult or new/worsening respiratory symptoms; (2) bilateral opacities seen on chest imaging, not fully explained by effusions, lobar/lung collapse, or nodules; (3) respiratory failure not fully explained by cardiac failure/fluid overload; (4) oxygenation impairment, defined as the ratio of partial pressure of arterial oxygen (PaO_2) to the fraction of inspired oxygen (FiO_2) below 300 mm Hg.

Inclusion and exclusion criteria are presented in Supplementary Table S1. We note that, during the data collection period, 1240 patients were hospitalized in our COVID-19 center; however, 825 patients were excluded according to exclusion criteria. Since there was an insufficient number of underweight patients (total of eight patients according to either BMI or BF% measurement), those patients were additionally excluded from further analysis.

2.2. Data Collection

Sociodemographic and medical history data were obtained using patients' electronic medical records (Health Informational System version 2, ComTrade, Kragujevac, Serbia). Arterial and peripheral venous blood for further analysis was routinely sampled at the time of admission.

Within 48 h of hospital admission, patients were measured on the TANITA BC-543 device (Tanita Corporation, Tokyo, Japan). According to the manufacturer's instructions, patients were measured in the morning, barefoot, in light clothing, before the first meal. In order to minimize the effect of acute infection and fever, patients were measured in an afebrile state.

Anthropometric parameters of interest were the following:

(I) BMI, calculated using the formula BMI $[kg/m^2]$ = BM $[kg]$/BH^2 $[m^2]$, where BM is the body mass expressed in kg (with 0.1 kg precision), and BH is body height expressed in m (with 0.01 m precision). According to BMI values, patients were categorized as (I) underweight < 18.5 kg/m^2, (II) normal weight 18.6–24.9 kg/m^2, (III) overweight 25–29.9 kg/m^2, (IV) class 1 obesity 30–34.9 kg/m^2, (V) class 2 obesity 35–39.9 kg/m^2, or (VI) class 3 obesity > 40 kg/m^2 [22].

(II) Body fat percentage (BF%), expressed as a percentage of the total mass (with 0.1% precision). According to BF% values, regarding age and sex, patients were categorized as (I) low BF%, (II) normal BF%, (III) high BF%, or (IV) very high BF% (age- and sex-adjusted cutoff values are presented in Table 1) [23].

(III) Visceral fat (VF) level, according to which patients were categorized as (I) normal (1–9), (II) high (10–14), or (III) very high ($\geq$15) [24].

Table 1. Age- and sex-adjusted cutoff values for BF% categories.

Sex	Age (Years)	BF% Categories			
		Low	Normal	High (Overweight)	Very High (Obesity)
Female	20–39	<21%	21–32.9%	33–39.5%	>39.5%
	40–59	<23%	23–33.9%	34–40%	>40%
	$\geq$60	24%	24–35.9%	36–41.5%	>41.5%
Male	20–39	<7%	7–19.9%	20–25%	>25%
	40–59	<10.5%	10.5–21.9%	22–27.5%	>27.5%
	$\geq$60	<12%	12–24.9%	25–30%	>30%

Abbreviations: BF%—Body fat percentage. BF% and VF levels were assessed using BIA analysis, by measuring the tissue's impedance to a low current electrical impulse.

2.3. Statistical Analysis

Statistical analysis was performed using the SPSS statistical package (version 25.0, IBM corporation, Armonk, NY, USA). Differences in quantitative data were tested using the Mann–Whitney U test. If applicable, continuous data were further transformed into a binary variable. When dividing continuous variables into categories, an accepted reference line or cutoff values given by ROC analysis (Supplementary Table S2) were used, depending on clinical applicability. After identifying the variables associated with primary outcome, uni- and multivariable binary logistic regression was performed. The strength of the relationship between examined variables and outcome was expressed as the odds ratio (OR) with 95% confidence interval (95% CI) for univariate, and as the adjusted odds ratio (aOR) with 95% CI for multivariate analysis. A p-value < 0.05 was considered significant.

3. Results

Our cohort consisted of 407 adult COVID-19 patients hospitalized at the University Clinical Center Kragujevac (Serbia), whose characteristics are presented in Table 2. During the hospitalization, 98.5% of patients required some form of oxygen support, 51.6% of patients required noninvasive/invasive ventilation, and 35.1% of patients developed ARDS, with a mortality rate of 17.4%. Younger age and female sex were associated with ARDS development, while patients with and without ARDS did not significantly differ in terms of comorbidities. In addition, patients who developed ARDS had a shorter period between disease onset and the need for inpatient treatment, more frequently required oxygen support upon admission, had a longer hospital stay, and had a higher mortality rate.

Table 2. Demographic and medical history data, with regard to ARDS development.

Cohort Characteristics		Frequency (Number of Cases) or Median Value (with IQR)			p-Value
		Cohort	No ARDS	ARDS	
Age [years]		68.0 (IQR 17.0)	68.5 (IQR 16.0)	66.0 (IQR 19.0)	0.006 *
Sex	Male	62.9% (n = 256)	68.9% (n = 182)	51.7% (n = 74)	0.001 *
	Female	37.1% (n = 151)	31.1% (n = 82)	48.3% (n = 69)	
COMORBIDITIES					
Arterial hypertension		68.1% (n = 277)	70.5% (n = 186)	63.6% (n = 91)	0.182
Diabetes mellitus		26.5% (n = 108)	25.4% (n = 67)	28.7% (n = 41)	0.482
Chronic kidney disease		14.7% (n = 60)	14.8% (n = 39)	14.7% (n = 21)	1.000
Neurological condition [1]		3.4% (n = 14)	3.8% (n = 10)	2.8% (n = 4)	0.778
Previous myocardial infarction		3.9% (n = 16)	3.8% (n = 10)	4.2% (n = 6)	0.797
Malignancy		6.1% (n = 25)	7.2% (n = 19)	4.2% (n = 6)	0.283
Obstructive lung disease [2]		3.2% (n = 13)	3.4% (n = 9)	2.8% (n = 4)	1.000
Charlson Comorbidity Index		3.0 (IQR 2.0)	3.0 (IQR 2.0)	3.0 (IQR 3.0)	0.052
DISEASE COURSE AND OUTCOME					
Time from disease onset to hospital admission [days]		6.0 (IQR 6.0)	7.0 (IQR 7.0)	6.0 (IQR 5.0)	0.003 *
ARDS development		35.1% (n = 143)	/	/	/
Mortality		17.4% (n = 71)	9% (n = 24)	44.1% (n = 63)	<0.001 *
Hospital stay [days]		17.0 (IQR 11.0)	14.5 (IQR 9.75)	21.0 (IQR 14.0)	<0.001 *
Oxygen support requirement on admission		92.9% (n = 378)	90.5% (n = 239)	97.2% (n = 139)	0.014 *

Abbreviations: ARDS—acute respiratory distress syndrome; IQR—interquartile range. * Statistical significance level at <0.05. [1] Neurological condition: the presence of history of stroke, brain tumor or malformation, vascular disease, dementia of any etiology, etc. [2] Obstructive lung disease: the presence of either chronic obstructive lung disease or bronchial asthma.

The prevalence of obesity was 37.9% according to BMI and 49.6% according to BF%, while 38.6% of patients had an excessive level of VF. (Figure 1) Furthermore, patients who developed ARDS more frequently had BMI above 30 kg/m^2 ($p < 0.001$), as well as very high body fat percentage ($p < 0.001$) and visceral fat level ($p < 0.001$).

The admission blood gas and laboratory analysis is presented in Table 3. Patients with ARDS, compared to those without, had significant differences in blood cell count (lower lymphocyte and higher granulocyte count), more impaired gas exchange (lower values of oxygen saturation (SaO$_2$) and partial oxygen pressure (PaO$_2$)), and more increased inflammatory biomarkers (including C-reactive protein (CRP), lactate dehydrogenase (LDH), and interleukin-6 (IL-6)).

After performing the univariate analysis, 11 variables were selected for the final binary logistic regression model. (Table 4) Six variables gave statistically significant contributions to the model: (1) very high BF (aOR 8.059), (2) SaO$_2$ < 87.5 (aOR 5.120), (3) IL-6 > 59.75 (aOR 4.089), (4) low lymphocyte count (aOR 2.880), (5) female sex (aOR 2.290), and (6) age < 68.5 years (aOR 1.976). The score was statistically significant (c^{11} = 178.54; $p < 0.001$), with a sensitivity of 76%, specificity of 87.7%, and C-index of 0.885 ($p < 0.001$) (Figure 2).

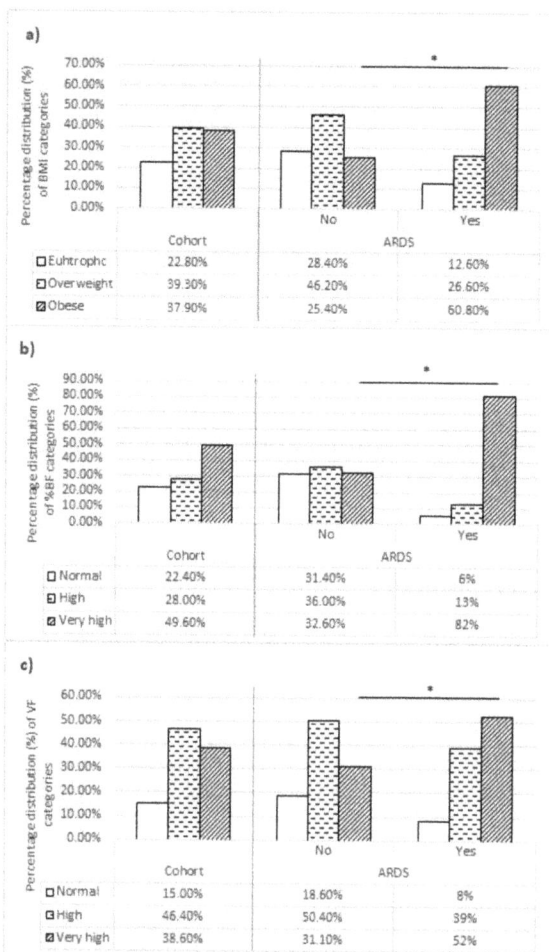

Figure 1. Percentage distribution of body composition categories for (**a**) BMI, (**b**) %BF, and (**c**) VF level, with regard to ARDS development. Abbreviations: ARDS—acute respiratory distress syndrome; BMI—body mass index; VF—visceral fat; %BF—body fat percentage. * Statistical significance at <0.05.

Table 3. Admission blood gas and laboratory analysis, with regard to ARDS development.

Blood Gas and Laboratory Analysis	Median Values (IQR)			p-Value
	Cohort	No ARDS	ARDS	
PaO$_2$ [kPa]	6.9 (IQR 1.4)	14.5 (IQR 9.75)	6.4 (IQR 1.2)	<0.001 *
SaO$_2$ [%]	88 (IQR 6)	89 (IQR 5)	86 (IQR 5)	<0.001 *
WBC [10^9/L]	8.2 (IQR 4.8)	8.2 (IQR 4.5)	8.3 (IQR 6.6)	0.751
Granulocyte count [10^9/L]	6.9 (IQR 4.9)	6.5 (IQR 4.85)	7.4 (IQR 4.1)	0.710
Granulocytes [%]	84.2 (IQR 11.7)	83 (IQR 12.2)	85.9 (IQR 10.8)	0.001 *
Lymphocyte count [10^9/L]	0.7 (IQR 0.5)	0.73 (IQR 0.57)	0.69 (IQR 0.43)	0.009 *
Lymphocytes [%]	9.1 (IQR 8.5)	9.5 (IQR 8.6)	8.5 (IQR 6.4)	0.036 *

Table 3. Cont.

Blood Gas and Laboratory Analysis	Median Values (IQR)			p-Value
	Cohort	No ARDS	ARDS	
RBC [10^{12}/L]	4.5 (IQR 0.7)	4.48 (IQR 0.81)	4.47 (IQR 0.69)	0.968
HGB [g/L]	134 (IQR 21)	134.5 (IQR 21.75)	133 (IQR 21)	0.081
PLT [10^9/L]	201 (IQR 113)	203.5 (IQR 108)	199 (IQR 115)	0.771
INR	1.08 (IQR 0.18)	1.08 (IQR 0.16)	1.07 (IQR 0.19)	0.079
aPTT [s]	31.4 (IQR 6.85)	31.5 (IQR 7)	33.3 (IQR 6.3)	0.917
Fibrinogen [g/L]	6.5 (IQR 2.15)	6.26 (IQR 2.06)	6.22 (IQR 2.09)	0.485
D-dimer [ug/mL]	0.93 (IQR 0.97)	0.97 (IQR 1.25)	0.85 (IQR 0.76)	0.159
Albumin [g/L]	36 (IQR 4)	36 (IQR 4)	36 (IQR 5)	0.337
AST [IU/L]	42 (IQR 35)	41 (IQR 31)	43 (IQR 41)	0.271
ALT [IU/L]	36 (IQR 36)	36 (IQR 38.25)	41 (IQR 40)	0.830
GGT [IU/L]	41 (IQR 65)	42 (IQR 65)	41 (IQR 64)	0.819
BUN [mmol/L]	7.8 (IQR 5.3)	8.4 (IQR 5.5)	7.1 (IQR 4.2)	0.054
Creatinine [mmol/L]	92 (IQR 41)	91 (IQR 42)	94 (IQR 40)	0.216
LDH [U/L]	773 (IQR 382)	702 (IQR 388)	890 (IQR 242)	<0.001 *
Ferritin [ug/L]	838 (IQR 745)	815 (IQR 792)	877 (IQR 746)	0.335
CK [U/L]	107(IQR 166)	91.5 (IQR 152.75)	156 (IQR 179)	0.001 *
CKMB [U/L]	18 (IQR 10)	18 (IQR 9)	18 (IQR 11)	0.386
CRP [mg/L]	99 (IQR 96.1)	96.6 (IQR 92.5)	108.7 (IQR 99.8)	0.009 *
PCT [ng/mL]	0.11 (IQR 0.18)	0.1 (IQR 0.17)	0.114 (IQR 0.18)	0.413
cTnI [ng/mL]	0.0038 (IQR 0.014)	0.00145 (IQR 0.0145)	0.006 (IQR 0.0127)	0.637
pro-BNP [pg/mL]	559 (IQR 880)	604 (IQR 959)	389 (IQR 895)	0.066
IL-6 [pg/mL]	58.7 (IQR 97)	47.4 (IQR 89.15)	89.8 (IQR 119.3)	<0.001 *

Abbreviations: ALT—alanine transaminase; aPTT—activated partial thromboplastin clotting time; AST—aspartate transaminase; BUN—blood urea nitrogen; CK—creatine kinase; CKMB—muscle–brain form of creatine kinase; CRP—C-reactive protein; D—D-dimer; GGT—gamma-glutamyl transferase; Gran—granulocyte; Hgb—hemoglobin; hsTnI—high-sensitivity troponin I; IL-6—interleukin 6; INR—international normalized ratio; LDH—lactate dehydrogenase; Lym—lymphocytes; NT pro-BNP—N-terminal pro-brain natriuretic peptide; PaO$_2$—partial pressure of oxygen; PCT—procalcitonin; PLT—platelets; RBC—red blood cells; SaO$_2$—oxygen saturation of blood; WBC—white blood cells. * Statistical significance level at <0.05.

Table 4. Crude and adjusted OR for variables available upon hospital admission with regard to predicting ARDS development of hospitalized COVID-19 patients.

Variable		Frequency of ARDS	Crude OR		Adjusted OR	
			OR (95% CI)	p-Value	OR (95% CI)	p-Value
PaO$_2$ [kPa]	≥6.85	20.5%	1	/	Excluded for multicollinearity **	
	<6.85	52.4%	4.282 (2.770–6.619)	<0.001 *		
SaO$_2$ [kPa]	≥87.5	18.9%	1	/	1	/
	<87.5	56.9%	5.670 (3.635–8.844)	<0.001 *	5.120 (2.758–9.505)	<0.001 *

Table 4. Cont.

Variable		Frequency of ARDS	Crude OR		Adjusted OR	
			OR (95% CI)	p-Value	OR (95% CI)	p-Value
Lymphocyte count [10^9/L]	≥1.20	14.9%	1	/	1	/
	<1.20	39.1%	3.662 (1.807–7.422)	<0.001 *	2.880 (1.218–6.809)	0.016 *
LDH [U/L]	≤793.5	24.8%	1	/	1	/
	>793.5	49.1%	2.934 (1.898–4.538)	<0.001 *	1.078 (0.580–2.002)	0.812
CK [U/L]	≤171	29.8%	1	/	1	/
	>171	45.0%	1.927 (1.257–2.955)	0.003 *	1.911 (0.978–3.733)	0.058
CRP [mg/L]	≤108.5	30.6%	1	/	1	/
	>108.5	40.9%	1.572 (1.039–2.376)	0.032 *	1.096 (0.594–2.024)	0.768
IL-6 [pg/mL]	≤59.75	21.6%	1	/	1	/
	>59.75	49.7%	3.586 (2.327–5.525)	<0.001 *	4.089 (2.136–7.826)	<0.001 *
Age [years]	≥68.5	29.8%	1	/	1	/
	<68.5	39.7%	1.554 (1.027–2.349)	0.037 *	1.976 (1.038–3.762)	0.038 *
Sex	Male	28.9%	1	/	1	/
	Female	45.7%	2.070 (1.361–3.147)	0.001 *	2.290 (1.158–4.529)	0.017 *
Need for oxygen therapy upon admission	No	13.8%	1	/	Excluded for multicollinearity **	
	Yes	36.8%	3.635 (1.239–10.661)	0.019 *		
BMI	<30	22.1%	1	/	Excluded for multicollinearity **	
	≥30	56.5%	4.568 (2.955–7.060)	<0.001 *		
BF%	Normal/High	13.2%	1	/	1	/
	Very high	57.4%	8.892 (5.439–14.538)	<0.001 *	8.059 (3.990–16.276)	<0.001 *
VF	Normal/High	27.2%	1	/	1	/
	Very high	47.8%	2.448 (1.610–3.722)	<0.001 *	1.159 (0.566–2.372)	0.686
Time from disease onset [days]	/	/	0.923 (0.877–0.970)	0.002 *	0.941 (0.867–1.020)	0.140

Abbreviations: aOR—adjusted OR; ARDS—acute respiratory distress syndrome; BMI—body mass index; BF%—body fat percentage; CI—confidence interval; CK—creatine kinase; CRP—C-reactive protein; VF—visceral fat; IL-6—interleukin 6; LDH—lactate dehydrogenase; OR—odds ratio; PaO$_2$—partial pressure of oxygen; SaO$_2$—oxygen saturation of the blood. * Statistical significance level at <0.5. ** Variables excluded due to the multicollinearity principle of multiple logistic regression.

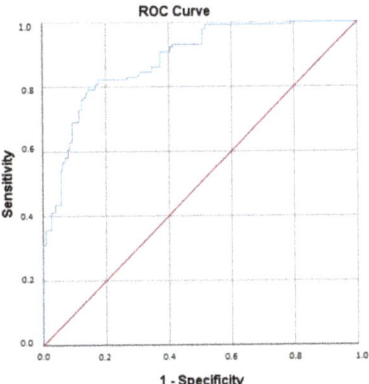

Figure 2. Receiver operator characteristics (ROC) curve of multiple regression analysis model in predicting ARDS. Legend: Blue line—ROC curve, red line—diagonal reference line.

4. Discussion

This study aimed to examine the impact of obesity on ARDS development and the likelihood of variables available upon admission to predict ARDS in hospitalized COVID-19 patients. Patients who developed ARDS had a shorter time from disease onset to hospital admission, and, with each day that passed from disease onset to hospital admission, the risk of ARDS development decreased by 7.7% (OR 0.923) [25].

The majority of patients had disturbed nutritional status according to all three anthropometric measurements (BMI, BF%, and VF). Body composition disturbances in hospitalized COVID-19 patients are not unexpected. Firstly, the high prevalence of obesity and obesity-related comorbidities has reached pandemic proportions [22], with consequences also noticeable in Serbia. According to research from 2006, 55.7% of the adult population in Serbia was overweight or obese [26]. Secondly, several studies have demonstrated that obesity is a significant risk factor for hospital admission [12–15]; therefore, it is somewhat expected to have a high prevalence of obesity among hospitalized COVID-19 patients. Furthermore, patients with BMI above 30 kg/m^2, very high BF%, and/or very high VF levels were at significantly higher risk of developing ARDS compared to nonobese patients (OR: 4.568, 8.892, and 2.448, respectively), which is in accordance with most of the literature data [12–14,18,27–32]. Obesity augments the risk of critical illness and mortality in SARS-CoV-2 infection through multiple mechanisms, including chronic inflammation, immune dysregulation, respiratory compromise, impaired pulmonary function, and endocrine and endothelial dysfunction [16,17,33]. However, the majority of mechanisms through which obesity can initiate the clinical deterioration of COVID-19 patients, especially in terms of inflammation and immune response dysregulation, are the effect of the adipose tissue. In obese patients, adipose tissue is responsible for chronic low-grade inflammation, characterized by increased production of cytokines and acute-phase reactants, as well as the macrophage accumulation, resulting in both innate and adaptive immune response impairment. Additionally, chronic inflammation in obese patients could potentially enhance the inflammatory response to COVID-19, resulting in a hyperinflammatory state and disease progression [16,17,34]. This could potentially explain why BF% was a stronger predictor of ARDS development compared to BMI, and why a very high BF% was the strongest independent predictor of ARDS (aOR 8.059) in a multiple regression analysis.

Interestingly, the VF level did not maintain statistical significance in a final regression model. This result could partially be explained by the inadequacy of BIA visceral fat assessment to differentiate adipose tissue between visceral and abdominal compartments [35].

In addition to obesity, the most common comorbidities in our cohort were arterial hypertension, diabetes mellitus, and chronic kidney disease. Despite literature data linking several comorbidities with clinical deterioration and worse outcomes in COVID-19 patients, no comorbidity showed a significant impact on ARDS development in our research [36]. Such differences could partially be explained by the characteristics of the comorbidities in the examined cohort, such as their prevalence, severity, duration, medication burden, and presence of disease-related complications. Therefore, the presence of well-controlled, uncomplicated comorbidities in our cohort could be a possible explanation for the absent impact of the most frequent comorbidities on the ARDS development. Additionally, patients initially hospitalized or requiring hospital treatment for non-COVID-19 pathology, with terminal stage of malignant disease, and with end-stage of renal disease were excluded from our study.

Among demographic characteristics, the female sex was shown to be an independent predictor of ARDS (aOR 2.290). Although the male sex is commonly linked with a higher risk of ICU admission and mortality in hospitalized COVID-19 patients [37,38], some explanations could include different cohort characteristics, more present high-risk behavior related to COVID-19, higher frequency of pre-existing comorbidities, differences in innate immune response, and different activity and expression of ACE 2 [39,40]. In addition, literature data advocate older age as ARDS and mortality risk factors in hospitalized COVID-19 patients [5,10,41]. However, our study singled out age below 68 years to be an independent predictor of ARDS (aOR 1.976). A possible explanation for such a result could be that older patients had a significantly higher mortality rate compared to those younger than 68 years (24.5% and 11.4%, respectively; $p = 0.001$). Thus, those patients experienced lethal outcome in greater numbers before ICU admittance and ARDS development/diagnosis.

With regard to gas exchange upon admission, patients who developed ARDS during the course of inpatient treatment more frequently required oxygen support upon admission and had more prominent hypoxemia, assessed as lower values of PaO_2 and SaO_2. Additionally, low SaO_2 ($\leq 87\%$) was the second strongest predictor of ARDS in the multiple regression analysis model. Such findings are of significant practical importance, since both PaO_2 and SaO_2 are affordable, widely used, and feasible indicators of hypoxemia's severity. Pronounced hypoxemia upon admission has been confirmed to be a significant risk factor for COVID-19 progression and lethal outcome [5,7,42]. The combined effects of capillary damage associated with COVID-19 affect tissue oxygenation in key organs. A vicious cycle ensues, as inflammation and hypoxia cause capillary function to deteriorate, which accelerates hypoxia-induced inflammation, oxidative stress, tissue damage, and ARDS [43].

With regard to laboratory analysis upon admission, patients with and without ARDS differed in several parameters. Firstly, patients who developed ARDS had significantly higher values of inflammatory biomarkers upon admission, including IL-6, CRP, and LDH. Furthermore, IL-6 > 59.75 pg/mL upon admission was an independent predictor of ARDS with an aOR of 4.089. A pronounced inflammatory response is considered to be one of the keystones of COVID-19 progression, and elevated inflammatory biomarkers are one of the most commonly advocated predictors of ICU admission and death [10,44,45]. Secondly, patients significantly differed in blood cell count. Clinical observation of lymphopenia has been apparent since the start of the COVID-19 pandemic and may be associated with worsening disease [46]. Our results are in accordance with the literature in that a low lymphocyte count in our cohort was singled out as an independent predictor of ARDS development (aOR 2.880).

Lastly, we singled out independent predictors of ARDS development and provided an ARDS risk assessment score relying on the parameters available upon hospital admission: y = 0.007 + (very high BF%) × 8.059 + (SaO_2 < 87.5%) × 5.120 + (IL6 > 59.75 pg/mL) × 4.089 + (low lymphocyte count) × 2.880 + (female sex) × 2.290 + (age < 68.5 years) × 1.976. The model had a C-index of 0.885 ($p < 0.001$), indicating a strong predictive model. Due to its high specificity (87.7%) and negative predictive value (86.6%), this model could have clinical importance as a "rule-out" tool in helping physicians define patients with a high risk of developing ARDS. Selecting predictors of worse outcomes and understanding the mechanisms responsible for the clinical deterioration of hospitalized COVID-19 patients has been the focus of scientific research for the past 2 years. More than 30 different parameters can be linked with ARDS development in COVID-19, and several risk assessment scores can be found [5–11,47–49]. However, the selection of predictors, as well as their cutoff and aOR values, significantly varies across the literature. Additionally, proposed predictive models differ in terms of accuracy (C-index according to ROC analysis), sensitivity, and specificity, which can greatly influence their potential utilization. These variations can be explained by differences in the statistical and methodological approach, patient characteristics, availability of examined parameters, health system organization, SARS-CoV-2 variant predominance, etc. Therefore, no specific model should be generally accepted irrespective of geographical, sociodemographic, patient structure, hospital equipment, and other important specifics. Instead, such research tends to extend the data to understand the mechanisms of COVID-19 progression and to point out that, in different settings, physicians can select patients with a higher risk of disease progression and death. In addition, to the authors' knowledge, this is the first registry to use admission BIA measurements in an ARDS prediction model. Despite their limitations, available and affordable BIA measurements gave the strongest independent predictor of ARDS development.

Our study had certain limitations. Firstly, active infection can potentially affect the BIA measurement, especially in the febrile state [50]. This limitation could, therefore, have been responsible for misinterpreting the body composition, in terms of a higher percentage of body fat. In order to minimize this effect, patients were measured within the first 48 h upon admission, in the absence of fever. Secondly, although BIA measurements provide satisfactory insight into total body fat and fat-free mass, this method has difficulties in distinguishing visceral from abdominal fat, for which computed tomography and magnetic resonance imaging remain the gold standard [35,51]. This could have been responsible for underestimating the individual impact of VF levels in our cohort. Lastly, the number of patients included may be insufficient for the generalization of the results. Therefore, we encourage fellow physicians and researchers to continue investigating BIA measurements in predicting COVID-19 outcome.

5. Conclusions

Obesity is an important risk factor for the clinical deterioration of hospitalized COVID-19 patients. Because of the insight into the total body and visceral fat, BIA measurements could be a useful and affordable tool in selecting COVID-19 patients with a high risk of developing ARDS.

Supplementary Materials: The following supporting information can be downloaded at: https://www.mdpi.com/article/10.3390/biomedicines11041199/s1, Table S1: Flowchart of patient enrolment; Table S2: Threshold values for continuous variables, according to the ROC analysis or laboratory reference lines.

Author Contributions: Conceptualization, Đ.S. and M.P. (Marina Petrović); methodology, N.Z. and I.Č.; validation, V.Z. and M.P. (Marina Petrović); formal analysis, V.S.; investigation, I.S., M.P. (Marija Popović), T.N., M.M. and M.P. (Mina Poskurica); resources, V.Z. and M.P. (Marina Petrović); writing—original draft preparation, T.N., M.M., M.P. (Mina Poskurica) and M.M.; writing—review and editing, N.Ć. and Đ.S.; supervision, V.Z. and I.Č.; project administration, D.T., A.D. and M.P. (Mina Poskurica). All authors have read and agreed to the published version of the manuscript.

Funding: This research received no external funding.

Institutional Review Board Statement: The study was conducted in accordance with the Declaration of Helsinki and approved by the Ethics Committee of University Clinical Center Kragujevac, Serbia (protocol number: 01/21/397; date of approval: 19 August 2021).

Informed Consent Statement: Informed consent was obtained from all subjects involved in the study.

Data Availability Statement: The data presented in this study are available on request from the corresponding author.

Acknowledgments: The authors would like to thank all physicians, nurses, and other team members of the University Clinical Center Kragujevac (Serbia) COVID-19 center for dedicated work over the past 3 years. The authors would like to thank Nela Đonović and Dragan Vasiljević for academic help in implementing and interpreting BIA measurements in clinical practice.

Conflicts of Interest: The authors declare no conflict of interest.

References

1. Rahman, S.; Montero, M.T.V.; Rowe, K.; Kirton, R.; Kunik, F., Jr. Epidemiology, pathogenesis, clinical presentations, diagnosis and treatment of COVID-19: A review of current evidence. *Expert Rev. Clin. Pharmacol.* **2021**, *14*, 601–621. [CrossRef] [PubMed]
2. Knoll, R.; Schultze, J.L.; Schulte-Schrepping, J. Monocytes and Macrophages in COVID-19. *Front. Immunol.* **2021**, *12*, 720109. [CrossRef] [PubMed]
3. Huang, C.; Wang, Y.; Li, X.; Ren, L.; Zhao, J.; Hu, Y.; Zhang, L.; Fan, G.; Xu, J.; Gu, X.; et al. Clinical features of patients infected with 2019 novel coronavirus in Wuhan, China. *Lancet* **2020**, *395*, 497–506. [CrossRef] [PubMed]
4. Zhou, F.; Yu, T.; Du, R.; Fan, G.; Liu, Y.; Liu, Z.; Xiang, J.; Wang, Y.; Song, B.; Gu, X.; et al. Clinical course and risk factors for mortality of adult inpatients with COVID-19 in Wuhan, China: A retrospective cohort study. *Lancet* **2020**, *395*, 1054–1062. [CrossRef]
5. Gallo Marin, B.; Aghagoli, G.; Lavine, K.; Yang, L.; Siff, E.J.; Chiang, S.S.; Salazar-Mather, T.P.; Dumenco, L.; Savaria, M.C.; Aung, S.N.; et al. Predictors of COVID-19 severity: A literature review. *Rev. Med. Virol.* **2021**, *31*, 1–10. [CrossRef]
6. Masvekar, R.R.; Kosa, P.; Jin, K.; Dobbs, K.; Stack, M.A.; Castagnoli, R.; Quaresima, V.; Su, H.C.; Imberti, L.; Notarangelo, L.D.; et al. Prognostic value of serum/plasma neurofilament light chain for COVID-19-associated mortality. *Ann. Clin. Transl. Neurol.* **2022**, *9*, 622–632. [CrossRef]
7. Petrilli, C.M.; Jones, S.A.; Yang, J.; Rajagopalan, H.; O'Donnell, L.; Chernyak, Y.; Tobin, K.A.; Cerfolio, R.J.; Francois, F.; Horwitz, L.I. Factors associated with hospital admission and critical illness among 5279 people with coronavirus disease 2019 in New York City: Prospective cohort study. *BMJ* **2020**, *369*, m1966. [CrossRef]
8. Xu, W.; Sun, N.N.; Gao, H.N.; Chen, Z.Y.; Yang, Y.; Ju, B.; Tang, L.L. Risk factors analysis of COVID-19 patients with ARDS and prediction based on machine learning. *Sci. Rep.* **2021**, *11*, 2933. [CrossRef]
9. Gujski, M.; Jankowski, M.; Rabczenko, D.; Gorynski, P.; Juszczyk, G. The Prevalence of Acute Respiratory Distress Syndrome (ARDS) and Outcomes in Hospitalized Patients with COVID-19-A Study Based on Data from the Polish National Hospital Register. *Viruses* **2022**, *14*, 76. [CrossRef]
10. Mesas, A.E.; Cavero-Redondo, I.; Alvarez-Bueno, C.; Sarria Cabrera, M.A.; Maffei de Andrade, S.; Sequi-Dominguez, I.; Martinez-Vizcaino, V. Predictors of in-hospital COVID-19 mortality: A comprehensive systematic review and meta-analysis exploring differences by age, sex and health conditions. *PLoS ONE* **2020**, *15*, e0241742. [CrossRef]
11. Statsenko, Y.; Al Zahmi, F.; Habuza, T.; Gorkom, K.N.; Zaki, N. Prediction of COVID-19 severity using laboratory findings on admission: Informative values, thresholds, ML model performance. *BMJ Open* **2021**, *11*, e044500. [CrossRef]
12. Popkin, B.M.; Du, S.; Green, W.D.; Beck, M.A.; Algaith, T.; Herbst, C.H.; Alsukait, R.F.; Alluhidan, M.; Alazemi, N.; Shekar, M. Individuals with obesity and COVID-19: A global perspective on the epidemiology and biological relationships. *Obes. Rev.* **2020**, *21*, e13128. [CrossRef]
13. Pranata, R.; Lim, M.A.; Yonas, E.; Vania, R.; Lukito, A.A.; Siswanto, B.B.; Meyer, M. Body mass index and outcome in patients with COVID-19: A dose-response meta-analysis. *Diabetes Metab.* **2021**, *47*, 101178. [CrossRef]
14. Chu, Y.; Yang, J.; Shi, J.; Zhang, P.; Wang, X. Obesity is associated with increased severity of disease in COVID-19 pneumonia: A systematic review and meta-analysis. *Eur. J. Med. Res.* **2020**, *25*, 64. [CrossRef]
15. Yang, J.; Hu, J.; Zhu, C. Obesity aggravates COVID-19: A systematic review and meta-analysis. *J. Med. Virol.* **2021**, *93*, 257–261. [CrossRef]
16. Sattar, N.; McInnes, I.B.; McMurray, J.J.V. Obesity Is a Risk Factor for Severe COVID-19 Infection: Multiple Potential Mechanisms. *Circulation* **2020**, *142*, 4–6. [CrossRef]
17. Kwok, S.; Adam, S.; Ho, J.H.; Iqbal, Z.; Turkington, P.; Razvi, S.; Le Roux, C.W.; Soran, H.; Syed, A.A. Obesity: A critical risk factor in the COVID-19 pandemic. *Clin. Obes.* **2020**, *10*, e12403. [CrossRef]
18. Watanabe, M.; Caruso, D.; Tuccinardi, D.; Risi, R.; Zerunian, M.; Polici, M.; Pucciarelli, F.; Tarallo, M.; Strigari, L.; Manfrini, S.; et al. Visceral fat shows the strongest association with the need of intensive care in patients with COVID-19. *Metabolism* **2020**, *111*, 154319. [CrossRef]
19. World Health Organization. *COVID-19 Clinical Management: Living Guidance*; World Health Organization: Geneva, Switzerland, 2021.
20. Battaglini, D.; Fazzini, B.; Silva, P.L.; Cruz, F.F.; Ball, L.; Robba, C.; Rocco, P.R.M.; Pelosi, P. Challenges in ARDS Definition, Management, and Identification of Effective Personalized Therapies. *J. Clin. Med.* **2023**, *12*, 1381. [CrossRef]
21. Force, A.D.T.; Ranieri, V.M.; Rubenfeld, G.D.; Thompson, B.T.; Ferguson, N.D.; Caldwell, E.; Fan, E.; Camporota, L.; Slutsky, A.S. Acute respiratory distress syndrome: The Berlin Definition. *JAMA* **2012**, *307*, 2526–2533. [CrossRef]
22. Obesity: Preventing and Managing the Global Epidemic. Report of a WHO Consultation. In *World Health Organization Technical Report Series*; World Health Organization: Geneva, Switzerland, 2000; Volume 894, p. 252.

23. Gallagher, D.; Heymsfield, S.B.; Heo, M.; Jebb, S.A.; Murgatroyd, P.R.; Sakamoto, Y. Healthy percentage body fat ranges: An approach for developing guidelines based on body mass index. *Am. J. Clin. Nutr.* **2000**, *72*, 694–701. [CrossRef] [PubMed]
24. *TANITA-Medical Product Guide*; TANITA: Arlington Heights, IL, USA, 2021.
25. Dreher, M.; Kersten, A.; Bickenbach, J.; Balfanz, P.; Hartmann, B.; Cornelissen, C.; Daher, A.; Stohr, R.; Kleines, M.; Lemmen, S.W.; et al. The Characteristics of 50 Hospitalized COVID-19 Patients with and Without ARDS. *Dtsch. Arztebl. Int.* **2020**, *117*, 271–278. [CrossRef] [PubMed]
26. Grujic, V.; Dragnic, N.; Radic, I.; Harhaji, S.; Susnjevic, S. Overweight and obesity among adults in Serbia: Results from the National Health Survey. *Eat. Weight Disord.* **2010**, *15*, e34–e42. [CrossRef] [PubMed]
27. Fernandez Crespo, S.; Perez-Matute, P.; Iniguez Martinez, M.; Fernandez-Villa, T.; Dominguez-Garrido, E.; Oteo, J.A.; Marcos-Delgado, A.; Flores, C.; Riancho, J.A.; Rojas-Martinez, A.; et al. Severity of COVID-19 attributable to obesity according to BMI and CUN-BAE. *Semergen* **2022**, *48*, 101840. [CrossRef] [PubMed]
28. Ogata, H.; Mori, M.; Jingushi, Y.; Matsuzaki, H.; Katahira, K.; Ishimatsu, A.; Enokizu-Ogawa, A.; Taguchi, K.; Moriwaki, A.; Yoshida, M. Impact of visceral fat on the prognosis of coronavirus disease 2019: An observational cohort study. *BMC Infect. Dis.* **2021**, *21*, 1240. [CrossRef]
29. Zhang, X.; Lewis, A.M.; Moley, J.R.; Brestoff, J.R. A systematic review and meta-analysis of obesity and COVID-19 outcomes. *Sci. Rep.* **2021**, *11*, 7193. [CrossRef]
30. Favre, G.; Legueult, K.; Pradier, C.; Raffaelli, C.; Ichai, C.; Iannelli, A.; Redheuil, A.; Lucidarme, O.; Esnault, V. Visceral fat is associated to the severity of COVID-19. *Metabolism* **2021**, *115*, 154440. [CrossRef]
31. Goehler, A.; Hsu, T.H.; Seiglie, J.A.; Siedner, M.J.; Lo, J.; Triant, V.; Hsu, J.; Foulkes, A.; Bassett, I.; Khorasani, R.; et al. Visceral Adiposity and Severe COVID-19 Disease: Application of an Artificial Intelligence Algorithm to Improve Clinical Risk Prediction. *Open Forum Infect. Dis.* **2021**, *8*, ofab275. [CrossRef]
32. Bunnell, K.M.; Thaweethai, T.; Buckless, C.; Shinnick, D.J.; Torriani, M.; Foulkes, A.S.; Bredella, M.A. Body composition predictors of outcome in patients with COVID-19. *Int. J. Obes.* **2021**, *45*, 2238–2243. [CrossRef]
33. Nikolic, M.; Simovic, S.; Novkovic, L.; Jokovic, V.; Djokovic, D.; Muric, N.; Bazic Sretenovic, D.; Jovanovic, J.; Pantic, K.; Cekerevac, I. Obesity and sleep apnea as a significant comorbidities in COVID-19—A case report. *Obes. Res. Clin. Pract.* **2021**, *15*, 281–284. [CrossRef]
34. Chait, A.; den Hartigh, L.J. Adipose Tissue Distribution, Inflammation and Its Metabolic Consequences, Including Diabetes and Cardiovascular Disease. *Front. Cardiovasc. Med.* **2020**, *7*, 22. [CrossRef]
35. Chaudry, O.; Grimm, A.; Friedberger, A.; Kemmler, W.; Uder, M.; Jakob, F.; Quick, H.H.; von Stengel, S.; Engelke, K. Magnetic Resonance Imaging and Bioelectrical Impedance Analysis to Assess Visceral and Abdominal Adipose Tissue. *Obesity* **2020**, *28*, 277–283. [CrossRef]
36. Yang, J.; Zheng, Y.; Gou, X.; Pu, K.; Chen, Z.; Guo, Q.; Ji, R.; Wang, H.; Wang, Y.; Zhou, Y. Prevalence of comorbidities and its effects in patients infected with SARS-CoV-2: A systematic review and meta-analysis. *Int. J. Infect. Dis.* **2020**, *94*, 91–95. [CrossRef]
37. Pijls, B.G.; Jolani, S.; Atherley, A.; Derckx, R.T.; Dijkstra, J.I.R.; Franssen, G.H.L.; Hendriks, S.; Richters, A.; Venemans-Jellema, A.; Zalpuri, S.; et al. Demographic risk factors for COVID-19 infection, severity, ICU admission and death: A meta-analysis of 59 studies. *BMJ Open* **2021**, *11*, e044640. [CrossRef]
38. Attaway, A.H.; Scheraga, R.G.; Bhimraj, A.; Biehl, M.; Hatipoglu, U. Severe covid-19 pneumonia: Pathogenesis and clinical management. *BMJ* **2021**, *372*, n436. [CrossRef]
39. Sharma, G.; Volgman, A.S.; Michos, E.D. Sex Differences in Mortality From COVID-19 Pandemic: Are Men Vulnerable and Women Protected? *JACC Case Rep.* **2020**, *2*, 1407–1410. [CrossRef]
40. Salah, H.M.; Mehta, J.L. Hypothesis: Sex-Related Differences in ACE2 Activity May Contribute to Higher Mortality in Men Versus Women With COVID-19. *J. Cardiovasc. Pharmacol. Ther.* **2021**, *26*, 114–118. [CrossRef]
41. Jimenez-Solem, E.; Petersen, T.S.; Hansen, C.; Hansen, C.; Lioma, C.; Igel, C.; Boomsma, W.; Krause, O.; Lorenzen, S.; Selvan, R.; et al. Developing and validating COVID-19 adverse outcome risk prediction models from a bi-national European cohort of 5594 patients. *Sci. Rep.* **2021**, *11*, 3246. [CrossRef]
42. Mejia, F.; Medina, C.; Cornejo, E.; Morello, E.; Vasquez, S.; Alave, J.; Schwalb, A.; Malaga, G. Oxygen saturation as a predictor of mortality in hospitalized adult patients with COVID-19 in a public hospital in Lima, Peru. *PLoS ONE* **2020**, *15*, e0244171. [CrossRef]
43. Ostergaard, L. SARS CoV-2 related microvascular damage and symptoms during and after COVID-19: Consequences of capillary transit-time changes, tissue hypoxia and inflammation. *Physiol. Rep.* **2021**, *9*, e14726. [CrossRef]
44. Del Valle, D.M.; Kim-Schulze, S.; Huang, H.H.; Beckmann, N.D.; Nirenberg, S.; Wang, B.; Lavin, Y.; Swartz, T.H.; Madduri, D.; Stock, A.; et al. An inflammatory cytokine signature predicts COVID-19 severity and survival. *Nat. Med.* **2020**, *26*, 1636–1643. [CrossRef] [PubMed]
45. Leisman, D.E.; Ronner, L.; Pinotti, R.; Taylor, M.D.; Sinha, P.; Calfee, C.S.; Hirayama, A.V.; Mastroiani, F.; Turtle, C.J.; Harhay, M.O.; et al. Cytokine elevation in severe and critical COVID-19: A rapid systematic review, meta-analysis, and comparison with other inflammatory syndromes. *Lancet Respir. Med.* **2020**, *8*, 1233–1244. [CrossRef] [PubMed]
46. Tan, L.; Wang, Q.; Zhang, D.; Ding, J.; Huang, Q.; Tang, Y.Q.; Wang, Q.; Miao, H. Lymphopenia predicts disease severity of COVID-19: A descriptive and predictive study. *Signal Transduct. Target Ther.* **2020**, *5*, 33. [CrossRef] [PubMed]

47. Sanchez-Ramirez, D.C.; Normand, K.; Zhaoyun, Y.; Torres-Castro, R. Long-Term Impact of COVID-19: A Systematic Review of the Literature and Meta-Analysis. *Biomedicines* **2021**, *9*, 900. [CrossRef]
48. Pelosi, P.; Tonelli, R.; Torregiani, C.; Baratella, E.; Confalonieri, M.; Battaglini, D.; Marchioni, A.; Confalonieri, P.; Clini, E.; Salton, F.; et al. Different Methods to Improve the Monitoring of Noninvasive Respiratory Support of Patients with Severe Pneumonia/ARDS Due to COVID-19: An Update. *J. Clin. Med.* **2022**, *11*, 1704. [CrossRef]
49. Ambrosino, P.; Lanzillo, A.; Maniscalco, M. COVID-19 and Post-Acute COVID-19 Syndrome: From Pathophysiology to Novel Translational Applications. *Biomedicines* **2021**, *10*, 47. [CrossRef]
50. Marini, E.; Buffa, R.; Contreras, M.; Magris, M.; Hidalgo, G.; Sanchez, W.; Ortiz, V.; Urbaez, M.; Cabras, S.; Blaser, M.J.; et al. Effect of influenza-induced fever on human bioimpedance values. *PLoS ONE* **2015**, *10*, e0125301. [CrossRef]
51. Xu, Z.; Liu, Y.; Yan, C.; Yang, R.; Xu, L.; Guo, Z.; Yu, A.; Cheng, X.; Ma, L.; Hu, C.; et al. Measurement of visceral fat and abdominal obesity by single-frequency bioelectrical impedance and CT: A cross-sectional study. *BMJ Open* **2021**, *11*, e048221. [CrossRef]

Disclaimer/Publisher's Note: The statements, opinions and data contained in all publications are solely those of the individual author(s) and contributor(s) and not of MDPI and/or the editor(s). MDPI and/or the editor(s) disclaim responsibility for any injury to people or property resulting from any ideas, methods, instructions or products referred to in the content.

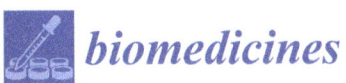

Article

Natural Course of COVID-19 and Independent Predictors of Mortality

Luana Orlando [1], Gianluca Bagnato [1,*], Carmelo Ioppolo [1], Maria Stella Franzè [1], Maria Perticone [2], Antonio Giovanni Versace [1], Angela Sciacqua [2], Vincenzo Russo [3], Arrigo Francesco Giuseppe Cicero [4], Alberta De Gaetano [1], Giuseppe Dattilo [1], Federica Fogacci [4], Maria Concetta Tringali [1], Pierpaolo Di Micco [5], Giovanni Squadrito [1] and Egidio Imbalzano [1]

1 Department of Clinical and Experimental Medicine, University of Messina, 98125 Messina, Italy
2 Department of Medical and Surgical Sciences, University Magna Græcia of Catanzaro, 88100 Catanzaro, Italy
3 Department of Medical Translational Sciences, Division of Cardiology, Monaldi Hospital, University of Campania "Luigi Vanvitelli", 80100 Naples, Italy
4 IRCCS Policlinico S. Orsola—Malpighi, Hypertension and Cardiovascular risk Research Center, DIMEC, University of Bologna, 40100 Bologna, Italy
5 Department of Medicine, PO Santa Maria delle Grazie Pozzuoli, 80100 Naples, Italy
* Correspondence: gianbagnato@gmail.com

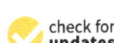

Citation: Orlando, L.; Bagnato, G.; Ioppolo, C.; Franzè, M.S.; Perticone, M.; Versace, A.G.; Sciacqua, A.; Russo, V.; Cicero, A.F.G.; De Gaetano, A.; et al. Natural Course of COVID-19 and Independent Predictors of Mortality. *Biomedicines* 2023, 11, 939. https://doi.org/10.3390/biomedicines11030939

Academic Editors: Elena Cecilia Rosca and Amalia Cornea

Received: 28 February 2023
Revised: 12 March 2023
Accepted: 13 March 2023
Published: 17 March 2023

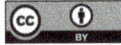

Copyright: © 2023 by the authors. Licensee MDPI, Basel, Switzerland. This article is an open access article distributed under the terms and conditions of the Creative Commons Attribution (CC BY) license (https://creativecommons.org/licenses/by/4.0/).

Abstract: Background: During the SARS-CoV-2 pandemic, several biomarkers were shown to be helpful in determining the prognosis of COVID-19 patients. The aim of our study was to evaluate the prognostic value of N-terminal pro-Brain Natriuretic Peptide (NT-pro-BNP) in a cohort of patients with COVID-19. Methods: One-hundred and seven patients admitted to the Covid Hospital of Messina University between June 2022 and January 2023 were enrolled in our study. The demographic, clinical, biochemical, instrumental, and therapeutic parameters were recorded. The primary outcome was in-hospital mortality. A comparison between patients who recovered and were discharged and those who died during the hospitalization was performed. The independent parameters associated with in-hospital death were assessed by multivariable analysis and a stepwise regression logistic model. Results: A total of 27 events with an in-hospital mortality rate of 25.2% occurred during our study. Those who died during hospitalization were older, with lower GCS and PaO_2/FiO_2 ratio, elevated D-dimer values, INR, creatinine values and shorter PT (prothrombin time). They had an increased frequency of diagnosis of heart failure ($p < 0.0001$) and higher NT-pro-BNP values. A multivariate logistic regression analysis showed that higher NT-pro-BNP values and lower PT and PaO_2/FiO_2 at admission were independent predictors of mortality during hospitalization. Conclusions: This study shows that NT-pro-BNP levels, PT, and PaO_2/FiO_2 ratio are independently associated with in-hospital mortality in subjects with COVID-19 pneumonia. Further longitudinal studies are warranted to confirm the results of this study.

Keywords: NT-pro-BNP; prothrombin time; PaO_2/FiO_2; COVID-19; biomarkers; SARS-CoV-2; coronavirus disease

1. Introduction

Two years after the outbreak of the coronavirus disease 2019 (COVID-19) pandemic, scientific progress and new vaccines has slowed mortality rates worldwide. However, in the first months, when the pandemic was announced in March 2020, the incidence of hospitalizations and mortality was very high. Patients with cardiovascular comorbidities, type 2 diabetes mellitus (T2DM), chronic kidney disease, cancer, pulmonary diseases, obesity, and those that are elderly were determined to have the most severe prognosis with the most significant mortality [1].

Although the main manifestations of COVID-19 are respiratory, septic and thromboembolic, other conditions such as brain damage, male infertility and pregnancy complications have been associated with severe acute respiratory syndrome coronavirus 2 (SARS-CoV-2), [2,3].

Among pregnancy complications, hypertensive disorders including preeclampsia and preeclampsia-like syndrome are associated with a dysregulated activity of the renin–angiotensin–aldosterone system. This disorder is common with COVID-19 and could be explained by high aldosterone levels causing hypertension and inflammation [4].

The cardiovascular system appears to be directly affected by numerous interactions with SARS-CoV-2, as suggested by the evidence of myocardial damage in children [5,6] and adult patients [7]. Several studies have investigated the possible correlation between cardiac biomarkers and the severity of COVID-19 disease [8–10] in order to identify one or more cut-off values to stratify patients for disease severity. Most of them show that B-type natriuretic peptide (BNP) as a predictive marker of the severity of COVID-19 disease [11]. Thus, genes and signaling pathways involved in the myocardium infected by SARS-CoV-2 were subsequently identified highlighting the mechanisms underlying cardiac damage [12]. Furthermore, numerous studies have revealed a key role for the angiotensin converting enzyme-2 (ACE2) receptor, whose physiological balance is altered by SARS-CoV-2, by activating angiotensin II (Ang II)/Ang II receptor type 1 (AT1R) pathways and by leading to severe disease complications [13,14]. The aim of our study was to evaluate the association between N-terminal fragment B-type natriuretic peptide (NT-pro-BNP) values and disease severity during the late phase of the pandemic, discovering a possible cut-off value to stratify the disease progression in COVID-19 patients.

2. Patients and Methods

This was a single center, retrospective, observational study. A total of 107 patients with a confirmed diagnosis of COVID-19, consecutively admitted between June 2022 and January 2023, at the COVID Division of the Hospital of the University of Messina, were enrolled in the study. The hospital is a large structure classified as a specialized second level hospital center serving an area of approximately 600,000 residents [15]. The diagnosis of SARS-CoV-2 infection was defined by using a Real-Time Polymerase Chain Reaction (RT-PCR) test, performed with oligonucleotide primers and probes drawn on conserved regions of the SARS-CoV-2 genome on biological material, collected by nasopharyngeal and oropharyngeal swabs. The swabs were repeated every 2–4 days to assess viral load clearance and the negativity of the test.

An anamnestic investigation, a complete objective examination, chest X-rays, and laboratory tests were recorded from each patient at hospital admission. The length of hospitalization was calculated from the date of admission to the hospital (in most cases corresponding to the date of diagnosis of COVID-19) to either discharge or in-hospital death. The presence of pre-existing cardiovascular diseases (e.g., arterial hypertension, coronary heart disease, heart failure) were recorded. The New York Heart Association (NYHA) classification was used to stratify patients with heart failure [16]. Treatments with Angiotensin-converting enzyme (ACE) inhibitors and Renin-Angiotensin-Aldosterone System (RAAS) inhibitors were recorded. Symptoms and signs of deep vein thrombosis (DVT) were sought in each patient both clinically and by performing bilateral compression ultrasonography (CUS), with the possible localization of venous thrombi and/or the development of a pulmonary embolism. Some patients underwent chest computed tomography (CT), including CT angiography or CT of the brain, abdomen, or limbs if required. The use of drugs for thromboprophylaxis was recorded, and it was specified whether the subject was treated with enoxaparin sodium or fondaparinux, vitamin K antagonists (VKAs), or non-vitamin K antagonists (NOACs). The partial pressure of oxygen (PaO_2) values, the fractional concentration of oxygen in inspired air (FiO_2) values, and the PaO_2/FiO_2 ratio were recorded at admission, as well as the oxygen-therapy required and the need for mechanical ventilation. The mean arterial pressure (MAP) was calculated at admission with the following formula: diastolic pressure +1/3 (systolic pressure—diastolic pressure).

The following laboratory tests were performed for each patient at admission: serum concentration of D-dimer, prothrombin time (PT), international normalized ratio (INR), fibrinogen, platelet count, serum creatinine, serum total bilirubin, NT-pro-BNP. The normal range of NT-pro-BNP in our laboratory was 0–300 ng/L.

Admission to the Intensive Care Unit (ICU) occurred in some patients due to the deterioration in vital functions and/or a worsening of the laboratory profile and/or instrumental evidence of signs of acute complications. The primary outcome of this study was in-hospital mortality, which was defined as death occurring during hospitalization.

No subject included in the study was asked for informed consent, since it was a non-interventional study and proposed as an anonymous retrospective analysis.

The study was conducted in accordance with the Declaration of Helsinki, and was approved by the or Ethics Committee of the University of Messina (protocol code 41-20; 04/05/2020).

Statistical Analysis

All statistical analyses were performed by IBM SPSS software (Version 26.0, SPSS, USA). The numerical data were expressed as mean and standard deviation (SD), whereas the categorical variables as a number and percentage. Examined continuous variables did not present a normal distribution as verified by a Kolmogorov–Smirnov test, and the non-parametric approach was consequently used. Accordingly, to compare the variables divided for survivors and deceased patients during hospitalization, the Mann–Whitney test was used for numerical variables. For categorical variables, the comparison between two groups was performed by Pearson's chi-square test. Univariate logistic regression analysis was used to identify predictors of death. Variables with a p value < 0.05 at univariate analysis were included in the multivariate logistic model. The results were expressed as odds ratio (OR) with a relative 95% confidence interval (CI) and p value. Furthermore, a stepwise regression model was designed to evaluate the potential independent predictors of mortality. The statistical significance level was set at a p value < 0.05.

3. Results

3.1. Patients' Characteristics

One hundred and seven COVID-19 patients [50 (46.7%) males/57 (53.3%) females with a mean age of 71.5 ± 16.1 years] that were consecutively hospitalized were enrolled in the study. The mean length of stay was 28.5 ± 17.3 days. During the hospitalization, four patients (3.7%) were transferred to the ICU and 27 (25.2%) died. Demographic, clinical, and biochemical characteristics of the study population are reported in Table 1. Thirty-four patients (31.8%) required oxygen-therapy at admission, and eight (7.5%) were treated with mechanical ventilation. The mean PaO_2/FiO_2 was 74.2 ± 20.2 mmHg, whereas the mean percentage of FiO_2 required was 26.4 ± 11.6. Sixty patients (56.1%) had a diagnosis of arterial hypertension, 16 (15%) had ischemic heart disease, and 55 (51.4%) had heart failure. Specifically, 7/55 patients (12.7%) were in NYHA class I, 14 (25.5%) were in NYHA class II, 14 (25.5%) were in NYHA class III, and 20 (36.4%) were in in NYHA class IV. Nineteen patients (17.8%) were under treatment with ACE inhibitors, and 31 (29%) were treated with RAAS inhibitors. At admission, the mean NT-pro-BNP value was 1954 ± 4941 pg/mL. During the hospitalization, serial compression ultrasonography (CUS) was performed in 50 patients (46.7%), and 13 patients (12.1%) underwent a chest CT scan. Only in three cases (2.8%) the instrumental investigation confirmed a diagnosis of deep venous thrombosis (DVT). The mean serum D-dimer levels recorded at admission was 1455 ± 1252 ng/mL. In particular, 27 patients (25.2%) had normal values (0–500 ng/mL), 29 (27.1%) 29 (27.1%) had mildly increased concentrations (500–1000 ng/mL), 35 (32.7%) had moderately elevated levels (1000–4000 ng/mL), and 16 (15%) were severely elevated (>4000 ng/mL). During the hospitalization, 103/107 (96.3%) patients underwent pharmacological thromboprophylaxis: 94/103 (87.9%) were treated with enoxaparin or fondaparinux, 3/103 (2.8%) were treated with VKAs, and 6/103 (5.6%) were treated with NOACs (rivaroxaban, apixaban, or edoxaban).

Table 1. Demographic and clinical characteristics of 107 COVID-19 patients included in the study.

Baseline Characteristics	Total (n = 107)	Survivors (n = 80)	Deceased (n = 27)	p
Male, n (%)	50 (46.7)	40 (50)	10 (37)	0.243
BMI, kg/m^2	23.48± 3.06	23.57 ± 2.99	23.11 ± 3.36	0.356
ICU, n (%)	4 (3.7)	3 (3.8)	1 (3.7)	0.991
Age, years	71.51 ± 16.14	68.13 ± 16.21	81.56 ± 11.1	**<0.0001**
Length of stays	28.45 ± 17.31	32.56 ± 15.83	16.29 ± 15.95	0.476
CUS, n (%)	50 (46.7)	37 (46.3)	13 (48.1)	0.864
DVT confirmed, n (%)	3 (2.8)	1 (1.3)	2 (7.4)	0.094
CT scan, n (%)	13 (12.1)	10 (12.5)	3 (11.1)	0.849
Drug thromboprophylaxis n (%)	103 (96.3)	77 (96.3)	26 (96.3)	0.991
Anticoagulant drugs, n (%) No therapy LMWH AVKs NOACs	 4 (3.7) 94 (87.9) 3 (2.8) 6 (5.6)	 3 (3.8) 70 (87.5) 2 (2.5) 5 (6.3)	 1 (3.7) 24 (88.9) 1 (3.7) 1 (3.7)	0.952
COVID-19 vaccination	19 (17.7)	13 (16.2)	6 (22.2)	0.482
Mechanical ventilation, n (%)	8 (7.5)	4 (5)	4 (14.8)	0.094
PaO$_2$/FiO$_2$ ratio	314 ± 115	342 ± 102	228 ± 113	**<0.001**
MAP, mmHg	87 ± 12.42	86.91 ± 11.98	87.25 ± 49.33	0.773
CCI	2.6 ± 1.3	2.3 ± 1.1	2.9 ± 1.7	0.334
Arterial hypertension, n (%)	60 (56.1)	42 (52.5)	18 (66.7)	0.200
Coronary heart disease, n (%)	16 (15.0)	11 (13.8)	5 (18.5)	0.548
ACE-Inhibitors, n (%)	19 (17.8)	14 (17.5)	5 (18.5)	0.905
RAAS, n (%)	31 (29.0)	22 (27.5)	9 (33.3)	0.563
Heart failure, n (%)	55 (51.4)	33 (41.3)	22 (81.5)	**<0.0001**
NYHA classes, n (%) Class I Class II Class III Class IV	 7 (12.7) 14 (25.5) 14 (25.5) 20 (36.4)	 6 (18.2) 12 (36.4) 9 (27.3) 6 (7.5)	 1 (4.5) 2 (9.1) 5 (22.7) 14 (63.6)	**0.004**
GCS	13.54 ±2.45	14.08 ± 2.11	11.96 ± 2.73	**<0.0001**

All numerical parameters are expressed as mean and standard deviations (SD). Bold characters identify statistically significant results. ICU: Intensive Care Unit. CUS: Compression Ultrasonography. VKA: Vitamin K Antagonist. DVT: Deep Venous thrombosis. CT: Computer tomography. DOACs: Direct Oral Anticoagulants SD: Standard Deviation PT: Prothrombin Time. INR: International Normalized Ratio. GCS: Glasgow Coma Scale. MAP: Mean Arterial Pression. CCI: Charlson Comorbidity index; p: p-value.

3.2. Comparison between Survivors and Deceased COVID-19 Patients

Next, we analyzed the study population after dividing them according to the outcome of interest as deceased (n = 27) and survivors (n = 80). As reported in Table 1, no statistically significant differences were observed concerning sex, BMI, MAP, presence of arterial hypertension, ischemic heart disease, treatment with ACE-inhibitors, or RAAS-inhibitors, bilirubin values, platelet count, fibrinogen levels, the presence of DVT signs (assessed by CUS or CT), and treatment with anticoagulants.

On the contrary, deceased patients were older, with lower GCS and a shorter length of hospitalization and more severe pulmonary involvement, as evidenced by the difference in PaO_2/FiO_2 values. Deceased patients had higher D-dimer values, shorter prothrombin time, higher INR and higher creatinine values at admission compared to survivors. Moreover, patients who died significantly differed from survivors with regard to the presence of heart failure with higher NYHA classes and higher NT-pro-BNP values (Tables 1 and 2).

Table 2. Biochemical characteristics of 107 COVID-19 patients included in the study.

	Baseline Characteristics	Survivors (n = 80)	Deceased (n = 27)	p
Creatinine, mg/dL	1.16 ± 1.22	0.93 ± 0.46	1.84 ± 2.91	**0.029**
Bilirubine, mg/dL	0.51 ± 0.27	0.49 ± 0.23	0.59 ± 0.35	0.182
NT-proBNP, pg/mL	1954 ± 4941	718 ± 1286	5616 ± 8712	**<0.0001**
D-dimer, ng/mL	1455 ± 1252	1276 ±1166	1988 ± 1367	**0.005**
D-Dimer classes, n (%)				
I (0–500 ng/mL)	27 (25.2%)	24 (30%)	3 (11.1%)	
II (500–1000 ng/mL)	29 (27.1%)	22 (27.5%)	7 (25.9%)	
III (1000–4000 ng/mL)	35 (32.7%)	25 (31.3%)	10 (37%)	
IV (>4000 ng/mL)	17 (15.0%)	9 (11.3%)	7 (25.9%)	
PT, seconds	81.1 ± 22.43	85.06 ± 19.61	69.29 ± 26.24	**0.002**
INR	1.31 ± 1.21	1.13 ± 0.30	1.84 ± 2.30	**0.001**
Platelet, n/mm^3	207.738 ± 80785	202.375 ± 77.733	190,000 ± 88.863	0.335

All numerical parameters are expressed as mean and standard deviations (SD). Bold characters identify statistically significant results. PT, prothrombin time; INR: International Nationalized Ratio.

3.3. Analysis of Independent Predictors of In-Hospital Death

We investigated the possible association between all parameters collected at admission and in-hospital mortality. Since age was significantly different between the groups, the initial univariate logistic regression was corrected for age. Upon univariate logistic regression analysis, mortality was significantly associated with lower PaO_2/FiO_2, lower PT values ($p = 0.004$), higher NT-pro-BNP values ($p = 0.001$), and lower Glasgow Coma Scale classes ($p = 0.001$). A multivariate stepwise logistic regression analysis showed that higher NT-pro-BNP values, lower PT values, and lower PaO_2/FiO_2 at admission were independent predictors of mortality during hospitalization. (Table 3).

Table 3. Age-adjusted univariate and multivariate stepwise backward logistic regression analysis of predictive factors for in-hospital mortality in patients with COVID-19.

	Univariate Analysis			Multivariate Analysis		
	Odds Ratio	CI 95%	p	Odds Ratio	CI 95%	p
D-Dimer			0.087	-	-	-
PT	0.964	0.941–0.988	**0.004**	0.958	0.927–0.990	**0.010**
INR			0.130			
Creatinine			0.083			
PaO_2/FiO_2 ratio	0.991	0.985–0.996	**0.001**	0.987	0.981–0.994	**0.001**
GCS	0.677	0.544–0.842	**0.001**			0.128
Heart failure			0.147	-	-	-
NYHA classes			0.055			
NT-pro-BNP	1.000	1.000–1.001	**0.026**	1.001	1.000–1.001	**0.004**

PT: prothrombin time. GCS: Glasgow Coma Scale.

4. Discussion

COVID-19 is known as a respiratory illness; however, current research suggests that SARS-CoV 2 has a direct cardiomyocyte tropism. As a result, myocarditis, the development of left ventricular systolic and diastolic dysfunction, and myocardial fibrosis might occur [17]. Due to the predominance and severity of pulmonary involvement, these individuals may also have right ventricular dysfunction. The inflammatory state caused by the action of the virus [18] induces the infiltration of the myocardium by inflammatory cells (monocytes, macrophages, lymphocytes, neutrophils), leading to myocarditis and consequently heart failure [19,20]. Myocarditis, as a result of an autoimmune response induced by the virus, could progress in structural cardiomyopathy [21], and could be associated with a poor prognosis when complicated by heart failure and left ventricular dysfunction [22,23]. This is particularly relevant considering that a recent meta-analysis compared fulminant myocarditis associated with COVID-19 infection versus COVID-19 vaccination. While this study reported a similarly high mortality rate and no differences in most biopsies/autopsies between these conditions, COVID-19 fulminant myocarditis was associated with a more aggressive course with more severe hemodynamic decompensation and more cardiac arrests [24].

This is particularly relevant, since an excess of myocardial injury may cause an increase in several cardiac biomarkers, such as NT-pro-BNP. NT-pro-BNP is a quantitative plasma biomarker reflecting hemodynamic cardiac stress that is usually caused by volume or pressure overload, and therefore plays a central role in the diagnosis and management of heart failure and cardiac function. Yet, seeing as its concentrations increase immediately after myocardial damage and improves as a consequence of clinical improvement, it represents a predictor of an adverse outcome in acute myocardial damage [25]. Myocardial injury, inflammation, interaction with angiotensin converting enzyme 2 (ACE2), or impairment of cardiac function with acute heart failure may be responsible for higher circulating natriuretic peptides in COVID-19 patients. Yang et al. retrospectively analyzed 203 patients with a confirmed diagnosis of SARS-CoV-2 infection and definite outcomes (discharge or death), consisting of 145 patients who recovered and 58 patients who died. In their analysis, 53% of the deceased had elevated NT-pro-BNP levels [26]. According to a recent meta-analysis involving 2248 patients, with the majority belonging to the early COVID-19 epidemic in China, NT-pro-BNP evaluation may help differentiate high-risk individuals [27]. Furthermore, as noted by Gao et al., patients with severe COVID-19 who have high NT-pro-BNP levels are more likely to be older, have greater levels of systemic inflammatory markers and heart damage markers, and have a poorer cumulative survival rate. After adjusting for relevant confounders, NT-pro-BNP was demonstrated to be an independent risk factor for in-hospital death in patients with severe COVID-19 [28]. According to other studies, it has been demonstrated that NT-pro-BNP levels were eight times higher at the time of hospitalization in deceased patients versus survivors. Therefore, despite the fact that cardiac injury is a common condition among hospitalized patients with COVID-19, high NT-pro-BNP levels were associated with a higher risk of in-hospital mortality [29]. Furthermore, numerous reports support the predictive role of NT-pro-BNP in the severity of the disease [30,31] in patients with and without pre-existing heart failure [32]. In line with previous studies, our results confirm that high NT-pro-BNP levels at admission increase the risk of in-hospital mortality and are very strong and independent indicators of mortality in COVID-19 patients. The routine measurements of cardiac biomarkers and especially NT-pro-BNP should be considered in COVID-19 patients. If confirmed by larger population studies, it might be possible to identify a cut-off value of this biomarker in order to stratify the population at higher risk of developing severe disease. The PaO_2/FiO_2 ratio is used to classify the severity of acute respiratory distress syndrome (ARDS), and is the most commonly used oxygenation index included in the sepsis management guidelines [33] and acute respiratory distress syndrome [34]. In a non-COVID-19 setting, PaO_2/FiO_2 is considered to be a predictor of unfavorable outcomes, as initially reported by Villar et al. [35], and subsequently verified in many additional studies, primarily from ICU settings [36,37]. Unexpectedly, despite being widely used in clinical practice, not many reports have previously investigated its ability to predict mortality in COVID-19 patients in critical care settings. In the context of COVID-19, the PaO_2/FiO_2 ratio has primarily been studied as an indicator of disease severity and as a predictor of mortality [38–40]. In this study, PaO_2/FiO_2 was an independent predictor of COVID-19 mortality. Therefore, our findings have the potential clinical relevance to support the use of a single PaO_2/FiO_2 ratio measurement at admission as an independent predictor of mortality. Prothrombin time (PT) levels are elevated in COVID-19 patients. Higher PT was noted in 183 individuals whose data were examined [41]. In addition, PT is reported to be higher in patients admitted to the ICU and in severe COVID-19 cases compared to those with mild disease [42,43].

5. Conclusions

In conclusion, our results suggest that there are multiple predictors of mortality among COVID-19 patients, and in particular our findings support that COVID-19 induces a systemic derangement involving not only the pulmonary system but also the coagulation cascade and the cardiovascular system. Thus, NT-pro-BNP, PaO_2/FiO_2, and PT could potentially serve as independent risk factors for predicting death in COVID-19 patients. It is worthy of note that clinicians might want to consider the aforementioned indicators and take action to reduce the mortality of COVID-19. Eventually, future confirmatory studies in larger prospective cohorts might prove useful for patients stratification into risk classes. This would allow to allocate patients to the appropriate intensity of care according to disease severity and adapt treatment regimen to the multifaceted systemic aspects of the disease.

Author Contributions: Conceptualization, L.O. and E.I.; methodology, L.O. and A.S.; software, G.B.; validation, E.I., V.R., M.P. and A.F.G.C.; formal analysis, G.B., A.D.G., M.C.T. and M.S.F.; investigation, C.I., F.F. and M.C.T.; resources, E.I. and A.G.V.; data curation, C.I., M.S.F. and A.S.; writing—original draft preparation, L.O., G.D., A.G.V., A.D.G., F.F. and M.P.; writing—review and editing, E.I., C.I., V.R., A.F.G.C., G.S., P.D.M. and G.B.; visualization, G.D. and M.S.F.; supervision, A.G.V., G.S., V.R., A.F.G.C., M.P., G.B., C.I. and P.D.M. All authors have read and agreed to the published version of the manuscript.

Funding: This research received no external funding.

Institutional Review Board Statement: The study was conducted in accordance with the Declaration of Helsinki, and approved by the Ethics Committee of the University of Messina (protocol code 41-20;04/05/2020).

Informed Consent Statement: Patient consent was waived due to the non-interventional nature of the study being an anonymous retrospective analysis.

Data Availability Statement: The data presented in this study are available on request from the corresponding author.

Conflicts of Interest: The authors declare that they have no conflict of interest.

References

1. Pepera, G.; Tribali, M.-S.; Batalik, L.; Petrov, I.; Papathanasiou, J. Epidemiology, risk factors and prognosis of cardiovascular disease in the Coronavirus Disease 2019 (COVID-19) pandemic era: A systematic review. *Rev. Cardiovasc. Med.* **2022**, *23*, 28. [CrossRef] [PubMed]
2. Delli Muti, N.; Finocchi, F.; Tossetta, G.; Salvio, G.; Cutini, M.; Marzioni, D.; Balercia, G. Could SARS-CoV-2 infection affect male fertility and sexuality? *APMIS* **2022**, *130*, 243–252. [CrossRef]
3. Marshall, M. How COVID-19 can damage the brain. *Nature* **2020**, *585*, 342–343. [CrossRef]
4. Tossetta, G.; Fantone, S.; Muti, N.D.; Balercia, G.; Ciavattini, A.; Giannubilo, S.R.; Marzioni, D. Preeclampsia and severe acute respiratory syndrome coronavirus 2 infection: A systematic review. *J. Hypertens.* **2022**, *40*, 1629–1638. [CrossRef] [PubMed]
5. Vukomanovic, V.; Krasic, S.; Prijic, S.; Petrovic, G.; Ninic, S.; Popovic, S.; Cerovic, I.; Ristic, S.; Nesic, D. Myocardial damage in multisystem inflammatory syndrome associated with COVID-19 in children and adolescents. *J. Res. Med. Sci.* **2021**, *26*, 113. [CrossRef] [PubMed]

6. Aeschlimann, F.A.; Misra, N.; Hussein, T.; Panaioli, E.; Soslow, J.H.; Crum, K.; Steele, J.M.; Huber, S.; Marcora, S.; Brambilla, P.; et al. Myocardial involvement in children with post-COVID multisystem inflammatory syndrome: A cardiovascular magnetic resonance based multicenter international study-the CARDOVID registry. *J. Cardiovasc. Magn. Reson.* **2021**, *23*, 140. [CrossRef]
7. Batta, Y.; King, C.; Johnson, J.; Haddad, N.; Boueri, M.; Haddad, G. Sequelae and Comorbidities of COVID-19 Manifestations on the Cardiac and the Vascular Systems. *Front. Physiol.* **2021**, *12*, 748972. [CrossRef]
8. Mueller, C.; Giannitsis, E.; Jaffe, A.S.; Huber, K.; Mair, J.; Cullen, L.; Hammarsten, O.; Mills, N.L.; Möckel, M.; Krychtiuk, K.; et al. Cardiovascular biomarkers in patients with COVID-19. *Eur. Heart J. Acute Cardiovasc. Care* **2021**, *10*, 310–319. [CrossRef]
9. Ruan, Q.; Yang, K.; Wang, W.; Jiang, L.; Song, J. Clinical predictors of mortality due to COVID-19 based on an analysis of data of 150 patients from Wuhan, China. *Intensive Care Med.* **2020**, *46*, 846–848. [CrossRef]
10. Xu, Z.; Shi, L.; Wang, Y.; Zhang, J.; Huang, L.; Zhang, C.; Liu, S.; Zhao, P.; Liu, H.; Zhu, L.; et al. Pathological findings of COVID-19 associated with acute respiratory distress syndrome. *Lancet Respir. Med.* **2020**, *8*, 420–422. [CrossRef]
11. Wungu, C.D.K.; Khaerunnisa, S.; Putri, E.A.C.; Hidayati, H.B.; Qurnianingsih, E.; Lukitasari, L.; Humairah, I. Meta-analysis of cardiac markers for predictive factors on severity and mortality of COVID-19. *Int. J. Infect. Dis.* **2021**, *105*, 551–559. [CrossRef] [PubMed]
12. Xie, L.M.; Huang, Y.F.; Liu, Y.L.; Liang, J.Q.; Deng, W.; Lin, G.L.; Luo, H.M.; Guo, X.G. Identification of the Hub Genes and the Signaling Pathways in Human iPSC-Cardiomyocytes Infected by SARS-CoV-2. *Biochem. Genet.* **2022**, *60*, 2052–2068. [CrossRef] [PubMed]
13. Beyerstedt, S.; Casaro, E.B.; Rangel, E.B. COVID-19: Angiotensin-converting enzyme 2 (ACE2) expression and tissue susceptibility to SARS-CoV-2 infection. *Eur. J. Clin. Microbiol. Infect. Dis.* **2021**, *40*, 905–919. [CrossRef]
14. Datta, P.K.; Liu, F.; Fischer, T.; Rappaport, J.; Qin, X. SARS-CoV-2 pandemic and research gaps: Understanding SARS-CoV-2 interaction with the ACE2 receptor and implications for therapy. *Theranostics* **2020**, *10*, 7448–7464. [CrossRef] [PubMed]
15. Laganà, P.; Facciolà, A.; Palermo, R.; Delia, S. Environmental Surveillance of Legionellosis within an Italian University Hospital-Results of 15 Years of Analysis. *Int. J. Environ. Res. Public Health* **2019**, *16*, 1103. [CrossRef]
16. McDonagh, T.A.; Metra, M.; Adamo, M.; Gardner, R.S.; Baumbach, A.; Böhm, M.; Burri, H.; Butler, J.; Čelutkienė, J.; Chioncel, O.; et al. 2021 ESC Guidelines for the diagnosis and treatment of acute and chronic heart failure. *Eur. Heart J.* **2021**, *42*, 3599–3726. [CrossRef]
17. Patone, M.; Mei, X.W.; Handunnetthi, L.; Dixon, S.; Zaccardi, F.; Shankar-Hari, M.; Watkinson, P.; Khunti, K.; Harnden, A.; Coupland, C.A.C.; et al. Risks of myocarditis, pericarditis, and cardiac arrhythmias associated with COVID-19 vaccination or SARS-CoV-2 infection. *Nat. Med.* **2022**, *28*, 410–422. [CrossRef]
18. Bagnato, G.; Imbalzano, E.; Aragona, C.O.; Ioppolo, C.; Di Micco, P.; La Rosa, D.; Costa, F.; Micari, A.; Tomeo, S.; Zirilli, N.; et al. New-Onset Atrial Fibrillation and Early Mortality Rate in COVID-19 Patients: Association with IL-6 Serum Levels and Respiratory Distress. *Medicina (Kaunas)* **2022**, *58*, 530. [CrossRef]
19. Adeghate, E.A.; Eid, N.; Singh, J. Mechanisms of COVID-19-induced heart failure: A short review. *Heart Fail Rev.* **2021**, *26*, 363–369. [CrossRef]
20. Bonaccorsi, I.; Carrega, P.; Rullo, E.V.; Ducatelli, R.; Falco, M.; Freni, J.; Miceli, M.; Cavaliere, R.; Fontana, V.; Versace, A.; et al. HLA-C*17 in COVID-19 patients: Hints for associations with severe clinical outcome and cardiovascular risk. *Immunol. Lett.* **2021**, *234*, 44–46. [CrossRef]
21. Tschöpe, C.; Ammirati, E.; Bozkurt, B.; Caforio, A.L.P.; Cooper, L.T.; Felix, S.B.; Hare, J.M.; Heidecker, B.; Heymans, S.; Hübner, N.; et al. Myocarditis and inflammatory cardiomyopathy: Current evidence and future directions. *Nat. Rev. Cardiol.* **2021**, *18*, 169–193. [CrossRef] [PubMed]
22. Gulizia, M.M.; Orso, F.; Mortara, A.; Lucci, D.; Aspromonte, N.; De Luca, L.; Di Tano, G.; Leonardi, G.; Navazio, A.; Pulignano, G.; et al. BLITZ-HF: A nationwide initiative to evaluate and improve adherence to acute and chronic heart failure guidelines. *Eur. J. Heart Fail* **2022**, *24*, 2078–2089. [CrossRef] [PubMed]
23. Ammirati, E.; Cipriani, M.; Moro, C.; Raineri, C.; Pini, D.; Sormani, P.; Mantovani, R.; Varrenti, M.; Pedrotti, P.; Conca, C.; et al. Clinical Presentation and Outcome in a Contemporary Cohort of Patients With Acute Myocarditis: Multicenter Lombardy Registry. *Circulation* **2018**, *138*, 1088–1099. [CrossRef] [PubMed]
24. Guglin, M.E.; Etuk, A.; Shah, C.; Ilonze, O.J. Fulminant Myocarditis and Cardiogenic Shock Following COVID-19 Infection Versus COVID-19 Vaccination: A Systematic Literature Review. *J. Clin. Med.* **2023**, *12*, 1849. [CrossRef] [PubMed]
25. Sangaralingham, S.J.; Kuhn, M.; Cannone, V.; Chen, H.H.; Burnett, J.C. Natriuretic peptide pathways in heart failure: Further therapeutic possibilities. *Cardiovasc. Res.* **2023**, *118*, 3416–3433. [CrossRef] [PubMed]
26. Yang, C.; Liu, F.; Liu, W.; Cao, G.; Liu, J.; Huang, S.; Zhu, M.; Tu, C.; Wang, J.; Xiong, B. Myocardial injury and risk factors for mortality in patients with COVID-19 pneumonia. *Int. J. Cardiol.* **2021**, *326*, 230–236. [CrossRef]
27. Sorrentino, S.; Cacia, M.; Leo, I.; Polimeni, A.; Sabatino, J.; Spaccarotella, C.A.M.; Mongiardo, A.; De Rosa, S.; Indolfi, C. B-Type Natriuretic Peptide as Biomarker of COVID-19 Disease Severity-A Meta-Analysis. *J. Clin. Med.* **2020**, *9*, 2957. [CrossRef]
28. Gao, L.; Jiang, D.; Wen, X.S.; Cheng, X.C.; Sun, M.; He, B.; You, L.N.; Lei, P.; Tan, X.W.; Qin, S.; et al. Prognostic value of NT-proBNP in patients with severe COVID-19. *Respir. Res.* **2020**, *21*, 83. [CrossRef]
29. Inciardi, R.M.; Adamo, M.; Lupi, L.; Cani, D.S.; Di Pasquale, M.; Tomasoni, D.; Italia, L.; Zaccone, G.; Tedino, C.; Fabbricatore, D.; et al. Characteristics and outcomes of patients hospitalized for COVID-19 and cardiac disease in Northern Italy. *Eur. Heart J.* **2020**, *41*, 1821–1829. [CrossRef]

30. Stefanini, G.G.; Chiarito, M.; Ferrante, G.; Cannata, F.; Azzolini, E.; Viggiani, G.; De Marco, A.; Briani, M.; Bocciolone, M.; Bragato, R.; et al. Early detection of elevated cardiac biomarkers to optimise risk stratification in patients with COVID-19. *Heart* **2020**, *106*, 1512–1518. [CrossRef]
31. Yoo, J.; Grewal, P.; Hotelling, J.; Papamanoli, A.; Cao, K.; Dhaliwal, S.; Jacob, R.; Mojahedi, A.; Bloom, M.E.; Marcos, L.A.; et al. Admission NT-proBNP and outcomes in patients without history of heart failure hospitalized with COVID-19. *ESC Heart Fail* **2021**, *8*, 4278–4287. [CrossRef] [PubMed]
32. Hermansyah, T.A.; Ginanjar, E.; Putri, V.H. Elevation of Cardiac Biomarkers in COVID-19 as a Major Determinant for Mortality: A Systematic Review. *Acta Med. Indones.* **2021**, *53*, 385–396.
33. Evans, L.; Rhodes, A.; Alhazzani, W.; Antonelli, M.; Coopersmith, C.M.; French, C.; Machado, F.R.; Mcintyre, L.; Ostermann, M.; Prescott, H.C.; et al. Surviving Sepsis Campaign: International Guidelines for Management of Sepsis and Septic Shock 2021. *Crit. Care Med.* **2021**, *49*, e1063–e1143. [CrossRef]
34. ARDS Definition Task Force; Ranieri, V.M.; Rubenfeld, G.D.; Thompson, B.T.; Ferguson, N.D.; Caldwell, E.; Fan, E.; Camporota, L.; Slutsky, A.S. Acute respiratory distress syndrome: The Berlin Definition. *JAMA* **2012**, *307*, 2526–2533. [PubMed]
35. Villar, J.; Blanco, J.; del Campo, R.; Andaluz-Ojeda, D.; Díaz-Domínguez, F.J.; Muriel, A.; Córcoles, V.; Suárez-Sipmann, F.; Tarancón, C.; González-Higueras, E.; et al. Assessment of PaO(2)/FiO(2) for stratification of patients with moderate and severe acute respiratory distress syndrome. *BMJ Open* **2015**, *5*, e006812. [CrossRef] [PubMed]
36. Feiner, J.R.; Weiskopf, R.B. Evaluating Pulmonary Function: An Assessment of PaO_2/FiO_2. *Crit. Care Med.* **2017**, *45*, e40–e48. [CrossRef]
37. Santus, P.; Radovanovic, D.; Saderi, L.; Marino, P.; Cogliati, C.; De Filippis, G.; Rizzi, M.; Franceschi, E.; Pini, S.; Giuliani, F.; et al. Severity of respiratory failure at admission and in-hospital mortality in patients with COVID-19: A prospective observational multicentre study. *BMJ Open* **2020**, *10*, e043651. [CrossRef]
38. Colaneri, M.; Sacchi, P.; Zuccaro, V.; Biscarini, S.; Sachs, M.; Roda, S.; Pieri, T.C.; Valsecchi, P.; Piralla, A.; Seminari, E.; et al. Clinical characteristics of coronavirus disease (COVID-19) early findings from a teaching hospital in Pavia, North Italy, 21 to 28 February 2020. *Euro. Surveill.* **2020**, *25*, 2000460. [CrossRef] [PubMed]
39. Gu, Y.; Wang, D.; Chen, C.; Lu, W.; Liu, H.; Lv, T.; Song, Y.; Zhang, F. PaO(2)/FiO(2) and IL-6 are risk factors of mortality for intensive care COVID-19 patients. *Sci. Rep.* **2021**, *11*, 7334. [CrossRef]
40. Bagnato, G.; La Rosa, D.; Ioppolo, C.; De Gaetano, A.; Chiappalone, M.; Zirilli, N.; Viapiana, V.; Tringali, M.C.; Tomeo, S.; Aragona, C.O.; et al. The COVID-19 Assessment for Survival at Admission (CASA) Index: A 12 Months Observational Study. *Front. Med. (Lausanne)* **2021**, *8*, 719976. [CrossRef]
41. Arachchillage, D.R.; Laffan, M. Abnormal coagulation parameters are associated with poor prognosis in patients with novel coronavirus pneumonia. *J. Thromb. Haemost.* **2020**, *18*, 1233–1234. [CrossRef] [PubMed]
42. Di Minno, M.N.D.; Calcaterra, I.; Lupoli, R.; Storino, A.; Spedicato, G.A.; Maniscalco, M.; Di Minno, A.; Ambrosino, P. Hemostatic Changes in Patients with COVID-19: A Meta-Analysis with Meta-Regressions. *J. Clin. Med.* **2020**, *9*, 2244. [CrossRef] [PubMed]
43. Baranovskii, D.S.; Klabukov, I.D.; Krasilnikova, O.A.; Nikogosov, D.A.; Polekhina, N.V.; Baranovskaia, D.R.; Laberko, L.A. Prolonged prothrombin time as an early prognostic indicator of severe acute respiratory distress syndrome in patients with COVID-19 related pneumonia. *Curr. Med. Res. Opin.* **2021**, *37*, 21–25. [CrossRef] [PubMed]

Disclaimer/Publisher's Note: The statements, opinions and data contained in all publications are solely those of the individual author(s) and contributor(s) and not of MDPI and/or the editor(s). MDPI and/or the editor(s) disclaim responsibility for any injury to people or property resulting from any ideas, methods, instructions or products referred to in the content.

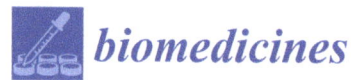

Article

Acute Kidney Injury Associated with Severe SARS-CoV-2 Infection: Risk Factors for Morbidity and Mortality and a Potential Benefit of Combined Therapy with Tocilizumab and Corticosteroids

Jose Iglesias [1,2,3,*], Andrew Vassallo [4], Justin Ilagan [1], Song Peng Ang [5], Ndausung Udongwo [1], Anton Mararenko [1], Abbas Alshami [1], Dylon Patel [6], Yasmine Elbaga [7] and Jerrold S. Levine [8,9]

1. Department of Medicine, Jersey Shore University Medical Center, Neptune, NJ 07753, USA
2. Department of Nephrology, Community Medical Center, RWJBarnabas Health, Toms River, NJ 08757, USA
3. Department of Medicine, Hackensack Meridian School of Medicine, Nutley, NJ 07110, USA
4. Department of Pharmacy, Community Medical Center, RWJBarnabas Health, Toms River, NJ 08757, USA
5. Department of Medicine, Community Medical Center, RWJBarnabas Health, Toms River, NJ 08757, USA
6. Hackensack Meridian School of Medicine, Nutley, NJ 07110, USA
7. Department of Pharmacy, Monmouth Medical Center Southern Campus, RWJBarnabas Health, 600 River Ave., Lakewood, NJ 08701, USA
8. Department of Medicine, Division of Nephrology, University of Illinois Chicago, Chicago, IL 60612, USA
9. Department of Medicine, Division of Nephrology, Jesse Brown Veterans Affairs Medical Center, Chicago, IL 60612, USA
* Correspondence: jiglesias23@gmail.com

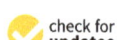

Citation: Iglesias, J.; Vassallo, A.; Ilagan, J.; Ang, S.P.; Udongwo, N.; Mararenko, A.; Alshami, A.; Patel, D.; Elbaga, Y.; Levine, J.S. Acute Kidney Injury Associated with Severe SARS-CoV-2 Infection: Risk Factors for Morbidity and Mortality and a Potential Benefit of Combined Therapy with Tocilizumab and Corticosteroids. *Biomedicines* 2023, 11, 845. https://doi.org/10.3390/biomedicines11030845

Academic Editors: Elena Cecilia Rosca and Amalia Cornea

Received: 4 February 2023
Revised: 3 March 2023
Accepted: 6 March 2023
Published: 10 March 2023

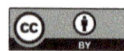

Copyright: © 2023 by the authors. Licensee MDPI, Basel, Switzerland. This article is an open access article distributed under the terms and conditions of the Creative Commons Attribution (CC BY) license (https://creativecommons.org/licenses/by/4.0/).

Abstract: Background: Acute kidney injury (AKI) is a common complication in patients with severe COVID-19. Methods: We retrospectively reviewed 249 patients admitted to an intensive care unit (ICU) during the first wave of the pandemic to determine risk factors for AKI. Demographics, comorbidities, and clinical and outcome variables were obtained from electronic medical records. Results: Univariate analysis revealed older age, higher admission serum creatinine, elevated Sequential Organ Failure Assessment (SOFA) score, elevated admission D-Dimer, elevated CRP on day 2, mechanical ventilation, vasopressor requirement, and azithromycin usage as significant risk factors for AKI. Multivariate analysis demonstrated that higher admission creatinine ($p = 0.0001$, OR = 2.41, 95% CI = 1.56–3.70), vasopressor requirement ($p = 0.0001$, OR = 3.20, 95% CI = 1.69–5.98), elevated admission D-Dimer ($p = 0.008$, OR = 1.0001, 95% CI = 1.000–1.001), and elevated C-reactive protein (CRP) on day 2 ($p = 0.033$, OR = 1.0001, 95% CI = 1.004–1.009) were independent risk factors. Conversely, the combined use of Tocilizumab and corticosteroids was independently associated with reduced AKI risk ($p = 0.0009$, OR = 0.437, 95% CI = 0.23–0.81). Conclusion: This study confirms the high rate of AKI and associated mortality among COVID-19 patients admitted to ICUs and suggests a role for inflammation and/or coagulopathy in AKI development. One should consider the possibility that early administration of anti-inflammatory agents, as is now routinely conducted in the management of COVID-19-associated acute respiratory distress syndrome, may improve clinical outcomes in patients with AKI.

Keywords: COVID-19; acute kidney injury; anti-inflammatory; Tocilizumab

1. Introduction

Severe COVID-19 disease, as caused by SARS-CoV-2 infection, results in a wide variety of renal injuries, manifesting as hematuria, proteinuria, tubular dysfunction, acute tubular necrosis, thrombotic microangiopathy (TMA), and/or collapsing glomerulopathy [1–3]. The incidence of acute kidney injury (AKI) with COVID-19 disease ranges from 0.5% to 36% among all infected patients and is much higher in patients requiring intensive care management [4–10]. The reasons for the variability in the development of AKI are not completely clear, and may be related to timing of diagnosis, severity of illness, differences in demographics, and definitions of AKI [10,11]. Aside from the development of COVID-19-associated respiratory distress syndrome (C19-ARDS), AKI in the setting of COVID-19 disease is the second most common cause of morbidity and mortality [5,12,13]. The prevalence of AKI in non-survivors of COVID-19 having C19-ARDS and infected with the Wuhan strain of the virus during the first wave of the pandemic was increased 2.5-fold compared to survivors of COVID-19 with C19-ARDS [12].

Although COVID-19 disease primarily impacts the respiratory tract, the enzyme angiotensin converting enzyme-2 (ACE-2), the primary receptor for SARS-CoV-2, is expressed by the endothelium of almost all extra-pulmonary organs, including the reproductive tract. Interaction of SARS-CoV-2 with the ACE-2 receptor leads to a pro-thrombotic hyper-inflammatory state as well as maladaptive hyper-activation of the innate immune system resulting in cytokine storm. In this respect, COVID-19 disease can be viewed as a multisystem disease, with both acute and chronic multiorgan dysfunction, including myocarditis, myocardial infarction, macrophage activation syndrome, arterial and venous thrombosis, encephalitis, stroke, thyroiditis, adrenal insufficiency, hepatitis, hepatic failure, preeclampsia, and sterility [14–18].

Moreover, infection with COVID-19 is associated with several pathophysiologic phases: an incubation phase, an early viremic phase (which may or may not be symptomatic), and an early inflammatory pulmonary phase occurring between seven and fourteen days after infection [19]. In some patients, this is followed by a progressive inflammatory pulmonary phase leading to the development of C19-ARDS and multiorgan dysfunction [19]. An imbalance among pro- and anti-anticoagulant factors, in part a result of hyper-inflammation and cytokine storm, produces a pro-thrombotic state characterized by disseminated intravascular coagulation, macro- and microvascular thrombotic events, and multiorgan failure [19].

A myriad of insults, each capable of causing AKI, can occur during severe COVID-19 infection. These include hyper-inflammation as a part of cytokine storm, septic-shock-associated hypoperfusion, ischemia, C19-ARDS-associated hypoxia, and vascular thrombosis [1,2,20–22]. Previous studies of COVID-19 patients found that the risk factors for developing AKI were similar to those identified in other groups of patients with critical illness, such as comorbidities, age, vasopressor requirement, and respiratory failure requiring mechanical ventilation [2,3,21–23]. What remains unclear is the impact and interaction of inflammatory-coagulopathic biomarkers and other clinical and laboratory variables on the development and mortality of COVID-19-associated AKI. In addition, few studies have included therapeutic agents among the variables examined. With this in mind, we evaluated the incidence, risk factors, and medical therapy associated with the development and outcome of AKI in patients with severe COVID-19 disease admitted to an intensive care unit (ICU).

2. Materials and Methods

To determine risk factors for the development of AKI in patients with severe COVID-19 infection, and to compare risk factors for mortality between patients with and without AKI, we conducted a retrospective analysis of 249 consecutive patients either admitted or transferred to the ICU of two community hospitals between 12 March 2020 and 17 June 2020. At the time of ICU entry, all patients manifested severe difficulty in breathing as evidenced by one or more of the following: respiratory rate greater than 30 breaths per minute, blood oxygen saturation of 93% or less on room air, PAO_2/FIO_2 ratio less than 300, and presence of lung infiltrates in more than half of the lung fields [24,25].

Inclusion criteria were age greater than 18, confirmed diagnosis of COVID-19 by a positive PCR test, and signs and symptoms of COVID-19 infection. Study baseline was the time of hospital admission. Patients with end-stage renal disease (ESRD) were excluded from the analysis. All patients received standard-of-care therapy. Management and timing of ventilator support, employment of C19-ARDS ventilator strategies, antibiotic use, antiviral therapy, anticoagulation, initiation of vasopressors, use of convalescent plasma, corticosteroid (CC) therapy, and Tocilizumab therapy were determined by the ICU physician and consultants.

All standard laboratory results were extracted from the electronic medical record and were performed according to standardized laboratory practices. D-Dimer levels were obtained using a latex agglutination photo-optical assay from a sample of citrated whole blood. C-reactive protein (CRP) levels were obtained from serum samples and analyzed incorporating a laser-nephelometric method. Missing values in the case of standard laboratory results were not imputed and accounted for less than 1% of all measurements. Missing biomarker data, including CRP, D-Dimer, and ferritin, were found to be missing completely at random (MCAR) by Little's MCAR test. Substituted values were inserted using an expectation maximization algorithm [26,27]. Missing biomarker data are reported in Supplementary Table S1.

Demographics, comorbidities, and clinical outcome variables were obtained from the electronic medical record or the patient's history and physical exam and entered into a de-identified database. Measurements obtained on admission included arterial blood gas (ABG), routine metabolic chemistries, CRP, D-Dimer, ferritin, WBC and differential, and all variables necessary to calculate a Sequential Organ Failure Assessment (SOFA) score on admission. Other collected data included the dates of admission, ICU transfer, and death; need for vasopressor therapy; need for mechanical ventilation; PAO2/FIO2 ratio; use of corticosteroid (CC) therapy; and use of azithromycin, hydroxychloroquine (HCQ), convalescent plasma, Tocilizumab, or heparin (low molecular weight or unfractionated) either as deep vein thrombosis (DVT) prophylaxis or anticoagulant therapy. If patients received both anticoagulant doses and thrombo-prophylactic doses of heparin, they were analyzed in the anticoagulant group.

AKI was defined according to Kidney Disease: Improving Global Outcomes (KDIGO) criteria, namely, an increase in serum creatinine value (SCr) by ≥ 0.3 mg/dL (≥ 26.5 µMol/L) within 48 h. Urine output was not considered. SCr on admission was used to assess the change in SCr [28–30]. For this study, AKI associated with COVID-19 is defined as AKI occurring during the first 7 days of admission. The consulting nephrologist determined the timing and indication for the initiation of renal replacement therapy (RRT).

All statistical analyses were performed with IBM SPSS 28 software (IBM SPSS Inc., Chicago, IL, USA). We performed both univariate and multivariate analyses. The primary outcome was development of AKI for patients admitted or transferred to the ICU during the index admission. Summary statistics were computed for patients who did or did not develop AKI and for survivors vs. non-survivors, as well as for various subgroups of those who did and did not develop AKI. Continuous variables were expressed as median with interquartile ranges (IQR) and compared by the Student's t-test or the Wilcoxon rank-sum test, as appropriate. Categorical variables were compared with Pearson's chi-squared test. Fisher's exact test was employed when indicated. Variables that were significant by univariate analysis at $p < 0.05$ were candidates for multivariate analysis. To determine risk factors that were independently associated with the outcome of AKI, we performed multivariate analysis by logistic regression with stepwise forward variable selection. Goodness of fit was determined by the Hosmer–Lameshow test. For continuous variables, the odds ratio (OR) represents the relative amount by which the odds ratio for the outcome variable increases or decreases when the independent variable is changed by exactly one unit. ORs and their 95% confidence intervals (95% CI) were determined by exponentiation of the beta coefficient and its upper and lower CI, respectively. If variables included imputed values for missing measurements, we performed multivariate analysis with and without these variables. Cox proportional hazards with forward variable selection was performed to determine variables independently predictive of the outcome of survival among all patients, and in those who did or did not develop AKI. For continuous variables, the hazard ratio (HR) represents the relative amount by which the probability of obtaining the outcome variable increases or decreases when the independent variable is changed by exactly one unit. HRs and their 95% CIs were determined by exponentiation of the regression coefficient and its upper and lower CI, respectively.

3. Results

3.1. Patient Characteristics

To evaluate risk factors for the development of AKI and its associated mortality, we retrospectively evaluated severe COVID-19 admissions (those patients requiring ICU admission or transfer). From 12 March 2020 to 17 June 2020, a total of 249 patients met the definition of severe COVID-19 infection; 90 (36%) were admitted directly to the ICU, and 159 (64%) were admitted to COVID-19 units and subsequently transferred to the ICU. The median age was 70 years (IQR 61, 80). There were 148 males (59%), and 177 patients were Caucasian (71%). The majority of patients had severe respiratory failure requiring mechanical ventilation (n = 173, 69%).

The mortality rate among these patients was 65% (162 patients). There was no significant difference in mortality between those directly admitted to the ICU (n = 56, 62%) vs. those transferred to the ICU (n = 106, 66%) (p = 0.48, OR = 0.82, 95% CI = 0.48–1.40). Likewise, there was no significant difference in the development of AKI between those directly admitted to the ICU (n = 40, 44%) and those transferred later (n = 79, 50%) (p = 0.43, OR = 0.8, 95% CI = 0.48–1.36). The median time to ICU transfer was three days (IQR 1, 5). For those patients not initially admitted to an ICU, there was no statistically significant difference in median time to ICU transfer between survivors and non-survivors (2 days (IQR 1, 4) vs. 3 days (IQR 1, 6), p = 0.1). Similarly, there was no significant difference in median time to ICU transfer between those who did and did not develop AKI (3 days (IQR 1, 6) vs. 3 days (IQR 1, 5), p = 0.17). As expected, patients directly admitted to the ICU had higher SOFA scores (6, IQR 3, 19) compared to those initially admitted to COVID-19 units (3, IQR 2, 5) (p = 0.00001).

3.2. Univariate Analysis of Risk Factors for AKI

Overall, 119 (48%) patients developed AKI, and 23 (19%) of these required RRT by the 7th day following hospital admission. Four additional patients developed AKI and required RRT later during their hospitalization (10–15 days). As the later development of AKI suggested an etiologic role for hospital-related factors distinct from initial COVID-19 infection, these patients were included in the non-AKI group. However, the inclusion of these late AKI patients in either group had no effect on the study's results. The admission characteristics of the entire group of patients with severe COVID-19 infection are given in Table 1. Univariate analysis revealed that older age, the need for mechanical ventilation, elevated SCr, and higher SOFA score were associated with the development of AKI (Table 1).

Therapeutic and pharmacologic interventions are given in Table 2 and Figure 1. In general, information on the timing, rationale, and route of administration of agents was available only for CC and Tocilizumab and is therefore not a part of the analysis. Among all severe COVID-19 patients, 152 (61%) required vasopressor support, 192 (77%) received HCQ, 87 (35%) received azithromycin, 26 (10%) received Tocilizumab alone without CC, 69 (27%) received CC alone without Tocilizumab, 92 (37%) received combination therapy with both Tocilizumab and CC, and 65 (26%) received convalescent plasma. Consistent with admission during the first wave of the pandemic, only six patients (2.4%) received Remdesivir. Full-dose heparin was administered in 126 (50%) patients, and thromboprophylactic doses were administered in 85 (34%) patients. By univariate analysis, the need for vasopressors (p = 0.009, OR = 2.58, 95% CI = 1.25–5.31) and the use of azithromycin (p = 0.04, OR = 1.74, 95% CI = 1.03–2.95) were associated with the development of AKI. Conversely, patients who received combination therapy with Tocilizumab and CC were less likely to develop AKI (p = 0.018, OR = 0.53, 95% CI = 0.31–0.90). The use of either Tocilizumab alone or CC alone as monotherapy was not associated with a reduced risk of AKI. Only the combination predicted a lower risk of AKI. There was no difference in the time of initiation of CC among patients with and without AKI (4 days (IQR 1, 14) versus

3 days (IQR 1, 8), $p = 0.56$). Similarly, there was no difference in the time of initiation of Tocilizumab among patients with and without AKI (4 days (IQR 2, 6) versus 3 days (IQR 1.5, 7), $p = 0.96$).

Table 1. COVID-19 ICU patients: characteristics of individuals with and without AKI.

	Non-AKI (n = 130)	AKI (n = 119)	p	OR	95% CI
Age	66 (58, 77)	73 (65, 82)	0.001		
Race (Caucasian)	88 (68%)	89 (75%)	0.22	1.41	0.81–2.46
BMI	29 (24, 33)	29 (24, 35)	0.62		
Sex (male)	71 (55%)	77 (65%)	0.10	1.52	0.91–2.53
Diabetes	35 (27%)	41 (35%)	0.19	1.42	0.83–2.40
CHF	13 (10%)	17 (14%)	0.28	1.51	0.70–3.30
CAD	32 (25%)	29 (24%)	0.96	0.99	0.55–1.80
COPD	33 (25%)	27 (23%)	0.62	0.86	0.48–1.55
CKD	11 (8%)	15 (13%)	0.28	1.56	0.69–3.60
HTN	65 (50%)	70 (60%)	0.26	1.42	0.86–2.30
Cirrhosis	2 (1.5%)	2 (1.7%)	1.0	1.09	0.15–7.9
Malignancy	14 (11%)	13 (11%)	0.96	1.01	0.45–2.26
CVA	13 (10%)	14 (12%)	0.65	1.2	0.53–2.7
Mechanical ventilation	79 (61%)	94 (79%)	0.002	2.42	1.38–4.20
Neutrophiles × 10^9/L	7.6 (4.4, 12)	7.6 (5, 13)	0.62		
Lymphocytes × 10^9/L	0.8 (0.5, 1.3)	0.8 (0.5, 1.2)	0.98		
Neutrophile/lymphocyte	8.8 (5.1, 16)	9.8 (5.2, 16)	0.64		
SCr (μmole/L)	84 (60, 127)	134.4 (97, 177)	0.00001		
Plts × 10^9/L	246 (136, 308)	230 (164, 301)	0.44		
Tbili (μmole/L)	9.41 (6.8, 13.7)	8.5 (6.8, 15.4)	0.97		
SOFA admit	3 (2, 6)	5 (3, 8)	0.00001		
PaO2/FIO2	200 (100, 286)	201 (94, 314)	0.95		
PaO2	9.4 (7.4, 12.4)	10 (8.6, 11)	0.64		
FIO2	0.36 (0.21, 1)	0.38 (0.23, 1)	0.72		

Abbreviations/legend: AKI = acute kidney injury, BMI= body mass index, CAD = coronary artery disease, CHF = congestive heart failure, CI = confidence interval, CKD = chronic kidney disease, COPD = chronic obstructive pulmonary disease, HD = hemodialysis, HTN = hypertension, OR = odds ratio, PaO2/FiO2 = ratio of partial pressure of oxygen to inspired concentration of oxygen, Plts = platelets, SCr= serum creatinine, SOFA = Sepsis-Related Organ Failure Assessment, TBili = total bilirubin.

Table 2. Pharmacological interventions in COVID-19 ICU patients with and without AKI.

	Non-AKI (n = 130)	AKI (n = 119)	p	OR	95% CI
Vasopressors	66 (50%)	86 (72%)	0.009	2.58	1.25–5.31
IV Ascorbic acid	79 (60%)	71 (60%)	0.85	0.95	0.59–1.60
Hydroxychloroquine	98 (78%)	94 (79%)	0.91	1.036	0.56–1.91
Azithromycin	37 (29%)	50 (42%)	0.040	1.74	1.030–2.95
Heparin full dose	72 (55%)	54 (45%)	0.13	0.67	0.41–1.10
Heparin DVT prophylaxis	37 (29%)	48 (40%)	0.06	1.69	1.002–2.38
Convalescent plasma	38 (29%)	27 (23%)	0.24	0.71	0.40–1.25
Remdesivir	5 (4%)	1 (0.9)	0.21	0.20	0.024–1.84
Tocilizumab	10 (7.7%)	16 (13.6%)	0.14	1.86	0.80–4.30
Corticosteroids only	39 (30%)	30 (25%)	0.39	0.80	0.46–1.40
Tocilizumab and steroids	57 (44%)	35 (29%)	0.018	0.53	0.31–0.90

Heparin full dose = anticoagulant dose of unfractionated or low molecular weight heparin. Heparin DVT prophylaxis = 5000 units sc every 8 h or low molecular weight heparin 30–40 mg daily. If patients received both anticoagulant and thrombo-prophylaxis doses during hospitalization they were analyzed in the full-dose group.

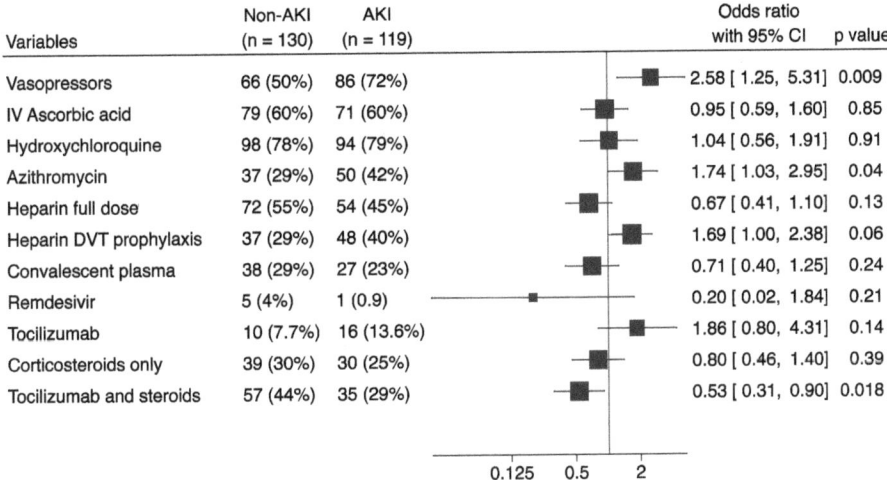

Figure 1. Forest plot depicting the effect of the indicated pharmacologic interventions on the odds ratio (OR) for developing AKI as determined by univariate analysis.

Finally, since endothelial dysfunction, thrombosis, and inflammation are common features of COVID-19 disease, we examined the levels of inflammatory and coagulopathic markers in these patients [31,32]. These data were available from the electronic record, as it was common practice during the first wave of the pandemic to obtain serial inflammatory and thrombotic biomarkers in patients with COVID-19. Patients who developed AKI were noted to have significantly higher levels of D-Dimer on day 1 (hospital admission) and of CRP on day 2 (Table 3). These results are consistent with the interaction of SARS-CoV-2 with ACE2 on vascular endothelial cells in nearly all organs of the body, leading to excessive circulating levels of angiotensin 2, a pro-inflammatory, pro-thrombotic, and vasoconstrictive molecule [31–33].

Table 3. Inflammatory and thrombotic markers in COVID-19 patients with and without AKI.

	Non-AKI (n = 130)	AKI (n = 119)	p
D-Dimer day 1 (ng/mL)	734 (510,1340)	1169 (470,3680)	0.049
D-Dimer day 2	727 (487,1592)	1380 (471,3680)	0.12
CRP day 1 (mg/L)	108 (52,172)	137 (84,178)	0.26
CRP day 2	105 (46,156)	128 (83,212)	0.026
Ferritin day 1 (ng/mL)	732 (450,1316)	1017 (536,1580)	0.20
Ferritin day 2	839 (524,1665)	906 (567,1756)	0.61

(Biomarker levels are expressed as median with interquartile ranges (IQR)). Abbreviations: CRP = C-reactive protein, AKI = acute kidney injury.

3.3. Multivariate Analysis of Risk Factors for the Development of AKI

Independent predictors of AKI development were identified by stepwise logistic regression with forward variable selection for all predictive variables identified by univariate analysis (Table 4 and Figure 2). Increased risk of AKI was associated with elevated admission SCr (p = 0.0001, OR = 2.406, 95% CI= 1.56–3.70), vasopressor requirement (p = 0.0001, OR = 3.188, 95% CI = 1.69–5.98), elevated D-Dimer on day 1 (p = 0.008, OR = 1.0001, 95% CI = 1.000–1.0010), and elevated CRP on day 2 (p = 0.033, OR = 1.004, 95% CI = 1.0001–1.009). In contrast, co-administration of Tocilizumab and CC was independently associated with a lower risk for development of AKI (p = 0.009, OR = 0.437, 95% CI = 0.23–0.81). Elevated SCr, vasopressor requirement, and lack of co-administration of Tocilizumab and CC remained significant independent risk factors for AKI development even when the biomarker variables with missing and imputed values were removed from the analysis.

Table 4. Multivariate analysis of risk factors for AKI.

	Beta	S.E	p	OR	95% CI
SCr	0.878	0.221	0.0001	2.406	1.56–3.70
Vasopressor requirement	1.159	0.321	0.0001	3.188	1.69–5.98
Tocilizumab plus CC	−0.827	0.317	0.009	0.437	0.23–0.81
D-Dimer day 1	0.000	0.000	0.008	1.0001	1.000–1.001
CRP day 2	0.004	0.002	0.033	1.004	1.0001–1.009

Abbreviations: 95% CI = 95% confidence interval, CC = corticosteroid therapy, CRP = C-reactive protein, OR = odds ratio, SCr = serum creatinine, S.E. = standard error. For categorical risk factors, the beta coefficient signifies the average change in outcome if that risk factor is present. In the case of continuous risk factors, it signifies the amount the outcome changes for a unit increase in the risk factor's value. Odds ratios and their 95% confidence intervals (95% CI) are determined by exponentiation of the beta coefficient and its upper and lower CI, respectively.

3.4. Univariate Analysis of Risk Factors for In-Hospital Mortality

We next examined the risk factors for in-hospital mortality among patients with severe COVID-19 infection. AKI development was associated with a 73% mortality, in contrast to a 56% mortality in patients not developing AKI. By univariate analysis, increased mortality was associated with older age, Caucasian race, presence of diabetes mellitus, presence of hypertension, development of AKI, requirement for RRT, need for mechanical ventilation, lower absolute lymphocyte count, elevated neutrophil to lymphocyte ratio, lower absolute platelet count, and elevated total bilirubin (Table 5).

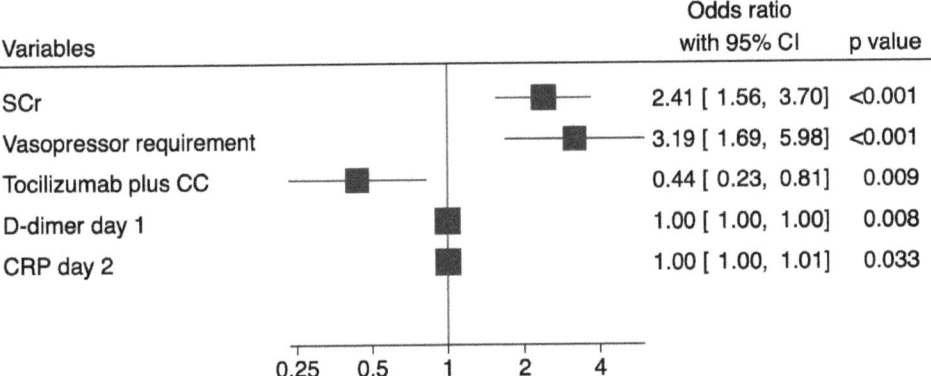

Figure 2. Forest plot depicting the impact of the indicated risk factors on the odds ratio (OR) for developing AKI as determined by logistic regression with stepwise forward variable selection. For continuous variables, the odds ratio (OR) represents the relative amount by which the odds ratio for the outcome variable increases or decreases when the independent variable is increased by exactly one unit.

Table 5. COVID-19 ICU patients: characteristics of survivors and non-survivors.

	Survivors (n = 87)	Non-Survivors (n = 162)	p	OR	95% CI
Age	66 (51, 75)	73 (63, 82)	0.00001		
Race (Caucasian)	54 (62%)	123 (76%)	0.021	1.9	1.09–3.40
BMI	28.9 (24, 33)	29 (24, 35)	0.62		
Sex (male)	50 (57%)	98 (60%)	0.64	1.06	0.66–1.92
Diabetes	18 (21%)	58 (36%)	0.014	2.1	1.16–3.90
CHF	8 (9%)	22 (14%)	0.30	1.56	0.66–3.60
CAD	18 (21%)	43 (26%)	0.30	1.38	0.74–2.6
COPD	22 (25%)	38 (23%)	0.74	0.9	0.50–1.6
CKD	8 (7%)	20 (12%)	0.18	1.90	0.73–4.90
HTN	39 (45%)	96 (59%)	0.029	1.80	1.06–3.0
AKI	31 (35%)	88 (54%)	0.005	2.14	1.25–3.70
Cirrhosis	0 (0%)	4 (2%)	0.3	0.64	0.58–0.7
Malignancy	7 (8%)	20 (12%)	0.39	1.61	0.65–3.97
CVA	9 (10%)	18 (11%)	0.85	1.1	0.46–2.52
Mechanical ventilation	43 (49%)	130 (80%)	0.00001	4.10	2.3–7.30
Dialysis *	3 (3.4%)	20 (12%)	0.022	3.94	1.13–13.6
Neutrophiles $\times 10^9$/L	8 (4.5, 13)	7.4 (5, 11.7)	0.67		
Lymphocytes $\times 10^9$/L	0.9 (0.6, 1.6)	0.7 (0.5, 1.1)	0.010		

Table 5. Cont.

	Survivors (n = 87)	Non-Survivors (n = 162)	p	OR	95% CI
Neutrophile/lymphocyte	7.6 (4.3, 14)	10 (6, 18.4)	0.03		
SCr µmoles/L	95.4 (55.2, 141.4)	106 (72.5, 155)	0.12		
Plts × 10^9/L	262 (195, 326)	226 (151, 279)	0.019		
Tbili (µmoles/L)	8.5 (5.1, 12)	10.3 (6.8, 16.4)	0.012		
SOFA	4 (2, 6)	4 (3, 7)	0.095		
PaO2/FIO2	231 (118, 310)	191 (79, 286)	0.051		
Pa02 KPa	9.7 (7.8, 13)	9.2 (7.3, 11.4)	0.14		
FI02	0.36 (0.29, 0.96)	0.40 (0.21, 1.0)	0.12		

Abbreviations: AKI = acute kidney injury, BMI = body mass index, CAD = coronary artery disease, CHF = congestive heart failure, CI = confidence interval, CKD = chronic kidney disease, COPD = chronic obstructive pulmonary disease, HD = hemodialysis, HTN = hypertension, OR = odds ratio, PaO2/FiO2 = ratio of partial pressure of oxygen to inspired concentration of oxygen, Plts = platelets, SCr = serum creatinine, SOFA = Sepsis-Related Organ Failure Assessment, TBili = total bilirubin. * Requirement for dialysis that developed within the first 7 days after hospital admission.

To determine the effect of AKI on mortality, we compared the risk factors for mortality between patients who did and did not develop AKI. For patients with AKI, an increase in mortality was associated with need for mechanical ventilation, lower absolute lymphocyte counts, elevated absolute neutrophil count, elevated neutrophil to lymphocyte ratio, lower admission SCr, and lower absolute platelet count (Table 6). For those not developing AKI, increased mortality was associated with increased age, need for mechanical ventilation, presence of several co-morbidities (diabetes mellitus, hypertension, coronary artery disease, and chronic kidney disease (CKD)), increased admission SCr, and increased total bilirubin (Table 7).

Table 6. Risk factors for mortality among COVID-19 ICU patients with AKI.

	Survivor (n = 31)	Non-Survivor (n = 88)	p	OR	95% CI
Age	69 (63, 77)	75 (65, 82)	0.1		
Race (Caucasian)	19 (63%)	69 (78%)	0.10	2.10	0.85–5.1
BMI	26 (24.32)	29 (25, 36)	0.10		
Sex (male)	18 (60%)	58 (66%)	0.50	1.20	0.52–3.0
Diabetes	11 (36%)	30 (34%)	0.80	0.89	0.38–2.10
CHF	5 (17%)	12 (14%)	0.70	0.8	0.25–2.50
CAD	9 (30%)	20 (23%)	0.40	0.68	0.27–1.70
COPD	33 (25%)	27 (33%)	0.67	0.88	0.49–1.58
CKD	6 (20%)	9 (10%)	0.16	0.6	0.23–1.50
HTN	18 (60%)	51 (58%)	0.84	0.9	0.39–2.10

Table 6. Cont.

	Survivor (n = 31)	Non-Survivor (n = 88)	p	OR	95% CI
Cirrhosis	0 (0%)	2 (2.3%)	1.0	0,75	0.66–0.82
Malignancy	4 (13%)	9 (10, 2%)	0.74	0.77	0.22–2.7
CVA	6 (19%)	8 (9%)	0.13	0.42	0.13–1.32
Mechanical ventilation	16 (53%)	77 (87%)	0.00001	6.1	2.30–16.0
Dialysis *	3 (9.7%)	20 (22.7%)	0.18	2.78	0.75–9.98
Neutrophiles $\times 10^9$/L	7.7 (4.6, 14)	7.5 (5.3, 13)	0.49		
Lymphocytes $\times 10^9$/L	1.0 (0.67, 1.9)	0.7 (0.5, 1.)	0.004		
Neutrophile/lymphocyte	7.30 (3.8, 12.6)	10.5 (6, 19)	0.009		
SCr µmole/L	159 (115, 256.4)	132.6 (88.4, 177.6)	0.04		
Plts $\times 10^9$/L	281 (212, 326)	223 (141, 277)	0.010		
Tbili µmole/L	6.8 (5.1, 13.7)	8.5 (6.8, 15.4)	0.12		
SOFA admit	4.5 (3, 8.5.5)	5 (3, 8)	0.80		
PaO2/FIO2	227 (122, 307)	200 (74, 313)	0.25		
Pa02 KPa	9.8 (8, 12)	9 (7.2, 11.3)	0.10		
FI02	0.34 (0.25, 0.96)	0.42 (0.21, 1)	0.40		

Abbreviations: AKI = acute kidney injury, BMI = body mass index, CAD = coronary artery disease, CHF = congestive heart failure, CI = confidence interval, CKD = chronic kidney disease, COPD = chronic obstructive pulmonary disease, HD = hemodialysis, HTN = hypertension, OR = odds ratio, PaO2/FIO2 = ratio of partial pressure of oxygen to inspired concentration of oxygen, Plts = platelets, SCr = serum creatinine, SOFA = Sepsis-Related Organ Failure Assessment, TBili = total bilirubin. * Requirement for dialysis that developed within the first 7 days after hospital admission.

Table 7. Risk factors for mortality among COVID-19 ICU patients without AKI.

	Survivor (n = 56)	Non-Survivor (n = 74)	p	OR	95% CI
Age	62 (44, 68)	70 (63, 80)	0.00001		
Race (Caucasian)	34 (60%)	54 (73%)	0.14	1.70	0.81–3.70
BMI	29 (26.34)	29 (24, 33)	0.52		
Sex (male)	31 (55%)	40 (54%)	0.88	0.95	0.47–1.90
Diabetes	7 (12%)	28 (38%)	0.001	4.3	1.70–11.0
CHF	3 (5.4%)	10 (13%)	0.13	2.8	0.72–10.5
CAD	9 (16%)	23 (31%)	0.049	2.40	1.0–5.70
COPD	13 (23%)	20 (27%)	0.6	1.22	0.54–2.70
CKD	0 (0%)	11 (15%)	0.003	9.9	1.20–79.0
HTN	21 (37%)	45 (61%)	0.005	2.79	1.36–5.70
Cirrhosis	0 (0%)	2 (2.7%)	0.50	0.56	0.48–0.65

Table 7. Cont.

	Survivor (n = 56)	Non-Survivor (n = 74)	p	OR	95% CI
Malignancy	3 (5.4%)	11 (15%)	0.095	3.1	0.82–11.6
CVA	3 (5.4%)	10 (13.5%)	0.15	2.76	0.72–10.4
Mechanical ventilation	26 (47%)	53 (71%)	0.005	2.90	1.4–6.0
Neutrophiles $\times 10^9$/L	8.6 (4.6, 15.0)	6.6 (4.4, 10.5)	0.22		
Lymphocytes $\times 10^9$/L	0.9 (0.5, 1.40)	0.7 (0.5, 1.2)	0.35		
Neutrophile/lymphocyte	8 (5, 15.3)	9 (6, 17)	0.64		
SCr (µmoles/L)	79.5 (53, 97)	88.4 (62, 123.8)	0.048		
Plts $\times 10^9$/L	248 (176, 330)	231 (164, 297)	0.30		
Tbili µmoles/L	49.2 (5.1, 12)	10.2 (7.7, 13.6)	0.03		
SOFA admit	3 (2.0.5.0)	4 (3, 6)	0.17		
PaO2/FIO2	230 (116, 309)	190 (98, 261)	0.12		
Pa02 KPa	9.7 (7.3, 12.7)	9.2 (7.4, 11.4)	0.53		
FI02	0.36 (0.21, 0.96)	0.40 (0.26, 1)	0.29		

Abbreviations: AKI = acute kidney injury, BMI = body mass index, CAD = coronary artery disease, CHF = congestive heart failure, CI = confidence interval, CKD = chronic kidney disease, COPD = chronic obstructive pulmonary disease, HD = hemodialysis, HTN = hypertension, OR = odds ratio, PaO2/FiO2 = ratio of partial pressure of oxygen to inspired concentration of oxygen, Plts = platelets, SCr = serum creatinine, SOFA = Sepsis-Related Organ Failure Assessment, TBili = total bilirubin.

The only pharmacologic intervention associated with increased mortality was the need for vasopressor support. This was true for the entire cohort (Table 8), as well as the subgroups with AKI (Table 9) and without AKI (Table 10). No inflammatory or thrombotic markers were associated with increased mortality (Table 11).

Table 8. Pharmacologic interventions in COVID-19 ICU survivors and non-survivors.

	Non-Survivor (n = 162)	Survivor (n = 87)	p	OR	95% CI
Vasopressors	119 (73%)	33 (38%)	0.00001	4.50	2.60–7.90
IV Ascorbic acid	99 (59%)	51 (59%)	0.70	1.1	0.66–1.89
Hydroxychloroquine	124 (78%)	68 (80%)	0.71	0.88	0.46–1.69
Azithromycin	63 (40%)	24 (28%)	0.071	1.69	0.97–3.0
Heparin full dose	79 (49%)	47 (54%)	0.51	0.80	0.48–1.36
Heparin DVT prophylaxis	54 (33%)	31 (36%)	0.8	0.90	0.52–1.60
Convalescent plasma	42 (26%)	23 (26%)	0.93	0.97	0.54–1.76
Remdesivir	6 (3%)	0 (0)	0.094	0.64	0.680.70
Tocilizumab	18 (11%)	8 (9.2%)	0.80	1.23	0.51–2.98
Corticosteroids only	44 (27%)	25 (28%)	0.47	0.80	0.48–1.40
Tocilizumab and steroids	55 (34%)	37 (42%)	0.18	0.69	0.40–1.86

Heparin full dose = anticoagulant dose of unfractionated or low molecular weight heparin. Heparin DVT prophylaxis = 5000 units sc every 8 h or low molecular weight heparin 30–40 mg daily. If patients received both anticoagulant and thrombo-prophylaxis doses during hospitalization they were analyzed in the full-dose group.

Table 9. Pharmacologic interventions in COVID-19 ICU survivors and non-survivors with AKI.

	Survivors (n = 31)	Non-Survivors (n = 88)	p	OR	95% CI
Vasopressors	14 (48%)	72 (82%)	0.00001	4.8	2.0–12.0
IV Ascorbic acid	21 (68%)	50 (57%)	0.28	0.62	0.26–1.48
Hydroxychloroquine	22 (71%)	72 (82%)	0.21	1.84	0.71–4.70
Azithromycin	11 (35%)	39 (44%)	0.39	1.44	0.62–3.37
Heparin full dose	18 (58%)	36 (41%)	0.09	0.50	0.22–1.15
Heparin DVT prophylaxis	11 (36%)	37 (41%)	0.090	0.50	0.22–3.10
Convalescent plasma	7 (23%)	20 (23%)	0.94	0.96	0.36–2.68
Remdesivir	0 (0%)	1 (0.9)	0.5	0.73	0.66–0.82
Tocilizumab	5 (16%)	11 (12%)	0.56	0.76	0.3–1.9
Corticosteroids only	9 (29%)	21 (23%)	0.57	1.12	0.52–2.4
Tocilizumab and steroids	12 (39%)	23 (26%)	0.18	0.56	0.23–1.33

Heparin full dose = anticoagulant dose of unfractionated or low molecular weight heparin. Heparin DVT prophylaxis = 5000 units sc every 8 h or low molecular weight heparin 30–40 mg daily. If patients received both anticoagulant and thrombo-prophylaxis doses during hospitalization they were analyzed in the full-dose group.

Table 10. Pharmacologic interventions in COVID-19 ICU survivors and non-survivors without AKI.

	Survivors (n = 56)	Non-Survivors (n = 74)	p	OR	95% CI
Vasopressors	18 (32%)	47 (63%)	0.00001	3.67	1.76–7.65
IV Ascorbic acid	30 (54%)	49 (66%)	0.14	1.70	0.83–3.50
Hydroxychloroquine	46 (85%)	52 (73%)	0.11	0.47	0.19–1.20
Azithromycin	13 (24%)	24 (34%)	0.21	1.65	0.75–3.64
Heparin full dose	29 (52%)	43 (58%)	0.47	1.29	0.64–2.60
Heparin DVT prophylaxis	20 (36%)	17 (44%)	0.10	0.53	0.25–1.20
Convalescent plasma	16 (28%)	22 (30%)	0.86	1.06	0.49–2.27
Remdesivir	0 (0%)	5 (6.8)	0.070	0.54	0.46–0.64
Tocilizumab	3 (5%)	7 (9%)	0.51	1.86	0.45–7.50
Corticosteroids only	16 (29%)	23 (31%)	0.75	1.12	0.69–1.66
Tocilizumab and steroids	25 (44%)	32 (43%)	0.87	0.94	0.47–1.90

Heparin full dose = anticoagulant dose of unfractionated or low molecular weight heparin. Heparin DVT prophylaxis = 5000 units sc every 8 h or low molecular weight heparin 30–40 mg daily. If patients received both anticoagulant and thrombo-prophylaxis doses during hospitalization they were analyzed in the full-dose group.

Table 11. Inflammatory and thrombotic markers in COVID-19 ICU survivors and non-survivors.

All ICU Patients	Survivors (n = 87)	Non-Survivors (n = 162)	p
D-Dimer day 1 (ng/mL)	636 (337,1502)	852 (520,2309)	0.069
D-Dimer day 2	1166 (548,3555)	691 (436,1743)	0.089
CRP day 1 (mg/L)	134 (90,204)	124 (61,175)	0.41
CRP day 2	123 (47,171)	115 (81,184)	0.38
Ferritin day 1 (ng/mL)	995 (352,1571)	790 (400,1460)	0.25
Ferritin day 2	987 (675,1888)	822 (462,1478)	0.12

Table 11. Cont.

ICU Patients without AKI	Survivors (n = 56)	Non-Survivors (n = 74)	p
D-Dimer day 1	629 (330,1033)	799 (632,1432)	0.092
D-Dimer day 2	900 (548,1814)	646 (481,839)	0.12
CRP day 1	130 (58,232)	103 (51,162)	0.35
CRP day 2	97 (38,157)	105 (73,152)	0.59
Ferritin day 1	735 (471,1347)	699 (416,1338)	0.80
Ferritin day 2	987 (691,1972)	748 (446,1374)	0.19
ICU Patients with AKI	Survivors (n= 31)	Non-Survivors (n = 88)	p
D-Dimer day 1	644 (335,3680)	1219 (500,3083)	0.71
D-Dimer day 2	2390 (543,3680)	1182 (419,3436)	0.28
CRP day 1	137 (93,169)	140 (21,185)	0.86
CRP day 2	140 (80,204)	122 (83,223)	0.89
Ferritin day 1	1390 (1003,2318)	923 (320,1542)	0.070
Ferritin day 2	1139 (657,2130)	993 (447,1590)	0.30

Abbreviations: CRP = C-reactive protein.

3.5. Multivariate Analysis of Risk Factors Associated with Mortality

Finally, to determine independent risk factors associated with mortality, we performed Cox proportional hazards analysis with forward variable selection (Table 12 and Figure 3). For the entire cohort of COVID-19 patients admitted to the ICU, only advanced age was independently associated with decreased survival (p = 0.00001, HR = 1.028, 95% CI = 1.016–1.041). For patients not developing AKI, increased age (p = 0.00001, HR = 1.044, 95% CI = 1.024–1.065) and CKD (p = 0.004, HR = 2.65, 95% CI = 1.37–5.1) were independently associated with decreased survival. For patients who developed AKI, surprisingly, the only independent risk factor was a lower SCr on admission (p = 0.011, HR = 0.79, 95% CI = 0.66–0.95).

Table 12. Multivariate Cox proportional hazards analysis of risk factors for mortality.

All ICU Patients	B	SE	p	HR	95% CI
Age	0.028	0.006	0.00001	1.028	1.016–1.041
ICU Patients with AKI					
SCr	−2.32	0.092	0.01	0.79	0.66–0.95
ICU Patients without AKI					
Age	0.043	0.01	0.00001	1.044	1.024–1.065
CKD	0.97	0.34	0.004	2.65	1.37–5.1

Abbreviations: 95% CI = 95% confidence interval, CKD = chronic kidney disease, HR = hazards ratio, SCr = serum creatinine, S.E. = standard error.

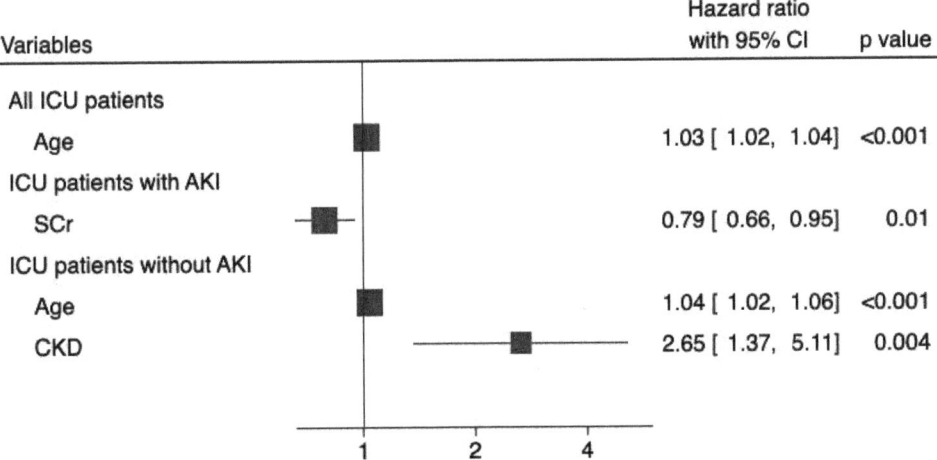

Figure 3. Forest plot depicting the impact of the indicated risk factors on the hazard ratio (HR) for mortality as determined by Cox proportional hazards with stepwise forward variable selection. For continuous variables, the hazard ratio (HR) represents the relative amount by which the probability of obtaining the outcome increases or decreases when the independent variable is changed by exactly one unit.

4. Discussion

Clinical experience with patients hospitalized from COVID-19 has demonstrated significant heterogeneity in the development of AKI [10,34]. Chinese and Italian studies reported the development of AKI in 0.5–29% of patients [1,2,6,11]. In contrast, data from the United States and other developed nations have demonstrated a much higher incidence of this complication [9,12,35,36]. In a large cohort of COVID-19 patients, Fisher et al. found that COVID-19 patients developed AKI at twice the rate of historical controls [12]. The same investigators observed a similarly increased rate of AKI over the same timeframe when COVID-19 patients were compared to those admitted without COVID-19 [12]. Moreover, AKI in the setting of COVID-19 tends to be more severe. As compared to historical controls, COVID-19 patients had a 2.6-fold higher mortality and an increased requirement for RRT [37,38]. A recent meta-analysis involving over 25,000 COVID-19 patients found a pooled incidence of AKI of 53% in those with severe disease [39]. Schaubroeck et al., in a multi-center study involving 1286 critically ill patients, observed the development of AKI in 85% of patients [7]. In an ICU cohort of 313 ICU patients, Lumlertgul et al. observed the development of AKI in 76% of patients [40]. The results of our retrospective study are in accord with these data. AKI occurred in 119 of 249 (48%) of COVID-19 patients requiring ICU admission. Of these 119 patients, 23 (19%) required RRT, and 88 died (74%). These findings are consistent with previous studies from the US and other developed nations demonstrating an incidence of AKI in 40–80% of patients admitted to the ICU [5,7,12,40,41].

Despite these differences in incidence and severity, no risk factors have been consistently identified that discriminate between AKI developing in the presence or absence of COVID-19 infection. Traditional risk factors for AKI have included older age, elevated SCr on admission, requirement for vasopressors, thrombo-inflammatory biomarkers, and comorbidities such as diabetes and hypertension. By univariate analysis, in agreement with past studies, we found that the development of AKI was associated older age, the need for mechanical ventilation, elevated admission SCr, higher SOFA score, vasopressor requirement, and elevated inflammatory and thrombotic biomarkers (Tables 1–3). Of these, an elevated SCr, vasopressor requirement, and elevated inflammatory and thrombotic biomarkers were independent predictors (Table 4 and Figure 2). The lack of influence of comorbidities on the development of AKI may be a consequence of the advanced age of patients in our study (median age of 70), for whom comorbidities were similarly common in both AKI and non-AKI patients. In their studies of ICU patients with C19-ARDS, Wang et al. and Piniero et al. also found that the presence of multiple co-morbidities was not associated with the development of AKI [42,43].

A critical question is whether COVID-19-associated AKI is a separate clinical entity from other causes of AKI [44–46]. Investigations into this question have yielded conflicting results. Autopsy and biopsy series of COVID-19 patients with AKI have demonstrated a wide variety of glomerular and tubular injuries [44,46–49]. The prominence of glomerular and thrombotic injury, including collapsing glomerulopathy and TMA, is striking, and typically absent in sepsis-mediated AKI [46,47,49,50]. Nonetheless, notably, for both septic and COVID-19-associated AKI, morphologic and molecular evidence implicates inflammation as the primary driver of injury [51]. Thus, postmortem pathologic and molecular gene expression analyses have revealed that tubular injury occurring during the course of COVID-19 infection bears many similarities to sepsis-mediated acute tubular necrosis (ATN) [47,51]. Similarities include mitochondrial injury and dysregulation, increased autophagy, increased ceramide signaling, abnormalities in oxidative phosphorylation, up-regulation of apoptotic and necroptotic pathways, and increased endothelial and microvascular inflammation [51]. In addition, proteomic and genomic evidence indicates that a large number of genes involved in immune and metabolic counter-regulatory pathways, such as Treg differentiation and Sirtuin signaling, are expressed in both septic ATN and COVID-19-associated AKI [51].

In contrast, Volbeda and colleagues evaluated non-autolytic post mortem biopsies of patients with severe COVID-19 infection and observed morphologically more severe tubular injury, significant thrombosis of peritubular capillaries, and a less intense inflammatory response [52]. In fact, transcript levels for the pro-inflammatory cytokines TNF-α, IL-6, and MMP8 in biopsies from COVID-19-associated AKI patients were comparable to those found in normal controls [47,52]. In addition, the transcript levels of several genes, normally down-regulated during states of decreased renal perfusion, were also down-regulated in biopsies of COVID-19-associated AKI. Taken together, these differences suggest that decreased renal perfusion, rather than intense inflammatory state, may be the driver in some cases of COVID-19-associated AKI [52].

Such heterogeneity of pathologic and molecular findings may be due to differences in the timing of biopsies or possibly the existence of different endotypes within COVID-19-associated AKI. Certainly, the existence of an inflammatory phenotype is supported by the Recovery trial, which showed that the administration of Tocilizumab, a monoclonal antibody directed against the IL-6 receptor, led to a decrease in severe AKI requiring RRT [53]. Additional studies have demonstrated that the use of CC decreases the incidence of severe AKI [54–56]. Our own data also favor a role for inflammation in the pathophysiology of COVID-19-associated AKI. In the multivariate analysis, not only was increased CRP on day 2 independently predictive of AKI, but also combined treatment with Tocilizumab and CC was associated with decreased development of AKI. Our data further suggest a role for thrombosis, as an elevated level of D-Dimer on day 1 was also an independent predictor of AKI. In accord with this finding, Jewell et al. observed in a large UK cohort that patients who developed AKI had a statistically significant increase in thromboembolic complications [13]. Moreover, a systematic review has shown the risk of both venous and arterial thromboembolism to be statistically significantly higher in those with COVID-19 infection relative to those without [57].

With regard to mortality, although a large number of patient characteristics and interventions were associated with increased mortality, including the development of AKI, the only independent predictor for the entire cohort was advanced age. The impact of age is especially noteworthy, given that the median age of both survivors and non-survivors was greater than 65 and the difference in their median ages was less than 10 years (66 and 73, respectively). It is pertinent to note that the independent effect of older age on mortality is an almost universal finding. While one may associate increasing age with frailty and increased comorbidities, this may not be the entire explanation. For example, cellular expression of ACE-2, the putative receptor for the COVID-19 virus, decreases with age. As ACE-2 is capable of cleaving the pro-inflammatory peptide angiotensin 2 into the anti-inflammatory and anti-oxidant peptide angiotensin (1–7), aging may be associated with an increased tendency for inflammation [58–61]. Similar changes in ACE-2 expression have been observed in patients with cardiovascular disease [59,62–65]. Thus, aging and underlying cardiovascular disease may represent pro-inflammatory conditions predisposing patients to increased complications during the clinical course of COVID-19 disease.

Among patients without AKI, CKD was an additional independent predictor of mortality. Surprisingly, among patients with AKI, the only independent predictor of mortality was a lower SCr on admission. We can only speculate on the reasons for this anomalous finding. For example, a lower SCr on admission may have masked recognition of AKI and led to later renal consultation, resuscitative efforts, and use of RRT. Alternatively, a lower SCr might have been a surrogate for wasting or poorer nutritional status.

The retrospective and observational nature of our study necessarily entails several weaknesses. First, its retrospective nature limited our ability to determine and adjust for all differences in baseline characteristics and comorbidities. Second, we were unable to obtain information on such important potential risk factors as urinary output, urinary sediment, or proteinuria. Third, there were insufficient data to adjust for titration or timing and dose of pharmacologic interventions and therapies. Fourth, the diagnosis of comorbidities such as CKD or coronary artery disease were based on ICD coding rather than independent assessment by a non-involved clinician. Fifth, our retrospective analysis poses the usual limitations of selection and introduction bias. Thus, the benefits of anti-inflammatory therapy with Tocilizumab and CC in preventing AKI are associational and need to be confirmed in prospective trials. Sixth, there were many missing data points for the biomarkers D-Dimer, CRP, and ferritin, thus making it difficult to draw robust conclusions regarding their role as risk factors in the development of AKI. As a result, we had to rely on imputed data. Employing the imputed values into the multivariate analysis should therefore be considered exploratory. Nonetheless, removing the imputed biomarker data from the multivariate analysis did not alter the remaining risk factors. Further studies are needed to elucidate the role of biomarkers as predictors of AKI in patients with COVID-19 disease. Finally, our study was conducted during the first wave of the pandemic, before vaccinations were available, and extrapolation of our data to current patients may not necessarily be possible.

Despite these limitations, a major strength of our study is its study population, which comes from a large community hospital and is thus clinically and demographically similar to elderly COVID-19 patients in the general population.

5. Conclusions

The current study confirms the high rates of AKI and mortality among COVID-19 patients admitted to an ICU. As seen with other causes of AKI, multivariate analysis demonstrated that an elevated SCr on admission and the need for vasopressors were independent predictors of the development of AKI in patients with severe COVID-19. In addition, elevations of CRP and D-Dimer, biomarkers for inflammation and thrombosis, respectively, were also associated with an increased risk for AKI, albeit the effect was of small magnitude. Notably, patients who received both CC and Tocilizumab, but not either alone, were less likely to develop AKI. As has been shown for the development of C-19 ARDS in severely ill COVID-19 patients, our data suggest a potential role for inflammation in the development of COVID-19-associated AKI. One should consider the possibility that early administration of anti-inflammatory agents, just as one performs in the management of C-19 ARDS, may improve clinical outcomes in patients with AKI.

Supplementary Materials: The following supporting information can be downloaded at: https://www.mdpi.com/article/10.3390/biomedicines11030845/s1, Table S1. Missing values of biomarkers.

Author Contributions: Conceptualization, J.I. (Jose Iglesias), A.V., J.S.L., J.I. (Justin Ilagan), N.U. and A.M.; methodology, J.I. (Jose Iglesias), J.S.L. and A.V.; data curation, J.I. (Jose Iglesias), A.V. and Y.E.; validation, J.I. (Jose Iglesias), J.S.L. and AV; formal analysis, S.P.A., J.I. (Jose Iglesias), A.V., J.S.L., J.I. (Justin Ilagan) and A.A.; investigation, J.I. (Jose Iglesias), A.V., J.S.L., J.I. (Justin Ilagan), N.U. and A.M.; data curation, J.I. (Jose Iglesias); writing—original draft preparation, J.I. (Jose Iglesias) and J.S.L.; writing—reviewing, J.I. (Jose Iglesias), J.S.L., A.V., S.P.A., D.P. and Y.E,. All authors have read and agreed to the published version of the manuscript.

Funding: This research received no external funding.

Institutional Review Board Statement: The study was conducted in accordance with the Declaration of Helsinki and approved by Medical Center Institutional Review Board (IRB # 20-005).

Informed Consent Statement: Informed consent was waived by the Community Medical Center Institutional Review Board as the study was deemed minimal risk to participants due to its retrospective nature and de-identified results.

Data Availability Statement: The data used in this study are protected under HIPPA and were not intended or allowed to be shared publicly, so due to the sensitive nature of the research supporting data are not available.

Acknowledgments: Jerrold S. Levine is employed by the Department of Veteran Affairs as a Staff Physician, Medical Service, Jesse Brown Veterans Affairs Medical Center, Chicago, IL. The views expressed in this manuscript are those of the author and do not necessarily reflect the position or policy of the Department of Veterans Affairs or the United States government.

Conflicts of Interest: The authors declare no conflict of interest.

References

1. Chávez-Valencia, V.; Orizaga-de-la-Cruz, C.; Lagunas-Rangel, F.A. Acute Kidney Injury in COVID-19 Patients: Pathogenesis, Clinical Characteristics, Therapy, and Mortality. *Diseases* **2022**, *10*, 53. [CrossRef]
2. Ahmadian, E.; Hosseiniyan Khatibi, S.M.; Razi Soofiyani, S.; Abediazar, S.; Shoja, M.M.; Ardalan, M.; Zununi Vahed, S. COVID-19 and Kidney Injury: Pathophysiology and Molecular Mechanisms. *Rev. Med. Virol.* **2021**, *31*, e2176. [CrossRef]
3. Ahmed, A.R.; Ebad, C.A.; Stoneman, S.; Satti, M.M.; Conlon, P.J. Kidney Injury in COVID-19. *World J. Nephrol.* **2020**, *9*, 18–32. [CrossRef] [PubMed]
4. El-Sayed, E.E.; Allayeh, A.K.; Salem, A.A.; Omar, S.M.; Zaghlol, S.M.; Abd-Elmaguid, H.M.; Abdul-Ghaffar, M.M.; ElSharkawy, M.M. Incidence of Acute Kidney Injury among COVID-19 Patients in Egypt. *Ren. Replace Ther.* **2021**, *7*, 32. [CrossRef]
5. Hirsch, J.S.; Ng, J.H.; Ross, D.W.; Sharma, P.; Shah, H.H.; Barnett, R.L.; Hazzan, A.D.; Fishbane, S.; Jhaveri, K.D. Acute Kidney Injury in Patients Hospitalized with COVID-19. *Kidney Int.* **2020**, *98*, 209–218. [CrossRef] [PubMed]
6. Guan, W.-J.; Ni, Z.-Y.; Hu, Y.; Liang, W.-H.; Ou, C.-Q.; He, J.-X.; Liu, L.; Shan, H.; Lei, C.-L.; Hui, D.S.C.; et al. Clinical Characteristics of Coronavirus Disease 2019 in China. *N. Engl. J. Med.* **2020**, *382*, 1708–1720. [CrossRef]
7. Schaubroeck, H.; Vandenberghe, W.; Boer, W.; Boonen, E.; Dewulf, B.; Bourgeois, C.; Dubois, J.; Dumoulin, A.; Fivez, T.; Gunst, J.; et al. Acute Kidney Injury in Critical COVID-19: A Multicenter Cohort Analysis in Seven Large Hospitals in Belgium. *Crit. Care* **2022**, *26*, 225. [CrossRef] [PubMed]
8. Mohamed, M.M.B.; Lukitsch, I.; Torres-Ortiz, A.E.; Walker, J.B.; Varghese, V.; Hernandez-Arroyo, C.F.; Alqudsi, M.; LeDoux, J.R.; Velez, J.C.Q. Acute Kidney Injury Associated with Coronavirus Disease 2019 in Urban New Orleans. *Kidney360* **2020**, *1*, 614–622. [CrossRef] [PubMed]
9. Rubin, S.; Orieux, A.; Prevel, R.; Garric, A.; Bats, M.-L.; Dabernat, S.; Camou, F.; Guisset, O.; Issa, N.; Mourissoux, G.; et al. Characterization of Acute Kidney Injury in Critically Ill Patients with Severe Coronavirus Disease 2019. *Clin. Kidney J.* **2020**, *13*, 354–361. [CrossRef]
10. Sabaghian, T.; Kharazmi, A.B.; Ansari, A.; Omidi, F.; Kazemi, S.N.; Hajikhani, B.; Vaziri-Harami, R.; Tajbakhsh, A.; Omidi, S.; Haddadi, S.; et al. COVID-19 and Acute Kidney Injury: A Systematic Review. *Front. Med.* **2022**, *9*, 705908. [CrossRef]
11. Gameiro, J.; Fonseca, J.A.; Oliveira, J.; Marques, F.; Bernardo, J.; Costa, C.; Carreiro, C.; Braz, S.; Lopes, J.A. Acute Kidney Injury in Hospitalized Patients with COVID-19: A Portuguese Cohort. *Nefrología* **2021**, *41*, 689–698. [CrossRef]
12. Fisher, M.; Neugarten, J.; Bellin, E.; Yunes, M.; Stahl, L.; Johns, T.S.; Abramowitz, M.K.; Levy, R.; Kumar, N.; Mokrzycki, M.H.; et al. AKI in Hospitalized Patients with and without COVID-19: A Comparison Study. *J. Am. Soc. Nephrol.* **2020**, *31*, 2145–2157. [CrossRef] [PubMed]

13. Jewell, P.D.; Bramham, K.; Galloway, J.; Post, F.; Norton, S.; Teo, J.; Fisher, R.; Saha, R.; Hutchings, S.; Hopkins, P.; et al. COVID-19-Related Acute Kidney Injury; Incidence, Risk Factors and Outcomes in a Large UK Cohort. *BMC Nephrol.* **2021**, *22*, 359. [CrossRef]
14. Elrobaa, I.H.; New, K.J. COVID-19: Pulmonary and Extra Pulmonary Manifestations. *Front. Public Health* **2021**, *9*, 711616. [CrossRef]
15. Gulati, A.; Pomeranz, C.; Qamar, Z.; Thomas, S.; Frisch, D.; George, G.; Summer, R.; DeSimone, J.; Sundaram, B. A Comprehensive Review of Manifestations of Novel Coronaviruses in the Context of Deadly COVID-19 Global Pandemic. *Am. J. Med. Sci.* **2020**, *360*, 5–34. [CrossRef]
16. Tossetta, G.; Fantone, S.; Delli Muti, N.; Balercia, G.; Ciavattini, A.; Giannubilo, S.R.; Marzioni, D. Preeclampsia and Severe Acute Respiratory Syndrome Coronavirus 2 Infection: A Systematic Review. *J. Hypertens.* **2022**, *40*, 1629–1638. [CrossRef]
17. Dale, L. Neurological Complications of COVID-19: A Review of the Literature. *Cureus* **2022**, *14*, e27633. [CrossRef]
18. Delli Muti, N.; Finocchi, F.; Tossetta, G.; Salvio, G.; Cutini, M.; Marzioni, D.; Balercia, G. Could SARS-CoV-2 Infection Affect Male Fertility and Sexuality? *APMIS* **2022**, *130*, 243–252. [CrossRef] [PubMed]
19. Griffin, D.O.; Brennan-Rieder, D.; Ngo, B.; Kory, P.; Confalonieri, M.; Shapiro, L.; Iglesias, J.; Dube, M.; Nanda, N.; In, G.K.; et al. The Importance of Understanding the Stages of COVID-19 in Treatment and Trials. *AIDS Rev.* **2021**, *23*, 40–47. [CrossRef] [PubMed]
20. Chaibi, K.; Dao, M.; Pham, T.; Gumucio-Sanguino, V.D.; Di Paolo, F.A.; Pavot, A.; Cohen, Y.; Dreyfuss, D.; Pérez-Fernandez, X.; Gaudry, S. Severe Acute Kidney Injury in Patients with COVID-19 and Acute Respiratory Distress Syndrome. *Am. J. Respir. Crit. Care Med.* **2020**, *202*, 1299–1301. [CrossRef]
21. Del Vecchio, L.; Locatelli, F. Hypoxia Response and Acute Lung and Kidney Injury: Possible Implications for Therapy of COVID-19. *Clin. Kidney J.* **2020**, *13*, 494–499. [CrossRef] [PubMed]
22. Diebold, M.; Zimmermann, T.; Dickenmann, M.; Schaub, S.; Bassetti, S.; Tschudin-Sutter, S.; Bingisser, R.; Heim, C.; Siegemund, M.; Osswald, S.; et al. Comparison of Acute Kidney Injury in Patients with COVID-19 and Other Respiratory Infections: A Prospective Cohort Study. *J. Clin. Med.* **2021**, *10*, 2288. [CrossRef]
23. Nardo, A.D.; Schneeweiss-Gleixner, M.; Bakail, M.; Dixon, E.D.; Lax, S.F.; Trauner, M. Pathophysiological Mechanisms of Liver Injury in COVID-19. *Liver Int.* **2021**, *41*, 20–32. [CrossRef]
24. Berlin, D.A.; Gulick, R.M.; Martinez, F.J. Severe COVID-19. *N. Engl. J. Med.* **2020**, *383*, 2451–2460. [CrossRef] [PubMed]
25. Wu, Z.; McGoogan, J.M. Characteristics of and Important Lessons from the Coronavirus Disease 2019 (COVID-19) Outbreak in China: Summary of a Report of 72,314 Cases from the Chinese Center for Disease Control and Prevention. *JAMA* **2020**, *323*, 1239–1242. [CrossRef]
26. Li, C. Little's Test of Missing Completely at Random. *Stata J.* **2013**, *13*, 795–809. [CrossRef]
27. Do, C.B.; Batzoglou, S. What Is the Expectation Maximization Algorithm? *Nat. Biotechnol.* **2008**, *26*, 897–899. [CrossRef]
28. Bernier-Jean, A.; Beaubien-Souligny, W.; Goupil, R.; Madore, F.; Paquette, F.; Troyanov, S.; Bouchard, J. Diagnosis and Outcomes of Acute Kidney Injury Using Surrogate and Imputation Methods for Missing Preadmission Creatinine Values. *BMC Nephrol.* **2017**, *18*, 141. [CrossRef]
29. Kellum, J.A.; Lameire, N. Diagnosis, Evaluation, and Management of Acute Kidney Injury: A KDIGO Summary (Part 1). *Crit. Care* **2013**, *17*, 204. [CrossRef] [PubMed]
30. Singbartl, K.; Kellum, J.A. AKI in the ICU: Definition, Epidemiology, Risk Stratification, and Outcomes. *Kidney Int.* **2012**, *81*, 819–825. [CrossRef]
31. Gómez-Mesa, J.E.; Galindo-Coral, S.; Montes, M.C.; Muñoz Martin, A.J. Thrombosis and Coagulopathy in COVID-19. *Curr. Probl. Cardiol.* **2021**, *46*, 100742. [CrossRef]
32. Asakura, H.; Ogawa, H. COVID-19-Associated Coagulopathy and Disseminated Intravascular Coagulation. *Int. J. Hematol.* **2021**, *113*, 45–57. [CrossRef] [PubMed]
33. Amraei, R.; Rahimi, N. COVID-19, Renin-Angiotensin System and Endothelial Dysfunction. *Cells* **2020**, *9*, 1652. [CrossRef] [PubMed]
34. Chen, Y.-T.; Shao, S.-C.; Hsu, C.-K.; Wu, I.-W.; Hung, M.-J.; Chen, Y.-C. Incidence of Acute Kidney Injury in COVID-19 Infection: A Systematic Review and Meta-Analysis. *Crit. Care* **2020**, *24*, 346. [CrossRef]
35. Hardenberg, J.-H.B.; Stockmann, H.; Eckardt, K.-U.; Schmidt-Ott, K.M. COVID-19 and acute kidney injury in the intensive care unit. *Nephrologe* **2021**, *16*, 20–25.e1. [CrossRef]
36. Ng, J.H.; Hirsch, J.S.; Hazzan, A.; Wanchoo, R.; Shah, H.H.; Malieckal, D.A.; Ross, D.W.; Sharma, P.; Sakhiya, V.; Fishbane, S.; et al. Outcomes Among Patients Hospitalized with COVID-19 and Acute Kidney Injury. *Am. J. Kidney Dis.* **2021**, *77*, 204–215.e1. [CrossRef]
37. Kolhe, N.V.; Fluck, R.J.; Selby, N.M.; Taal, M.W. Acute Kidney Injury Associated with COVID-19: A Retrospective Cohort Study. *PLOS Med.* **2020**, *17*, e1003406. [CrossRef] [PubMed]
38. McNicholas, B.A.; Rezoagli, E.; Simpkin, A.J.; Khanna, S.; Suen, J.Y.; Yeung, P.; Brodie, D.; Li Bassi, G.; Pham, T.; Bellani, G.; et al. Epidemiology and Outcomes of Early-Onset AKI in COVID-19-Related ARDS in Comparison with Non-COVID-19-Related ARDS: Insights from Two Prospective Global Cohort Studies. *Critical. Care* **2023**, *27*, 3. [CrossRef]
39. Fabrizi, F.; Alfieri, C.M.; Cerutti, R.; Lunghi, G.; Messa, P. COVID-19 and Acute Kidney Injury: A Systematic Review and Meta-Analysis. *Pathogens* **2020**, *9*, 1052. [CrossRef]

40. Lumlertgul, N.; Pirondini, L.; Cooney, E.; Kok, W.; Gregson, J.; Camporota, L.; Lane, K.; Leach, R.; Ostermann, M. Acute Kidney Injury Prevalence, Progression and Long-Term Outcomes in Critically Ill Patients with COVID-19: A Cohort Study. *Ann. Intensive Care* 2021, *11*, 123. [CrossRef]
41. Flythe, J.E.; Assimon, M.M.; Tugman, M.J.; Chang, E.H.; Gupta, S.; Shah, J.; Sosa, M.A.; Renaghan, A.D.; Melamed, M.L.; Wilson, F.P.; et al. Characteristics and Outcomes of Individuals with Pre-Existing Kidney Disease and COVID-19 Admitted to Intensive Care Units in the United States. *Am. J. Kidney Dis.* 2021, *77*, 190–203.e1. [CrossRef]
42. Piñeiro, G.J.; Molina-Andújar, A.; Hermida, E.; Blasco, M.; Quintana, L.F.; Rojas, G.M.; Mercadal, J.; Castro, P.; Sandoval, E.; Andrea, R.; et al. Severe Acute Kidney Injury in Critically Ill COVID-19 Patients. *J. Nephrol.* 2021, *34*, 285–293. [CrossRef]
43. Wang, F.; Ran, L.; Qian, C.; Hua, J.; Luo, Z.; Ding, M.; Zhang, X.; Guo, W.; Gao, S.; Gao, W.; et al. Epidemiology and Outcomes of Acute Kidney Injury in COVID-19 Patients with Acute Respiratory Distress Syndrome: A Multicenter Retrospective Study. *Blood Purif.* 2021, *50*, 499–505. [CrossRef]
44. Golmai, P.; Larsen, C.P.; DeVita, M.V.; Wahl, S.J.; Weins, A.; Rennke, H.G.; Bijol, V.; Rosenstock, J.L. Histopathologic and Ultrastructural Findings in Postmortem Kidney Biopsy Material in 12 Patients with AKI and COVID-19. *J. Am. Soc. Nephrol.* 2020, *31*, 1944–1947. [CrossRef] [PubMed]
45. Shetty, A.A.; Tawhari, I.; Safar-Boueri, L.; Seif, N.; Alahmadi, A.; Gargiulo, R.; Aggarwal, V.; Usman, I.; Kisselev, S.; Gharavi, A.G.; et al. COVID-19-Associated Glomerular Disease. *J. Am. Soc. Nephrol.* 2021, *32*, 33–40. [CrossRef] [PubMed]
46. Volbeda, M.; Jou-Valencia, D.; van den Heuvel, M.C.; Zijlstra, J.G.; Franssen, C.F.M.; van der Voort, P.H.J.; Moser, J.; van Meurs, M. Acute and Chronic Histopathological Findings in Renal Biopsies in COVID-19. *Clin. Exp. Med.* 2022, 1–12. [CrossRef]
47. Ng, J.H.; Bijol, V.; Sparks, M.A.; Sise, M.E.; Izzedine, H.; Jhaveri, K.D. Pathophysiology and Pathology of Acute Kidney Injury in Patients With COVID-19. *Adv. Chronic Kidney Dis.* 2020, *27*, 365–376. [CrossRef] [PubMed]
48. Santoriello, D.; Khairallah, P.; Bomback, A.S.; Xu, K.; Kudose, S.; Batal, I.; Barasch, J.; Radhakrishnan, J.; D'Agati, V.; Markowitz, G. Postmortem Kidney Pathology Findings in Patients with COVID-19. *J. Am. Soc. Nephrol.* 2020, *31*, 2158–2167. [CrossRef] [PubMed]
49. Tang, N.; Li, D.; Wang, X.; Sun, Z. Abnormal Coagulation Parameters Are Associated with Poor Prognosis in Patients with Novel Coronavirus Pneumonia. *J. Thromb. Haemost.* 2020, *18*, 844–847. [CrossRef]
50. Wu, H.; Larsen, C.P.; Hernandez-Arroyo, C.F.; Mohamed, M.M.B.; Caza, T.; Sharshir, M.; Chughtai, A.; Xie, L.; Gimenez, J.M.; Sandow, T.A.; et al. AKI and Collapsing Glomerulopathy Associated with COVID-19 and APOL 1 High-Risk Genotype. *J. Am. Soc. Nephrol.* 2020, *31*, 1688–1695. [CrossRef]
51. Alexander, M.P.; Mangalaparthi, K.K.; Madugundu, A.K.; Madugundu, A.K.; Moyer, A.M.; Adam, B.; Mengel, M.; Smrita, S.; Singh, S.; Singh, S.K.; et al. Acute Kidney Injury in Severe COVID-19 Has Similarities to Sepsis-Associated Kidney Injury: A Multi-Omics Study. *Mayo Clinic Proc.* 2021, *96*, 2561–2575. [CrossRef]
52. Volbeda, M.; Jou-Valencia, D.; van den Heuvel, M.C.; Knoester, M.; Zwiers, P.J.; Pillay, J.; Berger, S.P.; van der Voort, P.H.J.; Zijlstra, J.G.; van Meurs, M.; et al. Comparison of Renal Histopathology and Gene Expression Profiles between Severe COVID-19 and Bacterial Sepsis in Critically Ill Patients. *Crit. Care* 2021, *25*, 202. [CrossRef]
53. Tocilizumab in Patients Admitted to Hospital with COVID-19 (RECOVERY): A Randomised, Controlled, Open-Label, Platform Trial. *Lancet* 2021, *397*, 1637–1645. [CrossRef]
54. Orieux, A.; Khan, P.; Prevel, R.; Gruson, D.; Rubin, S.; Boyer, A. Impact of Dexamethasone Use to Prevent from Severe COVID-19-Induced Acute Kidney Injury. *Crit. Care* 2021, *25*, 249. [CrossRef] [PubMed]
55. Saggi, S.J.; Nath, S.; Culas, R.; Chittalae, S.; Burza, A.; Srinivasan, M.; Abdul, R.; Silver, B.; Lora, A.; Ibtida, I.; et al. Early Experience with Methylprednisolone on SARS-CoV-2 Infection in the African American Population, a Retrospective Analysis. *Clin. Med. Insights Circ. Respir. Pulm. Med.* 2020, *14*, 1–7. [CrossRef] [PubMed]
56. Dexamethasone in Hospitalized Patients with COVID-19. *N. Engl. J. Med.* 2021, *384*, 693–704. [CrossRef] [PubMed]
57. Malas, M.B.; Naazie, I.N.; Elsayed, N.; Mathlouthi, A.; Marmor, R.; Clary, B. Thromboembolism Risk of COVID-19 Is High and Associated with a Higher Risk of Mortality: A Systematic Review and Meta-Analysis. *EClinicalMedicine* 2020, *29*, 100639. [CrossRef]
58. Chen, J.; Jiang, Q.; Xia, X.; Liu, K.; Yu, Z.; Tao, W.; Gong, W.; Han, J.-D.J. Individual Variation of the SARS-CoV-2 Receptor ACE2 Gene Expression and Regulation. *Aging Cell* 2020, *19*, e13168. [CrossRef]
59. Monteonofrio, L.; Florio, M.C.; AlGhatrif, M.; Lakatta, E.G.; Capogrossi, M.C. Aging- and Gender-Related Modulation of RAAS: Potential Implications in COVID-19 Disease. *Vasc. Biol.* 2021, *3*, R1–R14. [CrossRef]
60. Zhu, H.; Zhang, L.; Ma, Y.; Zhai, M.; Xia, L.; Liu, J.; Yu, S.; Duan, W. The Role of SARS-CoV-2 Target ACE2 in Cardiovascular Diseases. *J. Cell. Mol. Med.* 2021, *25*, 1342–1349. [CrossRef]
61. Baker, S.A.; Kwok, S.; Berry, G.J.; Montine, T.J. Angiotensin-Converting Enzyme 2 (ACE2) Expression Increases with Age in Patients Requiring Mechanical Ventilation. *PLoS ONE* 2021, *16*, e0247060. [CrossRef]
62. Tikellis, C.; Thomas, M.C. Angiotensin-Converting Enzyme 2 (ACE2) Is a Key Modulator of the Renin Angiotensin System in Health and Disease. *Int. J. Pept.* 2012, *2012*, 256294. [CrossRef]
63. Bartleson, J.M.; Radenkovic, D.; Covarrubias, A.J.; Furman, D.; Winer, D.A.; Verdin, E. SARS-CoV-2, COVID-19 and the Aging Immune System. *Nat. Aging* 2021, *1*, 769–782. [CrossRef] [PubMed]

64. Keidar, S.; Kaplan, M.; Gamliel-Lazarovich, A. ACE2 of the Heart: From Angiotensin I to Angiotensin (1–7). *Cardiovasc. Res.* **2007**, *73*, 463–469. [CrossRef] [PubMed]
65. Oudit, G.Y.; Kassiri, Z.; Patel, M.P.; Chappell, M.; Butany, J.; Backx, P.H.; Tsushima, R.G.; Scholey, J.W.; Khokha, R.; Penninger, J.M. Angiotensin II-Mediated Oxidative Stress and Inflammation Mediate the Age-Dependent Cardiomyopathy in ACE2 Null Mice. *Cardiovasc. Res.* **2007**, *75*, 29–39. [CrossRef] [PubMed]

Disclaimer/Publisher's Note: The statements, opinions and data contained in all publications are solely those of the individual author(s) and contributor(s) and not of MDPI and/or the editor(s). MDPI and/or the editor(s) disclaim responsibility for any injury to people or property resulting from any ideas, methods, instructions or products referred to in the content.

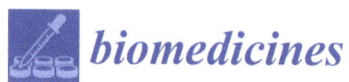

Review

COVID-19 in Elderly Patients Receiving Haemodialysis: A Current Review

Thomas McDonnell [1], Henry H. L. Wu [2,*], Philip A. Kalra [1,3] and Rajkumar Chinnadurai [1,3]

1. Department of Renal Medicine, Northern Care Alliance NHS Foundation Trust, Salford M6 8HD, UK
2. Renal Research Laboratory, Kolling Institute of Medical Research, Royal North Shore Hospital, The University of Sydney, Sydney, NSW 2065, Australia
3. Faculty of Biology, Medicine & Health, The University of Manchester, Manchester M1 7HR, UK
* Correspondence: honlinhenry.wu@health.nsw.gov.au; Tel.: +61-9926-4751

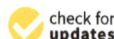

Citation: McDonnell, T.; Wu, H.H.L.; Kalra, P.A.; Chinnadurai, R. COVID-19 in Elderly Patients Receiving Haemodialysis: A Current Review. *Biomedicines* 2023, 11, 926. https://doi.org/10.3390/biomedicines11030926

Academic Editors: Elena Cecilia Rosca and Amalia Cornea

Received: 28 February 2023
Revised: 11 March 2023
Accepted: 14 March 2023
Published: 16 March 2023

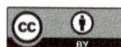

Copyright: © 2023 by the authors. Licensee MDPI, Basel, Switzerland. This article is an open access article distributed under the terms and conditions of the Creative Commons Attribution (CC BY) license (https://creativecommons.org/licenses/by/4.0/).

Abstract: There is an increased incidence of elderly adults diagnosed with kidney failure as our global aging population continues to expand. Hence, the number of elderly adults indicated for kidney replacement therapy is also increasing simultaneously. Haemodialysis initiation is more commonly observed in comparison to kidney transplantation and peritoneal dialysis for the elderly. The onset of the coronavirus 2019 (COVID-19) pandemic brought new paradigms and insights for the care of this patient population. Elderly patients receiving haemodialysis have been identified as high-risk groups for poor COVID-19 outcomes. Age, immunosenescence, impaired response to COVID-19 vaccination, increased exposure to sources of COVID-19 infection and thrombotic risks during dialysis are key factors which demonstrated significant associations with COVID-19 incidence, severity and mortality for this patient group. Recent findings suggest that preventative measures such as regular screening and, if needed, isolation in COVID-19-positive cases, alongside the fulfillment of COVID-19 vaccination programs is an integral strategy to reduce the number of COVID-19 cases and consequential complications from COVID-19, particularly for high-risk groups such as elderly haemodialysis patients. The COVID-19 pandemic brought about the rapid development and repurposing of a number of medications to treat patients in the viral and inflammatory stages of their disease. However, elderly haemodialysis patients were grossly unrepresented in many of these trials. We review the evidence for contemporary treatments for COVID-19 in this population to provide clinicians with an up-to-date guide. We hope our article increases awareness on the associations and impact of COVID-19 for the elderly haemodialysis population, and encourage research efforts to address knowledge gaps in this topical area.

Keywords: Coronavirus 2019; elderly patients; haemodialysis; risk factors; pathophysiology; prevention; management

1. Introduction

Emergence of the novel severe acute respiratory syndrome coronavirus 2 (SARS-CoV-2) in December 2019, responsible for the coronavirus 2019 (COVID-19) pandemic outbreak, has since had a profound impact on health systems globally [1]. While it was initially recognized as the cause of severe pneumonias, COVID-19 has since been found to have a range of extrapulmonary manifestations, including direct effects on the kidney [2–7]. The pandemic has also disproportionately affected vulnerable populations, such as elderly people and those affected by chronic medical conditions, in which chronic kidney disease (CKD) has been identified as a significant risk factor for morbidity and mortality following COVID-19 infection [8]. In particular, patients receiving haemodialysis face unique challenges, as they require frequent hospital visits and are at risk of COVID-19 exposure from other patients and clinical staff. As a consequence of frailty, multimorbidities and challenges relating to performing dialysis therapy at home, elderly patients requiring kidney replacement therapy are much more likely to receive haemodialysis compared to peritoneal dialysis or kidney transplantation [9]. This review discusses the risk factors and pathophysiological impact of COVID-19 infection in elderly people (i.e., people with age >65 years old) receiving haemodialysis, as well as the practical challenges of managing this patient population when they have a COVID-19 infection. We will explore the current preventative and pharmacological treatment options available to clinicians caring for this vulnerable patient group.

2. Risk Factors for Poor Clinical Outcomes in Elderly Haemodialysis Populations with COVID-19 Infection

Advancing age is associated with an increased likelihood of contracting COVID-19 infection, with adults above 80 years of age particularly being at greatest risk [8]. In addition, age is a major risk factor for progression towards having acute respiratory distress syndrome (ARDS) [10]. The hazard ratio (HR) for mortality also increases linearly with increasing age [11]. A significantly increased mortality risk is noticeable amongst those with pre-existing kidney disease, particularly those with dialysis-dependent kidney failure. The prevalence of COVID-19 infection is much higher in the CKD population. Outside of old age, CKD patients with an estimated glomerular filtration rate (eGFR) < 30 mL/min/1.73 m^2 is considered one of the strongest predictors for poor clinical outcomes [11,12]. Mortality rates are exacerbated in the dialysis population over 20 times compared to that expected of propensity-matched historic controls [13]. The risk of death following COVID-19 infection is further increased for an elderly population receiving dialysis [13,14]. There are various reasons which may explain these observed associations (Figure 1).

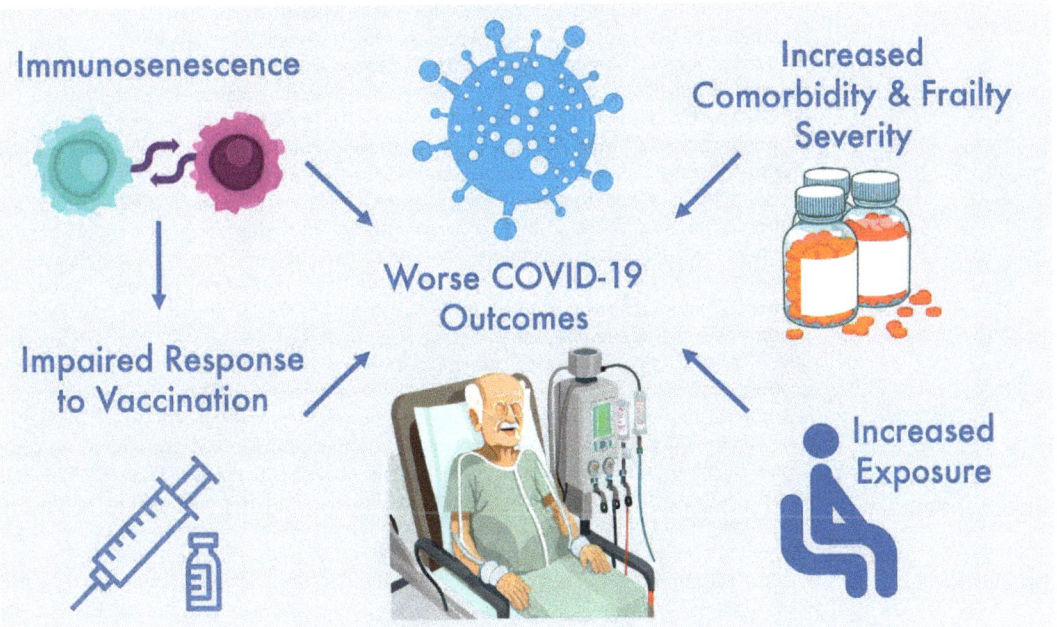

Figure 1. Risk factors for worsened clinical outcomes in elderly haemodialysis patients with COVID-19.

2.1. Increased Comorbidity Status and Frailty Severity

In a vast cohort study undertaken by National Health Service England, nearly 1000 COVID-19-related deaths were reviewed. Age by far was the greatest predictor of mortality, and most comorbidities were associated with increased mortality risk, particularly cardiovascular disease and diabetes. These are both common comorbidities amongst the dialysis population [11]. In another study involving nearly 500,000 dialysis patients in the United States, there were 60,090 patients identified with COVID-19 infection in which the greatest predictor of contracting COVID-19 and increased mortality was nursing home stay, regardless of the length of time the individual had been staying there. Additionally, the number of comorbidities and more importantly, the degree of burden and complications as a result of co-morbid status were all significant risk factors for COVID-19-related mortality [14]. These associations were found in observational studies involving long-term dialysis populations, where increased comorbid status and age correlated with worsened clinical outcomes and mortality rates [12,15]. It is difficult to pinpoint which underlying diseases in haemodialysis patients are more influential in leading towards poor clinical outcomes, due to the multidimensional factors which may contribute towards poor outcomes for this complex group of patients.

Frailty is a significant health burden for elderly patients with advanced CKD and those with kidney failure requiring dialysis treatment [16,17]. Frailty status was included as an important factor in guiding clinical decisions for patient management during early stages of the COVID-19 pandemic [18]. An age-related clinical syndrome characterized by a decline in physiologic reserve and decreased ability to respond to stressor events, frailty is associated with an increased risk of adverse outcomes including falls, hospitalization, poorer health-related quality of life and ultimately, earlier than expected death [19–22]. Frailty severity is influenced by numerous factors—poor nutrition. sarcopenia, infection and inflammation, cognitive impairment, reduced physical exercise threshold, vitamin D deficiency, metabolic acidosis and cellular senescence are all potential factors which accelerate the decline from fitness to frailty [23–28]. Whilst the data in relation to the impact of frailty status and frailty severity on outcomes of elderly haemodialysis patients are only emerging, the presence of COVID-19 infection likely adds further insult to the pathophysiological processes inherent to kidney disease and disrupts homeostatic responses during haemodialysis. These stressors would be more difficult to manage in complex and frail elderly individuals [29–32]. The management of frail patients receiving haemodialysis is challenging and unfortunately there is no 'one size fits all' approach. However, the timely identification of those with poor physical performance levels followed by arrangement of individualized and goal-based exercise programs showed promise [33]. Furthermore, non-pharmacological treatment to aid mood and manage depression has shown positive effects as well [34]. Though malnutrition is often associated with frailty and regular dietary assessments are recommended, there remains a paucity of studies examining the benefits of nutritional supplementation on frailty outcomes in the haemodialysis population at present [34]. Understanding the potential mechanisms of how acute COVID-19 infection affects the elderly dialysis-dependent population may bring further light into the impact of comorbidity and frailty status in this process. The natural history of COVID-19 infection is one manifesting with an initial viral stage, characterized by mild constitutional symptoms, lymphopenia and fever. This may progress to a more malign host inflammatory phase (cytokine storm) associated with ARDS, shock and high C-reactive protein (CRP) activity and the activity of other pro-inflammatory cytokines [35]. This phenomenon is more commonly observed in older age groups, and rarely observed in children and adolescents [36]. Current evidence suggests that elderly patients with COVID-19 infection are more likely to have a higher inflammatory state, with higher CRP levels, lymphopenia, neutrophilia and increased findings of multi lobe lung lesions on Computed Tomography scanning compared to their younger counterparts [37]. It is established that elderly patients and those with kidney failure have higher numbers of CD28 and CD4 null cells and advanced differentiated cells, which may result in the increased likelihood of cytokine storm and acute lung injury [38]. This may also be, in part, secondary to impaired airway clearance and reduced lung reserves in the elderly population affected by comorbidities and frailty.

2.2. Immunosenescence

Immunosenescence refers to the changes to the immune system that occur with aging, leading to an increased prevalence of infections, malignancy and autoimmune diseases [39]. Both T and B cells are involved in the process of immunosenescence. The decline in the number and functionality of naive T and B cells leads to an imbalance in the homeostatic mechanisms of the immune system and a decline in the ability to mount a primary immune response to new antigens. This increases the risk of infection and reduces the effectiveness of vaccines in elderly adults. There is a reduction in the number of both pre- and pro-B cells with aging, as well as impairment in the B-cell maturation process and number of immunoglobulins producing B cells [39]. Although there is a significant decrease in the production of B cells from the bone marrow, the number of peripheral B cells will remain constant, reflecting increased B-cell permanence [40]. The thymus is the primary site of T-cell development, and epithelial cells in the thymus are responsible for T-cell development. With advancing age, involution of the thymus is observed where there is a reduction in cellularity and in thymic epithelial space with a consequential decrease in T-cell output [39]. Not only will there be a decline in the number of T lymphocytes (CD4+ T cells and CD8+ T cells) in the circulation, but there will also be a decline in their ability to respond towards incoming pathogens [41]. T-cell clonal exhaustion is also observed, in which there is an impaired T-cell response to new antigens and declining ability to divide and multiply in response to new pathogens [42].

Immunosenescence is likely prevalent within the elderly haemodialysis population [43]. The percentage of newly formed 'naïve T cells' is reduced in the circulation with advancing age. This occurs due to a combination of reasons, predominantly explained by the reduction in thymic mass and consequently a reduced output of naïve T cells. Furthermore, the number of differentiated memory T cells increases as we age, and therefore decreases the proportion of naïve T cells in the body. Increased differentiation will also reduce T-cell telomere length [44]. When compared to healthy controls, the T-cell status of patients receiving dialysis is comparable to those up to 20 years more senior in age than themselves [45]. Acceleration in immune aging in the dialysis population is most probably caused by the manifestation of a pro-inflammatory state associated with advanced kidney disease. Accumulation of uremic toxins in kidney failure alongside increased oxidative stress leads to a build-up of pro-inflammatory cytokines such as CD4+ and CD28 as well as CD14+ and CD16++ monocyte populations [43]. The prevalence of senescent and exhausted lymphocyte phenotypes is also markedly increased. This form of accelerated immune aging in pro-inflammatory states, commonly referred to as 'inflammaging', explains why the elderly haemodialysis population is more susceptible to risk of infections including COVID-19. A depleted pool of naïve T cells may lead to a slower response to viral inoculation, considering lower numbers of naïve T cells are associated with worsened clinical outcomes and more severe COVID-19 infection [46,47]. Additionally, dialysis patents have a delayed viral clearance of SARS-CoV-2 following the resolution of acute symptoms, with time to a negative polymerase chain reaction (PCR) test being on average 7 days longer for a CKD compared to non-CKD populations [48]. For elderly haemodialysis patients with cytomegalovirus, this has further implications in the context of COVID-19 infection. Given the proportion of CD4 positive and CD28 negative T cells usually make up over 50% of the T-cell population in these groups, the excess pro-inflammatory cytokine activity here can result in greater likelihood of endothelial dysfunction and cytokine storm acutely progressing to systemic sepsis and organ failure if timely intervention is not provided [49].

2.3. Reduced Response to COVID-19 Vaccination

Not only are elderly haemodialysis patients at increased risk of contracting and having worse outcomes from COVID-19 infection, but their response to COVID-19 vaccination is also inferior compared with healthy controls [50]. This is an important point to consider, as there has been convincing evidence suggesting protective effects of COVID-19 vaccination with increased antibody levels post-vaccination. Following the first and second COVID-

19 vaccinations, healthy controls are expected to mount a threshold serological response 95% and 100% of the time. For dialysis patients, this is significantly reduced, at 45% and 89% [50]. Though for some dialysis patients, the threshold serological response could be reached, the overall antibody titre is still evidently lower in dialysis patients [51]. Considering these findings, elderly haemodialysis patients are at greater risk of poor serological response [52]. A lower antibody titre incurs lower protection during acute COVID-19 infection, particularly from the Omicron variant which is currently the most prevalent COVID-19 variant worldwide [53].

2.4. Increased Exposure to COVID-19 Infection

SARS-CoV-2 is a respiratory pathogen, spread via aerosolized droplets. It is highly contagious with an R0 of 2.2 with the degree of risk for infection related to exposure and proximity to an infected individual [15]. Many countries advocated quarantine and isolation measures as primary ways of reducing patient exposure to COVID-19 [54]. With the majority of dialysis-dependent kidney failure patients receiving in-centre haemodialysis, these patients present as a unique group in regard to their increased risk of COVID-19 exposure [55–57]. When the COVID-19 pandemic first hit, dialysis centres worldwide had to adapt quickly to protect this vulnerable cohort of patients and employ strategies to reduce their exposure to COVID-19 [58]. The increased risk of contracting COVID-19 and COVID-19 seropositivity amongst patients receiving in-centre haemodialysis is evident, with rates of infection double to those receiving home haemodialysis [59]. A study from the United Kingdom which screened COVID-19 seropositivity status amongst dialysis patients found 36.2% having positive serology (indicating prior infection) and 22.2% having a positive PCR test (though it should be noted that only 21% of the cohort received a PCR test) [60]. The mode of COVID-19 transmission in in-centre haemodialysis patients is predominantly horizontal (i.e., within dialysis shifts where they have interaction with healthcare workers and other dialysis patients) as opposed to vertical (i.e., from the preceding or following shift) [15]. The potential of COVID-19 transmission during shared transport to and from dialysis needs to be considered as another vector of transmission [61]. Though strategies of cohorting and isolating COVID-19 dialysis patients have been implemented during in-centre dialysis, the fact that elderly haemodialysis patients with COVID-19 infection remains seropositive for longer periods hinders the effects from these cohorting and isolation strategies. With over 60% of elderly haemodialysis patients remaining PCR positive for at least 20 days following COVID-19 infection, many of these patients remain infectious for longer periods and are at increased risk of infecting other in-centre haemodialysis patients [62]. Whilst elderly haemodialysis patients remain seropositive for longer, this does not appear to confer adequate protection from re-infection. In the general population with known prior COVID-19 infection, there is a 90% reduction of having a second COVID-19 infection following the first episode, in comparison with a reduction of just 45% for the dialysis population [52].

2.5. Risks of Thrombotic Complications

COVID-19 is known to induce a state of hypercoagulability and endothelial dysfunction that correlates with the degree of inflammation [63]. This mechanism does pose an additional health burden for the haemodialysis population who are already at greater risk of thrombosis through exposure to the extracorporeal dialysis circuit. Data on whether there is a significantly increased risk of thrombosis in the elderly population compared to younger persons receiving haemodialysis remain unestablished, but numerous studies have documented catheter, circuit, and arterial venous fistula thrombosis in patients with COVID-19 infection [64–67]. This can lead to delays in dialysis treatment, excess blood loss and other complications which may impact upon the elderly haemodialysis population more significantly, particularly those living with multimorbidities and more severe levels of frailty [65–67]. At the moment, there are no published studies which have evaluated the modification of anticoagulation strategies during intermittent haemodialysis for COVID-

19-positive patients, though increasing anticoagulation should be considered during active COVID-19 infection to reduce the risk of thrombosis.

3. Prevention Strategies for COVID-19 in Elderly Haemodialysis Patients

There were increased efforts to implement COVID-19 preventative measures specific to elderly haemodialysis patients, due to the increase risk of these patients contracting COVID-19 from their frequent contact and interactions with other dialysis patients and healthcare staff if receiving in-centre dialysis and a high-case fatality from COVID-19 compared to the general population.

3.1. Regular Screening

Strategies to prevent patient-to-patient transmission of COVID-19 may include the implementation of regular screening programs. Two types of screening programs can be employed: symptom-based screening followed by specific testing or a universal screening program. The screening process can vary based on the type of test used, such as nasal polymerase chain reaction (PCR), antigen testing or serum antibody testing, and screening programs may also differ based on the frequency of screening.

The International Society of Nephrology COVID-19 guidelines has recommended symptom-based testing as a method to identify and reduce the transmission of COVID-19 in patients with CKD, in particular those receiving dialysis [68]. A study conducted in the United Kingdom during the early phase of the pandemic (from 2 March 2020 to 13 April 2020) reported outcomes from employing a symptom-based testing program. PCR testing was performed if patients reported high-risk symptoms or the presence of fever. Of all the tests performed, 65.6% were positive for SARS-CoV-2. These patients were then separated from asymptomatic patients in an isolation unit. This high proportion of positive tests raises the question of whether symptom-based testing is too insensitive to pick up all COVID-19 infections, particularly since asymptomatic COVID-19 infections have been reported in between 10% and 50% of the dialysis community [60,69–72].

In another study that used the widely available rapid antigen tests (RAT), 277 haemodialysis patients were screened from 15 February 2021 to 15 November 2021. Thirty-eight tests were returned positive, but only five (14%) cases were subsequently confirmed as COVID-19 positive by PCR testing. Over this period, 6.4% of the haemodialysis population had contracted COVID-19, with routine RAT picking up 27.7% of the cases [73]. A similar study conducted from December 2021 to March 2022 used RAT to screen 220 haemodialysis patients, and 8.5% of asymptomatic patients returned a positive test over this time period (93% were subsequently confirmed COVID-19 positive by PCR testing). Symptomatic patients were screened with a PCR test, and of those who tested positive on PCR, RAT picked up 54% of cases as being COVID-19 positive [74].

Although RAT is able to identify asymptomatic COVID-19-positive cases and is cheaper to perform compared with PCR testing, it may not be sensitive enough to pick up an adequate number of cases. Data on PCR screening programs in haemodialysis populations are less well documented, but in one study, 200 patients were screened using PCR testing over a five-day period in early 2020 in a dialysis unit in France. Of these, 19% of patients had a positive result returned from their PCR test, and of those with a positive test result, 10% were asymptomatic [70]. If readily available, a universal PCR test screening program is more likely to pick up a greater number of COVID-19 cases than RAT, though the imperfect nature of PCR testing to identify COVID-19 cases has also been considered. One study sampled serum samples of 356 patients receiving dialysis, in which 129 patients were SARS-CoV-2 antibody positive. In this patient cohort, 40% of patients were asymptomatic from COVID-19 symptoms and of the 42 patients who had a negative PCR test result, eight were SARS-CoV-2 antibody positive [72].

It should be acknowledged that the clinical phenotype of COVID-19 has changed over time through the natural history and evolution of the virus and the increased delivery of vaccination. Esposito and colleagues highlighted that a cohort of COVID-19 haemodialysis patients in September 2021–February 2022, when compared to COVID-19 haemodialysis patients in March-December 2020 experienced less severe illness, though there were greater frequencies of asymptomatic disease [75]. This has likely impacted on the effectiveness of symptom-based screening programs. Ultimately, the cost-effectiveness of a screening system relies not only on the sensitivity of the test used, but also on the prevalence of the disease in focus. During the peak points of COVID-19 prevalence, a symptom-based screening program is unlikely to be adequate enough to capture all cases due to the high prevalence of asymptomatic COVID-19 infection. This may be adequate in times of low COVID-19 prevalence, though a dynamic and responsive screening system adapted to understanding the local prevalence of COVID-19 infection would be ideal. This philosophy of implementing COVID-19 screening strategies has been endorsed by many health systems, in which weekly PCR testing was recommended in areas where there are available resources during times of high community prevalence of COVID-19 [76].

3.2. Cohorting and Isolation Strategies

Once COVID-19-positive individuals receiving haemodialysis have been identified, it is important to cohort infected patients together to prevent a further spread of COVID-19 around the dialysis unit. The timeframe which presents the greatest risk of COVID-19 infection spread is within a dialysis session in which there are COVID-19-positive patients, in which horizontal transmission is commonly observed particularly in small in-centre dialysis venues where there are the greatest rates of infectious transmission [15]. There are variable reports in regard to the impact of shared transport to and from in-centre dialysis as a vector of COVID-19 infection spread. Some studies noted a significant association whilst other studies have not, though it has been recommended that patients should use private transport to and from in-centre dialysis if possible [15,77]. It is acknowledged that this may be challenging for many elderly haemodialysis patients who are unable to drive to and from in-centre dialysis due to their functional limitations, and many may not have family support to transport them to and from care facilities for dialysis [78].

The time recommended for elderly haemodialysis patients to remain isolated if COVID-19-positive test results were found is also longer than the general population. This is based on findings that the average time to a first negative test for kidney failure patients is 7 days longer than someone without kidney failure [48]. Over 65% of dialysis patients have a positive COVID-19 PCR test at 20 days [62]. Given increasing age has been noted to be an independent factor for lengthier viral clearance, it is suggested that the time spent on quarantine should be longer for these patient groups, or until a negative PCR test result is established [79]. It is difficult to prove whether positive COVID-19 PCR test results represent an active, transmissible infectious process or is simply reflecting the legacy of prior disease. Karoui and colleagues recommend the discontinuation of patient isolation once their COVID-19 vital load is lower than <1,000,000 copies/mL [52].

3.3. COVID-19 Vaccination

While most haemodialysis patients experience a durable immune response following a full COVID-19 vaccination schedule that is comparable to the general population, there is evidence to suggest that those with higher initial antibody titres exhibit a more prolonged response [80–83]. When reviewed after a second vaccination dose, reduced responses have been observed in haemodialysis patients as indicated by lower peak antibody levels compared to the general population [46,82]. A lower level of immunity is greatest amongst elderly individuals receiving haemodialysis [46,82]. However, a third COVID-19 vaccination dose has been demonstrated to have elicited increased and adequate peak antibody levels for this patient group [84]. These findings underscore the importance of ongoing surveillance for immune responses to COVID-19 vaccination in elderly haemodialysis patients, and highlights the clinical advantages of a third COVID-19 vaccination dose for them. Ongoing work in this area may inform future vaccination strategies for this vulnerable population.

In the current landscape of vaccine development for the prevention of COVID-19, two principal categories of vaccines have emerged: mRNA vaccines and adenovirus vector vaccines. The former includes the BNT162b2 (Pfizer-BioNTech) and mRNA-1273 vaccines (Moderna), while the latter encompasses the AZD1222 (AstraZeneca) and Ad26.COV2.S vaccines (Johnson & Johnson). The mRNA vaccines function by delivering genetic instructions for producing the viral spike protein to the host cell through the use of lipid nanoparticles, while the adenovirus vector vaccines rely on the use of modified adenoviruses to deliver genetic material for spike protein production to the host cell. Though both types of vaccines have demonstrated efficacy and safety in clinical trials involving the general population, and their widespread use has played a pivotal role in mitigating the ongoing COVID-19 pandemic, emerging data suggest that antibody responses to COVID-19 vaccination may differ amongst the various vaccination brands in elderly haemodialysis patients.

The adenovirus vector vaccine AZD1222 (AstraZeneca) has demonstrated reduced immunogenicity in patients receiving haemodialysis, in comparison to the mRNA BNT162b2 (Pfizer-BioNTech) vaccine [85]. Whilst three doses of the BNT162b2 vaccine have demonstrated adequate antibody response against the Omicron variant (the most prevalent strain of COVID-19 at present), the threshold is met in only 50% of cases when this vaccine is given to haemodialysis patients as a booster on top of two prior administered AZD1222 (AstraZeneca) vaccines [86]. Additionally, antibody responses are lower in haemodialysis patients given the adenovirus vector Ad26.COV2.S (Johnson & Johnson) vaccine compared to either mRNA vaccines [47]. Regardless, it would seem appropriate to vaccinate elderly haemodialysis patients with an mRNA COVID-19 vaccine. If either mRNA vaccine is available, then the mRNA-1273 (Moderna) appears to be the superior option, though a higher dose of the BNT162b2 (Pfizer-BioNTech) vaccine may also be suitable for dialysis patients in its absence.

In regard to the frequency of COVID-19 vaccination for elderly haemodialysis patients, previous studies have demonstrated that antibody levels in the general population following COVID-19 vaccination begin to decline approximately six months post-inoculation, with subsequent increased risk of infection but providing continued protection against risk of complications leading to hospitalization and mortality [87,88]. There is evidence of an earlier and more significant decrease in immunogenicity amongst dialysis patients, despite previous investigations not including matched control comparisons [89]. De Vriese and colleagues conducted a comparative study between responses to the BNT162b2 (Pfizer-BioNTech) and mRNA-1273 (Moderna) vaccines in dialysis-dependent and healthy control groups. Their study revealed suboptimal humoral and cellular immunities in dialysis patients at 24 weeks. While initial responses were stronger in the mRNA-1273 vaccine compared to the BNT162b2 vaccine, the cellular response was still attenuated at 24 weeks in haemodialysis patients. Notably, those with prior exposure to COVID-19 exhibited the greatest antibody response, with the vaccine brand received concluded to be of secondary importance [90]. This waning of antibody titres at an earlier point in the dialysis population raises awareness to consider more frequent booster vaccination programs, to prevent increased risks of COVID-19 infection in an at-risk patient population such as elderly persons receiving haemodialysis.

4. Treatment Strategies for Elderly Haemodialysis Patients Infected with COVID-19

Numerous medications have been proposed or developed during the pandemic in an effort to find treatment options for COVID-19, and to explore how patient outcomes could be improved. In a broad sense, therapeutics could be classified into two categories: antiviral and anti-inflammatory treatments. Antiviral treatments are aimed towards patients in the pre-hospital setting, during the early viral replication phases of their disease course. In contrast, anti-inflammatory treatments are intended for patients acutely unwell in the hospital setting, typically those requiring oxygen therapy, and those who exhibit signs of pneumonitis, with the goal of attenuating the cytokine/hyperinflammatory response. Due to the rapid emergence and evolution of COVID-19 pandemic data, discussion of all antiviral treatments that have been developed during the pandemic is beyond the scope of our review, as many antiviral treatments were eventually found to be ineffective and the Omicron variant with its numerous mutations in the spike protein has rendered many previous treatments obsolete. We will focus on treatment options that have received approval from the Centers for Disease Control and Prevention (CDC), the National Institutes of Health (NIH) and the National Institute for Health and Care Excellence (NICE) and discuss key trial findings, as well as evidence in relation to their use, efficacy and adverse effects within the context of elderly patients, patients with kidney disease and those receiving haemodialysis (Table 1).

Table 1. Summary of potential antiviral and anti-inflammatory treatment options for elderly haemodialysis populations with COVID-19.

Drug	Mechanism of Action	Outcome	Key Trials	Mean Age (years) of Study Participants in Key Trials	Recently Published/Ongoing Trials Studying for Use in Haemodialysis Populations
Antiviral Treatment (Administered in Pre-Hospital Patients Not on O_2 Therapy)					
Nirmatrelvir and ritonavir (Paxlovid)	Boosted 3cl protease inhibitor	Reduced risk of hospitalisation for COVID-19 or death from any cause	EPIC-HR (2022)	45.0 (18–86)	PANORAMIC (currently recruiting)
Remdesivir	Incorporation into viral RNA and termination of RNA transcription.	COVID-19-related hospitalisation	PINETREE (2022)	50.0 ± 15.0	Jeong-Hoon and colleagues (2022)
Molnupiravir	Prodrug of N-hydroxycytidine (NHC), a nucleoside analogue	Reduced the risk of hospitalisation or death from any cause	MOVe-OUT (2022) Fischer (2021)	42.0 (18–90)	Poznansk and colleagues (2022)
Anti-inflammatory treatment (administered in hospitalized patients)					
Dexamethasone	Glucocorticoid	Reduced all-cause mortality and discharge from hospital.	RECOVERY trial (2021)	66.9 ± 15.4	-
Tocilizumab/sarilumab	IL-6 inhibitors	Reduced all-cause mortality	REMAP-CAP (2021) RECOVERY (2021)	61.5 ± 12.5 63.3 ± 13.7	-
Baricitinib	JAK inhibitor	Reduced mortality and progression to invasive mechanical ventilation	RECOVERY (2022)	58.5 ± 15.4	Drug is not recommended for patients receiving dialysis

4.1. Nirmatrelvir and Ritonavir (Paxlovid)

Nirmatrelvir and ritonavir (Paxlovid) is a boosted 3cl protease inhibitor. It has been trialed in the EPIC-HR study which was a randomized trial which administered 300 mg of oral nirmatrelvir and 100 mg of oral ritonavir every 12 h for 5 days, or a placebo in non-vaccinated COVID-19-positive patients pre-hospital admission. The primary outcome of the study was risk of hospital admission or death from any cause [91]. The study included a provisory that patients had to have at least one established risk factor for developing severe disease following COVID-19 infection, in which the list of risk factors included age > 60 years old and CKD. However, the EPIC-HR study did not describe the proportion of dialysis patients involved, nor provided data on eGFR from the included patients. Though the median age of study participants was 45 years old, when subgroup analysis was completed for those > 65 years old, effect size did appear to have increased in elderly patients. Haemodialysis is unlikely to significantly clear nirmatrelvir from the circulation. To achieve effective blood concentrations for enzyme inhibition, a dose of 300 mg nirmatrelvir (with 100 mg ritonavir) on day 1, followed by 150 mg nirmatrelvir (with 100 mg ritonavir) administered daily after haemodialysis during dialysis days has been proposed [92,93]. However, as nirmatrelvir is a potent inhibitor of CYP3A4, caution should be exercised when administering it to patients receiving medications and other treatments which are metabolized by this enzyme. It is of note that kidney transplant recipients taking tacrolimus may have nirmatrelvir levels 10-fold higher than normal levels, and careful evaluation of the risks and benefits in this context is needed [92]. The PANORAMIC trial is an ongoing study which aims to assess the benefits of nirmatrelvir and ritonavir for those testing positive for COVID-19, and is open towards recruiting patients with CKD and kidney failure including those who are dialysis dependent [94].

4.2. Remdesivir

Remdesivir functions via its incorporation into viral RNA and termination of RNA transcription. This drug was trialed in the PINETREE study, a randomized controlled trial in which intravenous remdesivir (200 mg on day 1 and 100 mg daily on days 2 and 3) was compared with a placebo in non-vaccinated patients in pre-hospital settings [95]. The primary outcome was determining whether remdesivir reduced risk of hospital admission or death from any cause. Similar to the previous trial for nirmatrelvir and ritonavir, the included patients had to have at least one risk factor for developing severe disease following COVID-19 infection, which includes age > 60 and CKD. It was documented in the PINETREE study that only 2.5% of study participants had CKD whilst there were no dialysis patients included. The mean age was 50 years old. The effect size of remdesivir when compared to nirmatrelvir and ritonavir appears to be less, whilst another disadvantage of the drug is that it could only be administered as an intravenous preparation.

In another retrospective cohort study conducted between January and March 2022, 118 haemodialysis inpatients with positive COVID-19 tests were evaluated [96]. The mean age of the cohort was 68.5 ± 12.8 years. A total of 44 patients (37.3%) were administered with a loading dose of 100 mg and a maintenance dose of 50 mg for the next 2 to 4 days post-dialysis during dialysis days. The authors found that the remdesivir group had a lower risk of composite mortality and aggravation of disease severity, despite a higher level of disease severity at hospitalization compared to the non-remdesivir group. More importantly, there were no statistically significant differences between the two groups in terms of adverse events related to treatment. It should be considered that this study was retrospective in nature and as such, it may be subject to certain limitations, including potential bias in the selection of patients and incomplete data. Ultimately, study findings seem to suggest that remdesivir may be safely administered as an alternative option if nirmatrelvir and ritonavir is not available or when the patient is taking a calcineurin inhibitor.

4.3. Molnupinavir

Molnupinavir is a prodrug of N-hydroxycytidine (NHC), a nucleoside analogue. It has been trialed in two randomized clinical trials—the MOVe-OUT trial and another study by Fischer and colleagues compared clinical outcomes in pre-hospital non-vaccinated patients taking 800 mg of molnupiravir for 5 days versus placebo [97,98]. The primary outcome was the risk of hospitalization or death from any cause. There were some differences in the conclusions of these two studies, with the MOVe-OUT trial displaying improvement in the primary outcome with molnupiravir use whilst the study by Fischer and colleagues only found improvements in reducing viral load. Amongst the MOVe-OUT trial study participants who received molnupiravir, only 5.3% were diagnosed with CKD in which patients on haemodialysis were excluded from study participation. The median age of study participants in the MOVe-OUT trial was 42 years old. There were no statistically significant differences in study outcomes between molnupiravir and placebo treatment in a sub-group analysis for patients > 60 years old.

There are few studies which investigated the efficacy of molnupiravir in the context of the dialysis population. Poznansk and colleagues presented a retrospective cohort study reporting on the use of molnupiravir in 20 dialysis patients with positive COVID-19 test results [99]. These patients received a regimen of 800 mg of molnupiravir twice daily for 5 days. Their study also included an additional 16 transplant patients, who did not experience any serious side effects or drug interactions with their immunosuppressive therapy. The authors noted that the symptoms of COVID-19 amongst the dialysis patients improved rapidly or resolved within 24–48 h of starting treatment, though there were no matched controls in this study. Further investigation on the use of molnupiravir in the dialysis setting is required, though initial results are promising for its use as a safe home therapy for haemodialysis patients with positive COVID-19 status including those receiving simultaneous immunosuppressive treatment.

4.4. Dexamethasone

The RECOVERY trial aimed to evaluate the effectiveness of administering 6mg of dexamethasone for 10 days to adult patients diagnosed with COVID-19 infection [100]. Among adult patients requiring supplemental oxygen, corticosteroid treatment was shown to decrease all-cause mortality, increase hospital discharge rates, and potentially reduce the need for invasive mechanical ventilation and mortality within 28 days of treatment initiation compared to usual care or a placebo. The mean age of the study population was 66.9 ± 15.4 years, with 23% of patients being over the age of 80. Patients undergoing haemodialysis were excluded from the RECOVERY trial, although 8% had an eGFR <30 mL/min/1.73 m^2. Another retrospective analysis of haemodialysis patients with COVID-19 infection receiving dexamethasone did not demonstrate a clear clinical benefit [101]. However, this retrospective study was limited by its methodology, and it remains in current recommendations that haemodialysis patients with COVID-19 infection requiring oxygen support should receive steroid treatment.

4.5. IL-6 Inhibitors—Tocilizumab and Sarilumab

The interleukin-6 (IL-6) inhibitors, tocilizumab and sarilumab, have demonstrated reductions in all-cause mortality amongst hospitalized adults with COVID-19 when used with the standard care that was described in the RECOVERY and REMAP-CAP trials [102,103]. Tocilizumab and sarilumab is recommended for patients hospitalized with COVID-19 who require oxygen and have evidence of severe inflammation, as defined by CRP levels >75 or rapidly increasing oxygen requirements. However, the use of these IL-6 inhibitors comes with a significant risk of bacterial infection, and patients with suspected bacterial infection should not receive IL-6 inhibitors. In REMAP-CAP, the mean age of the study participants was 61.5 ± 12.5 years, and in RECOVERY, this was 63.3 ± 13.7 years, with 11% of patients aged >80 years. In REMAP-CAP, 9.6% of patients were labeled as having CKD, but no information on eGFR or dialysis dependency was provided. Current data on the use of IL-6 inhibitors for treating dialysis patients with positive COVID-19 status are limited, although a study from Japan assessing tocilizumab in patients with kidney failure and rheumatoid arthritis has demonstrated an acceptable safety profile [104]. Further work is needed to validate the consideration of IL-6 inhibitor use for this patient population, particularly elderly patients receiving dialysis.

4.6. Baricitinib

Baricitinib, a Janus kinase (JAK) inhibitor, was shown to be beneficial for hospitalized patients diagnosed with COVID-19 infection in the RECOVERY trial [105]. Importantly, clinical benefit was observed if baricitinib was administered in addition to steroids and IL-6 inhibitors, and the majority of patients (95% of patients) were already receiving steroids whilst 23% received tocilizumab. The mean age of the study cohort was 61.5 ± 12.5 years, with 8% being age >80 years. Only 2% had an eGFR < 30 mL/min/1.73 m^2 and unfortunately, the use of baricitinib is currently not recommended for patients on dialysis. A phase 2 trial is currently underway to investigate its use in patients with diabetic kidney disease [106].

4.7. Other Novel Therapies

The PROTECT-V (PROphylaxis for paTiEnts at risk of COVID-19 infecTion) study is a clinical trial aimed at evaluating the effectiveness of intranasal niclosamide prophylaxis in preventing COVID-19 infection [107]. Niclosamide, originally used for the treatment of tapeworm, has been shown to exhibit antiviral activity against SARS-CoV-2 in cell culture studies. The PROTECT-V trial will also evaluate the effectiveness of sotrovimab, a human IgG1κ monoclonal antibody that targets the spike protein of SARS-CoV-2, which is administered as a single infusion. This study is actively recruiting dialysis patients, given their increased risk of having poor clinical outcomes following acute COVID-19 infection is more well established, though they have previously been excluded from large-scale clinical trials.

5. Conclusions

Evidence regarding the associations between COVID-19 and clinical outcomes in dialysis patients, particularly the elderly haemodialysis population, has certainly increased since the onset of the pandemic. Our understanding of the various factors which contribute towards increased risks of contracting COVID-19 infection and disease severity for this vulnerable patient population has been broadened with the emergence of basic and clinical trial research within this topical area. Widening the recruitment and sub-study of the elderly haemodialysis population in ongoing COVID-19 clinical trials over time may further inform the long-term implications of COVID-19 for this patient group. It is encouraging that at a local, national and international level, there have been preliminary data to establish directive guidance for the prevention and medical treatment of COVID-19 infection in dialysis patients. Figure 2 outlines components of a pragmatic COVID-19 management approach for elderly patients receiving haemodialysis considering the currently available evidence. Nevertheless, there remains limited data in regard to the efficacy and adverse event profile of measures specifically for the elderly haemodialysis cohort. Going forward, further studies considering the unique challenges faced by these individuals compared to the general population and kidney disease patients who have received or are receiving other forms of kidney replacement therapy are required.

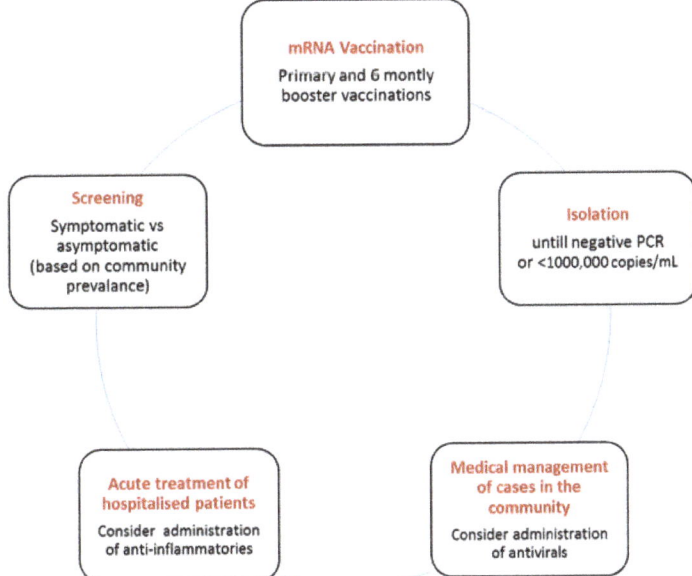

Figure 2. A pragmatic COVID-19 management approach for elderly patients receiving haemodialysis.

Author Contributions: Conceptualization, H.H.L.W., P.A.K. and R.C.; investigation, T.M.; resources, T.M. and H.H.L.W.; writing—original draft preparation, T.M.; writing—review and editing, H.H.L.W., P.A.K. and R.C.; visualization, H.H.L.W., P.A.K. and R.C.; supervision, P.A.K. and R.C.; project administration, H.H.L.W. All authors have read and agreed to the published version of the manuscript.

Funding: This research received no external funding.

Institutional Review Board Statement: Not applicable.

Informed Consent Statement: Not applicable.

Data Availability Statement: No new data were created for this article.

Conflicts of Interest: The authors declare no conflict of interest.

References

1. Zhu, N.; Zhang, D.; Wang, W.; Li, X.; Yang, B.; Song, J.; Zhao, X.; Huang, B.; Shi, W.; Lu, R.; et al. Novel Coronavirus from Patients with Pneumonia in China, 2019. *N. Engl. J. Med.* **2020**, *382*, 727–733. [CrossRef] [PubMed]
2. Gu, J.; Han, B.; Wang, J. COVID-19: Gastrointestinal manifestations and potential fecal–oral transmission. *Gastroenterology* **2020**, *158*, 1518–1519. [CrossRef] [PubMed]
3. Varatharaj, A.; Thomas, N.; Ellul, M.A.; Davies, N.W.; Pollak, T.A.; Tenorio, E.L.; Sultan, M.; Easton, A.; Breen, G.; Zandi, M.; et al. Neurological and neuropsychiatric complications of COVID-19 in 153 patients: A UK-wide surveillance study. *Lancet Psychiatry* **2020**, *7*, 875–882. [CrossRef]
4. He, W.; Chen, L.; Chen, L.; Yuan, G.; Fang, Y.; Chen, W.; Wu, D.; Liang, B.; Lu, X.; Ma, Y.; et al. COVID-19 in persons with haematological cancers. *Leukemia* **2020**, *34*, 1637–1645. [CrossRef] [PubMed]
5. Dhakal, B.P.; Sweitzer, N.K.; Indik, J.H.; Acharya, D.; William, P. SARS-CoV-2 infection and cardiovascular disease: COVID-19 heart. *Heart Lung Circ.* **2020**, *29*, 973–987. [CrossRef]
6. Jeyalan, V.; Storrar, J.; Wu, H.H.L.; Ponnusamy, A.; Sinha, S.; Kalra, P.A.; Chinnadurai, R. Native and transplant kidney histopathological manifestations in association with COVID-19 infection: A systematic review. *World J. Transplant.* **2021**, *11*, 480–502. [CrossRef]
7. Kunutsor, S.K.; Laukkanen, J.A. Renal complications in COVID-19: A systematic review and meta-analysis. *Ann. Med.* **2020**, *52*, 345–353. [CrossRef]
8. Verity, R.; Okell, L.C.; Dorigatti, I.; Winskill, P.; Whittaker, C.; Imai, N.; Cuomo-Dannenburg, G.; Thompson, H.; Walker, P.G.; Fu, H.; et al. Estimates of the severity of coronavirus disease 2019: A model-based analysis. *Lancet Infect. Dis.* **2020**, *20*, 669–677. [CrossRef]
9. US Renal Data System. *USRDS 2022 Annual Data Report: Chronic Kidney Disease*; National Institutes of Health, National Institute of Diabetes and Digestive and Kidney Diseases: Bethesda, MD, USA, 2022; Volume 2022.
10. Wu, C.; Chen, X.; Cai, Y.; Zhou, X.; Xu, S.; Huang, H.; Zhang, L.; Zhou, X.; Du, C.; Zhang, Y.; et al. Risk Factors Associated With Acute Respiratory Distress Syndrome and Death in Patients With Coronavirus Disease 2019 Pneumonia in Wuhan, China. *JAMA Intern. Med.* **2020**, *180*, 934–943. [CrossRef]
11. Williamson, E.J.; Walker, A.J.; Bhaskaran, K.; Bacon, S.; Bates, C.; Morton, C.E.; Curtis, H.J.; Mehrkar, A.; Evans, D.; Inglesby, P.; et al. Factors associated with COVID-19-related death using OpenSAFELY. *Nature* **2020**, *584*, 430–436. [CrossRef]
12. Gasparini, M.; Khan, S.; Patel, J.M.; Parekh, D.; Bangash, M.N.; Stümpfle, R.; Shah, A.; Baharlo, B.; Soni, S.; Collaborators Brett, S. Renal impairment and its impact on clinical outcomes in patients who are critically ill with COVID-19: A multicentre observational study. *Anaesthesia* **2021**, *76*, 320–326. [CrossRef] [PubMed]
13. Jager, K.J.; Kramer, A.; Chesnaye, N.C.; Couchoud, C.; Sánchez-Álvarez, J.E.; Garneata, L.; Collart, F.; Hemmelder, M.H.; Ambühl, P.; Kerschbaum, J.; et al. Results from the ERA-EDTA Registry indicate a high mortality due to COVID-19 in dialysis patients and kidney transplant recipients across Europe. *Kidney Int.* **2020**, *98*, 1540–1548. [CrossRef] [PubMed]
14. Salerno, S.; Messana, J.M.; Gremel, G.W.; Dahlerus, C.; Hirth, R.A.; Han, P.; Segal, J.H.; Xu, T.; Shaffer, D.; Jiao, A.; et al. COVID-19 Risk Factors and Mortality Outcomes Among Medicare Patients Receiving Long-term Dialysis. *JAMA Netw. Open* **2021**, *4*, e2135379. [CrossRef]
15. Corbett, R.W.; Blakey, S.; Nitsch, D.; Loucaidou, M.; McLean, A.; Duncan, N.; Ashby, D.R. Epidemiology of COVID-19 in an Urban Dialysis Center. *J. Am. Soc. Nephrol.* **2020**, *31*, 1815–1823. [CrossRef]
16. Bao, Y.; Dalrymple, L.; Chertow, G.M.; Kaysen, G.A.; Johansen, K.L. Frailty, dialysis initiation, and mortality in end-stage renal disease. *Arch. Intern. Med.* **2012**, *172*, 1071–1077. [CrossRef] [PubMed]
17. Sy, J.; Johansen, K.L. The impact of frailty on outcomes in dialysis. *Curr. Op. Nephrol. Hypertens.* **2017**, *26*, 537–542. [CrossRef] [PubMed]
18. Hewitt, J.; Carter, B.; Vilches-Moraga, A.; Quinn, T.J.; Braude, P.; Verduri, A.; Pearce, L.; Stechman, M.; Short, R.; Price, A.; et al. The effect of frailty on survival in patients with COVID-19 (COPE): A multicentre, European, observational cohort study. *Lancet Public Health* **2020**, *5*, e444–e451. [CrossRef]

19. De Vries, O.J.; Peeters, G.M.; Lips, P.T.; Deeg, D.J. Does frailty predict increased risk of falls and fractures? A prospective population-based study. *Osteoporos. Int.* **2013**, *24*, 2397–2403. [PubMed]
20. Theou, O.; Sluggett, J.K.; Bell, J.S.; Lalic, S.; Cooper, T.; Robson, L.; Morley, J.E.; Rockwood, K.; Visvanathan, R. Frailty, hospitalization, and mortality in residential aged care. *J. Gerontol. A Biol. Sci. Med. Sci.* **2018**, *73*, 1090–1096. [CrossRef]
21. Chang, Y.W.; Chen, W.L.; Lin, F.G.; Fang, W.H.; Yen, M.Y.; Hsieh, C.C.; Kao, T.W. Frailty and its impact on health-related quality of life: A cross-sectional study on elder community-dwelling preventive health service users. *PLoS ONE* **2012**, *7*, e38079. [CrossRef]
22. Nixon, A.C.; Bampouras, T.M.; Pendleton, N.; Woywodt, A.; Mitra, S.; Dhaygude, A. Frailty and chronic kidney disease: Current evidence and continuing uncertainties. *Clin. Kidney J.* **2018**, *11*, 236–245. [CrossRef] [PubMed]
23. Carrero, J.J.; Stenvinkel, P.; Cuppari, L.; Ikizler, T.A.; Kalantar-Zadeh, K.; Kaysen, G.; Mitch, W.E.; Price, S.R.; Wanner, C.; Wang, A.Y.; et al. Etiology of the protein-energy wasting syndrome in chronic kidney disease: A consensus statement from the International Society of Renal Nutrition and Metabolism (ISRNM). *J. Renal. Nutr.* **2013**, *23*, 77–90. [CrossRef]
24. Kim, J.C.; Kalantar-Zadeh, K.; Kopple, J.D. Frailty and protein-energy wasting in elderly patients with end stage kidney disease. *J. Am. Soc. Nephrol.* **2013**, *24*, 337–351. [CrossRef] [PubMed]
25. Beddhu, S.; Baird, B.C.; Zitterkoph, J.; Neilson, J.; Greene, T. Physical activity and mortality in chronic kidney disease (NHANES III). *Clin. J. Am. Soc. Nephrol.* **2009**, *4*, 1901–1906. [CrossRef] [PubMed]
26. Górriz, J.L.; Molina, P.; Bover, J.; Barril, G.; Martín-de Francisco, Á.L.; Caravaca, F.; Hervás, J.; Piñera, C.; Escudero, V.; Molinero, L.M. Characteristics of bone mineral metabolism in patients with stage 3-5 chronic kidney disease not on dialysis: Results of the OSERCE study. *Nefrología* **2013**, *33*, 46–60.
27. Walston, J.; Hadley, E.C.; Ferrucci, L.; Guralnik, J.M.; Newman, A.B.; Studenski, S.A.; Ershler, W.B.; Harris, T.; Fried, L.P. Research agenda for frailty in older adults: Toward a better understanding of physiology and etiology: Summary from the American Geriatrics Society/National Institute on Aging Research Conference on Frailty in Older Adults. *J. Am. Geriatr. Soc.* **2006**, *54*, 991–1001. [CrossRef]
28. McAdams-DeMarco, M.A.; Law, A.; Salter, M.L.; Boyarsky, B.; Gimenez, L.; Jaar, B.G.; Walston, J.D.; Segev, D.L. Frailty as a novel predictor of mortality and hospitalization in individuals of all ages undergoing hemodialysis. *J. Am. Geriatr. Soc.* **2013**, *61*, 896–901. [CrossRef]
29. Johansen, K.L.; Dalrymple, L.S.; Delgado, C.; Chertow, G.M.; Segal, M.R.; Chiang, J.; Grimes, B.; Kaysen, G.A. Factors associated with frailty and its trajectory among patients on hemodialysis. *Clin. J. Am. Soc. Nephrol.* **2017**, *12*, 1100–1108. [CrossRef]
30. Kular, D.; Ster, I.C.; Sarnowski, A.; Lioudaki, E.; Braide-Azikiwe, D.C.; Ford, M.L.; Makanjuola, D.; Rankin, A.; Cairns, H.; Popoola, J.; et al. The characteristics, dynamics, and the risk of death in COVID-19 positive dialysis patients in London, UK. *Kidney360* **2020**, *1*, 1226–1243. [CrossRef]
31. Hendra, H.; Vajgel, G.; Antonelou, M.; Neradova, A.; Manson, B.; Clark, S.G.; Kostakis, I.D.; Caplin, B.; Salama, A.D. Identifying prognostic risk factors for poor outcome following COVID-19 disease among in-centre haemodialysis patients: Role of inflammation and frailty. *J. Nephrol.* **2021**, *34*, 315–323. [CrossRef]
32. Chinnadurai, R.; Ogedengbe, O.; Agarwal, P.; Money-Coomes, S.; Abdurrahman, A.Z.; Mohammed, S.; Kalra, P.A.; Rothwell, N.; Pradhan, S. Older age and frailty are the chief predictors of mortality in COVID-19 patients admitted to an acute medical unit in a secondary care setting-a cohort study. *BMC Geriatr.* **2020**, *20*, 409. [CrossRef] [PubMed]
33. Matsuzawa, R.; Roshanravan, B. Management of physical frailty in patients requiring hemodialysis therapy. *Contrib. Nephrol.* **2018**, *196*, 101–109. [PubMed]
34. Mayes, J.; Young, H.M.; Blacklock, R.M.; Lightfoot, C.J.; Chilcot, J.; Nixon, A.C. Targeted Non-Pharmacological Interventions for People Living with Frailty and Chronic Kidney Disease. *Kidney Dial.* **2022**, *2*, 245–261. [CrossRef]
35. Siddiqi, H.K.; Mehra, M.R. COVID-19 illness in native and immunosuppressed states: A clinical–therapeutic staging proposal. *J. Heart Lung Transplant.* **2020**, *39*, 405–407. [CrossRef]
36. Tan, L.Y.; Komarasamy, T.V.; RMTBalasubramaniam, V. Hyperinflammatory Immune Response and COVID-19: A Double Edged Sword. *Front. Immunol.* **2021**, *12*, 3981. [CrossRef] [PubMed]
37. Liu, K.; Chen, Y.; Lin, R.; Han, K. Clinical features of COVID-19 in elderly patients: A comparison with young and middle-aged patients. *J. Infect.* **2020**, *80*, e14–e18. [CrossRef] [PubMed]
38. Stangou, M.J.; Fylaktou, A.; Ivanova-Shivarova, M.I.; Theodorou, I. Editorial: Immunosenescence and Immunoexhaustion in Chronic Kidney Disease and Renal Transplantation. *Front. Med.* **2022**, *9*, 772. [CrossRef]
39. Aw, D.; Silva, A.B.; Palmer, D.B. Immunosenescence: Emerging challenges for an ageing population. *Immunology* **2007**, *120*, 435–446. [CrossRef]
40. Huppert, F.; Solomou, W.; O'Connor, S.; Morgan, K.; Sussams, P.; Brayne, C. Aging and lymphocyte subpopulations: Whole-blood analysis of immune markers in a large population sample of healthy elderly individuals. *Exp. Gerontol.* **1998**, *33*, 593–600. [CrossRef]
41. Pawelec, G.; Barnett, Y.; Forsey, R.; Frasca, D.; Globerson, A.; McLeod, J.; Caruso, C.; Franceschi, C.; Fülöp, T.; Gupta, S.; et al. T cells and aging, January 2002 update. *Front. Biosci.* **2002**, *7*, 1056–1183. [CrossRef]
42. Rodriguez, I.J.; Lalinde Ruiz, N.; Llano León, M.; Martínez Enríquez, L.; Montilla Velásquez, M.D.P.; Ortiz Aguirre, J.P.; Rodríguez Bohórquez, O.M.; Velandia Vargas, E.A.; Hernández, E.D.; Parra López, C.A. Immunosenescence Study of T Cells: A Systematic Review. *Front. Immunol.* **2021**, *11*, 3460. [CrossRef] [PubMed]

43. Betjes, M.G.H. Immune cell dysfunction and inflammation in end-stage renal disease. *Nat. Rev. Nephrol.* **2013**, *9*, 255–265. [CrossRef]
44. Betjes, M.G.; Langerak, A.W.; Klepper, M.; Litjens, N.H. A very low thymus function identifies patients with substantial increased risk for long-term mortality after kidney transplantation. *Immun. Ageing.* **2020**, *17*, 4. [CrossRef] [PubMed]
45. Meijers, R.W.; Litjens, N.H.; de Wit, E.A.; Langerak, A.W.; van der Spek, A.; Baan, C.C.; Weimar, W.; Betjes, M.G. Uremia causes premature ageing of the T cell compartment in end-stage renal disease patients. *Immun. Ageing* **2012**, *9*, 19. [CrossRef]
46. Bensouna, I.; Caudwell, V.; Kubab, S.; Acquaviva, S.; Pardon, A.; Vittoz, N.; Bozman, D.F.; Hanafi, L.; Faucon, A.L.; Housset, P. SARS-CoV-2 Antibody Response After a Third Dose of the BNT162b2 Vaccine in Patients Receiving Maintenance Hemodialysis or Peritoneal Dialysis. *Am. J. Kidney Dis.* **2022**, *79*, 185–192.e1. [CrossRef]
47. Mulhern, J.G.; Fadia, A.; Patel, R.; Ficociello, L.H.; Willetts, J.; Dahne-Steuber, I.A.; Pollan, M.C.; Mullon, C.; DeLisi, J.; Johnson, C.; et al. Humoral response to MRNA versus an adenovirus vector-based SARS-CoV-2 vaccine in dialysis patients. *Clin. J. Am. Soc. Nephrol.* **2021**, *16*, 1720–1722. [CrossRef] [PubMed]
48. O'Sullivan, E.D.; Lees, J.S.; Howie, K.L.; Pugh, D.; Gillis, K.A.; Traynor, J.P.; Macintyre, I.; Mark, P.B. Prolonged SARS-CoV-2 viral shedding in patients with chronic kidney disease. *Nephrology* **2021**, *26*, 328–332. [CrossRef] [PubMed]
49. De Biasi, S.; Meschiari, M.; Gibellini, L.; Bellinazzi, C.; Borella, R.; Fidanza, L.; Gozzi, L.; Iannone, A.; Lo Tartaro, D.; Mattioli, M.; et al. Marked T cell activation, senescence, exhaustion and skewing towards TH17 in patients with COVID-19 pneumonia. *Nat. Commun.* **2020**, *11*, 3434. [CrossRef]
50. Carr, E.J.; Kronbichler, A.; Graham-Brown, M.; Abra, G.; Argyropoulos, C.; Harper, L.; Lerma, E.V.; Suri, R.S.; Topf, J.; Willicombe, M.; et al. Review of Early Immune Response to SARS-CoV-2 Vaccination Among Patients With CKD. *Kidney Int. Rep.* **2021**, *6*, 2292–2304. [CrossRef]
51. Van Praet, J.; Reynders, M.; De Bacquer, D.; Viaene, L.; Schoutteten, M.K.; Caluwé, R.; Doubel, P.; Heylen, L.; De Bel, A.V.; Van Vlem, B.; et al. Predictors and dynamics of the humoral and cellular immune response to SARS-CoV-2 mRNA vaccines in hemodialysis patients: A multicenter observational study. *J. Am. Soc. Nephrol.* **2021**, *32*, 3208–3220. [CrossRef]
52. El Karoui, K.; de Vriese, A.S. COVID-19 in dialysis: Clinical impact, immune response, prevention, and treatment. *Kidney Int.* **2022**, *101*, 883–894. [CrossRef] [PubMed]
53. Khoury, D.S.; Steain, M.; Triccas, J.A.; Sigal, A.; Davenport, M.P.; Cromer, D. A meta-analysis of Early Results to predict Vaccine efficacy against Omicron. *medRxiv* **2021**. [CrossRef]
54. Rocklöv, J.; Sjödin, H.; Wilder-Smith, A. COVID-19 outbreak on the Diamond Princess cruise ship: Estimating the epidemic potential and effectiveness of public health countermeasures. *J. Travel Med.* **2020**, *27*, taaa030. [CrossRef] [PubMed]
55. Alfano, G.; Ferrari, A.; Magistroni, R.; Fontana, F.; Cappelli, G.; Basile, C. The frail world of haemodialysis patients in the COVID-19 pandemic era: A systematic scoping review. *J. Nephrol.* **2021**, *34*, 1387–1403. [CrossRef] [PubMed]
56. Tofighi, M.; Asgary, A.; Merchant, A.A.; Shafiee, M.A.; Najafabadi, M.M.; Nadri, N.; Aarabi, M.; Heffernan, J.; Wu, J. Modelling COVID-19 transmission in a hemodialysis centre using simulation generated contacts matrices. *PLoS ONE* **2021**, *16*, e0259970. [CrossRef] [PubMed]
57. Taji, L.; Thomas, D.; Oliver, M.J.; Ip, J.; Tang, Y.; Yeung, A.; Cooper, R.; House, A.A.; McFarlane, P.; Blake, P.G. COVID-19 in patients undergoing long-term dialysis in Ontario. *CMAJ* **2021**, *193*, E278–E284. [CrossRef] [PubMed]
58. Ikizler, T.A.; Kliger, A.S. Minimizing the risk of COVID-19 among patients on dialysis. *Nat. Rev. Nephrol.* **2020**, *16*, 311–313. [CrossRef]
59. Couchoud, C.; Bayer, F.; Ayav, C.; Béchade, C.; Brunet, P.; Chantrel, F.; Frimat, L.; Galland, R.; Hourmant, M.; Laurain, E.; et al. Low incidence of SARS-CoV-2, risk factors of mortality and the course of illness in the French national cohort of dialysis patients. *Kidney Int.* **2020**, *98*, 1519–1529. [CrossRef]
60. Clarke, C.; Prendecki, M.; Dhutia, A.; Ali, M.A.; Sajjad, H.; Shivakumar, O.; Lightstone, L.; Kelleher, P.; Pickering, M.C.; Thomas, D.; et al. High Prevalence of Asymptomatic COVID-19 Infection in Hemodialysis Patients Detected Using Serologic Screening. *J. Am. Soc. Nephrol.* **2020**, *31*, 1969–1975. [CrossRef]
61. Rincon, A.; Moreso, F.; Lopez-Herradon, A.; Fernández-Robres, M.A.; Cidraque, I.; Nin, J.; Mendez, O.; Lopez, M.; Pajaro, C.; Satorra, A.; et al. The keys to control a COVID-19 outbreak in a haemodialysis unit. *Clin. Kidney J.* **2020**, *13*, 542–549. [CrossRef]
62. Shaikh, A.; Zeldis, E.; Campbell, K.N.; Chan, L. Prolonged SARS-CoV-2 Viral RNA Shedding and IgG Antibody Response to SARS-CoV-2 in Patients on Hemodialysis. *Clin. J. Am. Soc. Nephrol.* **2021**, *16*, 290–292. [CrossRef] [PubMed]
63. Abou-Ismail, M.Y.; Diamond, A.; Kapoor, S.; Arafah, Y.; Nayak, L. The hypercoagulable state in COVID-19: Incidence, pathophysiology, and management. *Thromb. Res.* **2020**, *194*, 101–115. [CrossRef] [PubMed]
64. Zhang, Y.; Yi, J.; Zhang, R.; Peng, Y.; Dong, J.; Sha, G. Risk factors for arteriovenous fistula thrombus development: A systematic review and meta-analysis. *Kidney Blood Pres. Res.* **2022**, *47*, 643–653. [CrossRef] [PubMed]
65. Grenon, E.; Canet, E. High incidence of circuit clotting in critically ill COVID-19 patients treated with renal replacement therapy. *J. Am. Soc. Nephrol.* **2021**, *32*, 1823–1824. [CrossRef]
66. Khoo, B.Z.E.; Lim, R.S.; See, Y.P.; Yeo, S.C. Dialysis circuit clotting in critically ill patients with COVID-19 infection. *BMC Nephrol.* **2021**, *22*, 141. [CrossRef]
67. Desbuissons, G.; Michon, A.; Attias, P.; Burbach, M.; Diaconita, M.; Karie-Guiges, S.; Novelli, L.; Abou Rjeili, M.; Awad, S.; Besse, F.; et al. Arteriovenous fistulas thrombosis in hemodialysis patients with COVID-19. *J. Vasc. Access* **2022**, *23*, 412–415. [CrossRef]

68. Kliger, A.S.; Silberzweig, J. Mitigating Risk of COVID-19 in Dialysis Facilities. *Clin. J. Am. Soc. Nephrol.* **2020**, *15*, 707–709. [CrossRef]
69. Yau, K.; Muller, M.P.; Lin, M.; Siddiqui, N.; Neskovic, S.; Shokar, G.; Fattouh, R.; Matukas, L.M.; Beaubien-Souligny, W.; Thomas, A.; et al. COVID-19 Outbreak in an Urban Hemodialysis Unit. *Am. J. Kidney Dis.* **2020**, *76*, 690–695.e1. [CrossRef]
70. Tang, H.; Tian, J.B.; Dong, J.W.; Tang, X.T.; Yan, Z.Y.; Zhao, Y.Y.; Xiong, F.; Sun, X.; Song, C.X.; Xiang, C.G.; et al. Serologic Detection of SARS-CoV-2 Infections in Hemodialysis Centers: A Multicenter Retrospective Study in Wuhan, China. *Am. J. Kidney Dis.* **2020**, *76*, 490–499.e1. [CrossRef]
71. Creput, C.; Fumeron, C.; Toledano, D.; Diaconita, M.; Izzedine, H. COVID-19 in Patients Undergoing Hemodialysis: Prevalence and Asymptomatic Screening During a Period of High Community Prevalence in a Large Paris Center. *Kidney Med.* **2020**, *2*, 716–723.e1. [CrossRef]
72. Poulikakos, D.; Chinnadurai, R.; Mcgee, Y.; Gray, S.; Clough, T.; Clarke, N.; Murphy, T.; Wickens, O.; Mitchell, C.; Darby, D.; et al. A Quality Improvement Project to Minimize COVID-19 Infections in Patients Receiving Haemodialysis and the Role of Routine Surveillance Using Nose and Throat Swabs for SARS-CoV-2 rRT-PCR and Serum Antibody Testing. *Nephron* **2022**, *146*, 335–342. [CrossRef]
73. Alfano, G.; Scarmignan, R.; Morisi, N.; Fontana, F.; Giovanella, S.; Ligabue, G.; Rofrano, L.; Gennari, W.; Pecorari, M.; Gregorini, M.; et al. COVID-19 Rapid Antigen Test Screening in Patients on Hemodialysis. *Int. J. Nephrol.* **2022**, *2022*, 4678717. [CrossRef] [PubMed]
74. Alfano, G.; Scarmignan, R.; Amurri, A.; Fontana, F.; Giovanella, S.; Ligabue, G.; Gennari, W.; Pecorari, M.; Sarti, M.; Guaraldi, G.; et al. Weekly Rapid Antigen Test Screening for COVID-19 in Patients on Hemodialysis. *In Vivo* **2022**, *36*, 2823–2827. [CrossRef] [PubMed]
75. Esposito, P.; Picciotto, D.; Cappadona, F.; Russo, E.; Falqui, V.; Conti, N.E.; Parodi, A.; Mallia, L.; Cavagnaro, S.; Battaglia, Y.; et al. The evolving scenario of COVID-19 in hemodialysis patients. *Int. J. Environ. Res. Public Health* **2022**, *19*, 10836. [CrossRef] [PubMed]
76. KQuIP COVID-19 Patient Safety Workstream. Recommendations for Minimising the Risk of Transmission of SARS-CoV-2 (COVID-19) in UK Adult Haemodialysis Units. KQuIP COVID-19 HD Ensuring Patient Safety Work Stream. 14 January 2022; Version 4. Available online: https://ukkidney.org/sites/renal.org/files/Recommendations%20to%20minimise%20risk%20of%20transmission%20of%20COVID-19%20in%20UK%20adult%20haemodialysis%20units%2014th%20January%202022.pdf (accessed on 1 February 2023).
77. Goodlad, C.; Collier, S.; Davenport, A. Spread of Covid-19 in hemodialysis centres; the effects of ventilation and communal transport. *Artif. Organs* **2022**, *46*, 2453–2459. [CrossRef]
78. Fox, V.; Poulikakos, D. Travel arrangements in hemodialysis patients during the COVID-19 pandemic including London-style "black cabs" for transfer to a designated isolation unit. *Hemodial. Int.* **2021**, *25*, 563–564. [CrossRef]
79. Yan, D.; Liu, X.Y.; Zhu, Y.N.; Huang, L.; Dan, B.T.; Zhang, G.J.; Gao, Y.H. Factors associated with prolonged viral shedding and impact of lopinavir/ritonavir treatment in hospitalised non-critically ill patients with SARS-CoV-2 infection. *Eur. Respir. J.* **2020**, *56*, 2000799. [CrossRef]
80. Sakhi, H.; Dahmane, D.; Attias, P.; Kofman, T.; Bouvier, M.; Lapidus, N.; Fourati, S.; El Karoui, K.; Mondor NephroCov Study Group. Kinetics of anti-SARS-CoV-2 IgG antibodies in hemodialysis patients six months after infection. *J. Am. Soc. Nephrol.* **2021**, *32*, 1033–1036. [CrossRef]
81. Speer, C.; Schaier, M.; Nusshag, C.; Töllner, M.; Buylaert, M.; Kälble, F.; Reichel, P.; Grenz, J.; Süsal, C.; Zeier, M.; et al. Longitudinal Humoral Responses after COVID-19 Vaccination in Peritoneal and Hemodialysis Patients over Twelve Weeks. *Vaccines* **2021**, *9*, 1130. [CrossRef]
82. Nacasch, N.; Cohen-Hagai, K.; Benchetrit, S.; Zitman-Gal, T.; Einbinder, Y.; Erez, D.; Hornik-Lurie, T.; Goldman, S.; Tanasiychuk, T.; Frajewicki, V.; et al. Comparison of long-term antibody response to mRNA SARS-CoV-2 vaccine among peritoneal dialysis and hemodialysis patients. *Nephrol. Dial. Transplant.* **2022**, *37*, 602–604. [CrossRef]
83. Hsu, C.M.; Weiner, D.E.; Manley, H.J.; Aweh, G.N.; Ladik, V.; Frament, J.; Miskulin, D.; Argyropoulos, C.; Abreo, K.; Chin, A.; et al. Seroresponse to SARS-CoV-2 Vaccines among Maintenance Dialysis Patients over 6 Months. *Clin. J. Am. Soc. Nephrol.* **2022**, *17*, 403–413. [CrossRef] [PubMed]
84. Frantzen, L.; Thibeaut, S.; Moussi-Frances, J.; Indreies, M.; Kiener, C.; Saingra, Y.; Santini, J.; Stroumza, P.; El-Haik, Y.; Cavaillé, G. COVID-19 vaccination in haemodialysis patients: Good things come in threes … . *Nephrol. Dial. Transplant.* **2021**, *36*, 1947–1949. [CrossRef] [PubMed]
85. Carr, E.J.; Wu, M.; Harvey, R.; Wall, E.C.; Kelly, G.; Hussain, S.; Howell, M.; Kassiotis, G.; Swanton, C.; Gandhi, S.; et al. Neutralising antibodies after COVID-19 vaccination in UK haemodialysis patients. *Lancet* **2021**, *398*, 1038–1041. [CrossRef] [PubMed]
86. Carr, E.J.; Wu, M.; Harvey, R.; Billany, R.E.; Wall, E.C.; Kelly, G.; Howell, M.; Kassiotis, G.; Swanton, C.; Gandhi, S.; et al. Omicron neutralising antibodies after COVID-19 vaccination in haemodialysis patients. *Lancet* **2022**, *399*, 800–802. [CrossRef]
87. Levin, E.G.; Lustig, Y.; Cohen, C.; Fluss, R.; Indenbaum, V.; Amit, S.; Doolman, R.; Asraf, K.; Mendelson, E.; Ziv, A.; et al. Waning Immune Humoral Response to BNT162b2 Covid-19 Vaccine over 6 Months. *N. Engl. J. Med.* **2021**, *385*, e84. [CrossRef]

88. Chemaitelly, H.; Tang, P.; Hasan, M.R.; AlMukdad, S.; Yassine, H.M.; Benslimane, F.M.; Al Khatib, H.A.; Coyle, P.; Ayoub, H.H.; Al Kanaani, Z.; et al. Waning of BNT162b2 vaccine protection against SARS-CoV-2 infection in Qatar. *N. Engl. J. Med.* **2021**, *385*, e83. [CrossRef]
89. Angel-Korman, A.; Peres, E.; Bryk, G.; Lustig, Y.; Indenbaum, V.; Amit, S.; Rappoport, V.; Katzir, Z.; Yagil, Y.; Iaina, N.L.; et al. Diminished and waning immunity to COVID-19 vaccination among hemodialysis patients in Israel: The case for a third vaccine dose. *Clin. Kidney J.* **2022**, *15*, 226–234. [CrossRef]
90. De Vriese, A.S.; Van Praet, J.; Reynders, M.; Heylen, L.; Viaene, L.; Caluwé, R.; Schoutteten, M.; De Bacquer, D. Longevity and Clinical Effectiveness of the Humoral and Cellular Responses to SARS-CoV-2 Vaccination in Hemodialysis Patients. *Kidney Int. Rep.* **2022**, *7*, 1103–1107. [CrossRef]
91. Hammond, J.; Leister-Tebbe, H.; Gardner, A.; Abreu, P.; Bao, W.; Wisemandle, W.; Baniecki, M.; Hendrick, V.M.; Damle, B.; Simón-Campos, A.; et al. Oral Nirmatrelvir for High-Risk, Nonhospitalized Adults with COVID-19. *N. Engl. J. Med.* **2022**, *386*, 1397–1408. [CrossRef]
92. Hiremath, S.; McGuinty, M.; Argyropoulos, C.; Brimble, K.S.; Brown, P.A.; Chagla, Z.; Cooper, R.; Hoar, S.; Juurlink, D.; Treleaven, D.; et al. Prescribing Nirmatrelvir/Ritonavir for COVID-19 in Advanced CKD. *Clin. J. Am. Soc. Nephrol.* **2022**, *17*, 1247–1250. [CrossRef]
93. Lingscheid, T.; Kinzig, M.; Krüger, A.; Müller, N.; Bölke, G.; Tober-Lau, P.; Münn, F.; Kriedemann, H.; Witzenrath, M.; Sander, L.E.; et al. Pharmacokinetics of Nirmatrelvir and Ritonavir in COVID-19 Patients with End-Stage Renal Disease on Intermittent Hemodialysis. *Antimicrob. Agents Chemother.* **2022**, *66*, e01229-22. [CrossRef] [PubMed]
94. Lee, T.C.; Boulware, D.R. Ongoing Need for Clinical Trials and Contemporary End Points for Outpatient COVID-19. *Ann. Intern. Med.* **2023**, *176*, 137–138. [CrossRef]
95. Gottlieb, R.L.; Vaca, C.E.; Paredes, R.; Mera, J.; Webb, B.J.; Perez, G.; Oguchi, G.; Ryan, P.; Nielsen, B.U.; Brown, M.; et al. Early Remdesivir to Prevent Progression to Severe COVID-19 in Outpatients. *N. Engl. J. Med.* **2022**, *386*, 305–315. [CrossRef]
96. Lim, J.H.; Park, S.D.; Jeon, Y.; Chung, Y.K.; Kwon, J.W.; Jeon, Y.H.; Jung, H.Y.; Park, S.H.; Kim, C.D.; Kim, Y.L.; et al. Clinical Effectiveness and Safety of Remdesivir in Hemodialysis Patients with COVID-19. *Kidney Int. Rep.* **2022**, *7*, 2522–2525. [CrossRef] [PubMed]
97. Jayk Bernal, A.; Gomes da Silva, M.M.; Musungaie, D.B.; Kovalchuk, E.; Gonzalez, A.; Delos Reyes, V.; Martín-Quirós, A.; Caraco, Y.; Williams-Diaz, A.; Brown, M.L.; et al. Molnupiravir for Oral Treatment of COVID-19 in Nonhospitalized Patients. *N. Engl. J. Med.* **2022**, *386*, 509–520. [CrossRef] [PubMed]
98. Fischer, W.; Eron, J.J., Jr.; Holman, W.; Cohen, M.S.; Fang, L.; Szewczyk, L.J.; Sheahan, T.P.; Baric, R.; Mollan, K.R.; Wolfe, C.R.; et al. Molnupiravir, an oral antiviral treatment for COVID-19. *medRxiv* **2021**, 2021-06. [CrossRef]
99. Poznański, P.; Augustyniak-Bartosik, H.; Magiera-Żak, A.; Skalec, K.; Jakuszko, K.; Mazanowska, O.; Janczak, D.; Krajewska, M.; Kamińska, D. Molnupiravir When Used Alone Seems to Be Safe and Effective as Outpatient COVID-19 Therapy for Hemodialyzed Patients and Kidney Transplant Recipients. *Viruses* **2022**, *14*, 2224. [CrossRef] [PubMed]
100. RECOVERY Trial Collaborators. Dexamethasone in Hospitalized Patients with COVID-19. *N. Engl. J. Med.* **2021**, *384*, 693–704. [CrossRef]
101. Toçoglu, A.; Dheir, H.; Demirci, T.; Kurt, R.; Salihi, S.; Yaylaci, S.; Çakar, G.Ç.; Toptan, H.; Karabay, O.; Sipahi, S. The effectiveness of dexamethasone on the prognosis of dialysis patients with severe COVID-19. *Rev. Assoc. Med. Bras.* **2021**, *67*, 1299–1304. [CrossRef]
102. RECOVERY Trial Collaborators. Tocilizumab in patients admitted to hospital with COVID-19 (RECOVERY): A randomised, controlled, open-label, platform trial. *Lancet* **2021**, *397*, 1637–1645.
103. RECOVERY Trial Collaborators. Interleukin-6 Receptor Antagonists in Critically Ill Patients with COVID-19. *N. Engl. J. Med.* **2021**, *384*, 1491–1502. [CrossRef] [PubMed]
104. Mori, S.; Yoshitama, T.; Hidaka, T.; Hirakata, N.; Ueki, Y. Effectiveness and safety of tocilizumab therapy for patients with rheumatoid arthritis and renal insufficiency: A real-life registry study in Japan (the ACTRA-RI study). *Ann. Rheum. Dis.* **2015**, *74*, 627–630. [CrossRef] [PubMed]
105. RECOVERY Trial Collaborators. Baricitinib in patients admitted to hospital with COVID-19 (RECOVERY): A randomised, controlled, open-label, platform trial and updated meta-analysis. *Lancet* **2022**, *400*, 359–368. [CrossRef] [PubMed]
106. A Study to Test Safety and Efficacy of Baricitinib in Participants With Diabetic Kidney Disease—Full Text View—ClinicalTrials.gov. Available online: https://www.clinicaltrials.gov/ct2/show/NCT01683409 (accessed on 17 February 2023).
107. PROphylaxis for paTiEnts at Risk of COVID-19 infecTion -V—Full Text View—ClinicalTrials.gov. Available online: https://clinicaltrials.gov/ct2/show/NCT04870333 (accessed on 17 February 2023).

Disclaimer/Publisher's Note: The statements, opinions and data contained in all publications are solely those of the individual author(s) and contributor(s) and not of MDPI and/or the editor(s). MDPI and/or the editor(s) disclaim responsibility for any injury to people or property resulting from any ideas, methods, instructions or products referred to in the content.

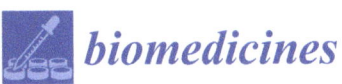

Article

Elevated Serum Urea-to-Creatinine Ratio and In-Hospital Death in Patients with Hyponatremia Hospitalized for COVID-19

Giuseppe Regolisti [1,2], Paola Rebora [3], Giuseppe Occhino [3], Giulia Lieti [4], Giulio Molon [5], Alessandro Maloberti [4,6], Michela Algeri [6], Cristina Giannattasio [4,6], Maria Grazia Valsecchi [3] and Simonetta Genovesi [4,7,*]

[1] Clinica e Immunologia Medica, Azienda Ospedaliero-Universitaria di Parma, 43100 Parma, Italy; giuseppe.regolisti@unipr.it
[2] Department of Medicine and Surgery, University of Parma, 43126 Parma, Italy
[3] Bicocca Bioinformatics, Biostatistics and Bioimaging Centre-B4, School of Medicine and Surgery, Milano-Bicocca University, 20126 Milan, Italy; paola.rebora@unimib.it (P.R.); giuseppe.occhino@unimib.it (G.O.); grazia.valsecchi@unimib.it (M.G.V.)
[4] School of Medicine and Surgery, Milano-Bicocca University, 20126 Milan, Italy; g.lieti@campus.unimib.it (G.L.); alessandro.maloberti@unimib.it (A.M.); cristina.giannattasio@unimib.it (C.G.)
[5] Cardiology Department, Istituto Ricovero Cura Carattere Scientifico (IRCCS) Sacro Cuore Don Calabria Hospital, Negrar di Valpolicella, 37024 Verona, Italy; giulio.molon@sacrocuore.it
[6] Cardiology 4, Cardio Center, ASST-GOM Niguarda, Niguarda Hospital, 20162 Milan, Italy; michela.algeri@ospedaleniguarda.it
[7] Istituto Auxologico Italiano, Istituto Ricovero Cura Carattere Scientifico (IRCCS), 20135 Milan, Italy
* Correspondence: simonetta.genovesi@unimib.it; Tel.: +39-335243910

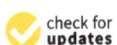

Citation: Regolisti, G.; Rebora, P.; Occhino, G.; Lieti, G.; Molon, G.; Maloberti, A.; Algeri, M.; Giannattasio, C.; Valsecchi, M.G.; Genovesi, S. Elevated Serum Urea-to-Creatinine Ratio and In-Hospital Death in Patients with Hyponatremia Hospitalized for COVID-19. Biomedicines 2023, 11, 1555. https://doi.org/10.3390/biomedicines11061555

Academic Editors: Elena Cecilia Rosca and Amalia Cornea

Received: 17 April 2023
Revised: 23 May 2023
Accepted: 25 May 2023
Published: 27 May 2023

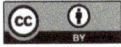

Copyright: © 2023 by the authors. Licensee MDPI, Basel, Switzerland. This article is an open access article distributed under the terms and conditions of the Creative Commons Attribution (CC BY) license (https://creativecommons.org/licenses/by/4.0/).

Abstract: Hyponatremia is associated with adverse outcomes in hospitalized patients. An elevated value of the serum urea-to-creatinine ratio (UCR) has been proposed as a proxy of hypovolemia. The aim of this study was to investigate the relationship between the UCR and in-hospital death in patients hospitalized with COVID-19 and hyponatremia. We studied 258 patients admitted for COVID-19 between January 2020 and May 2021 with serum sodium at < 135 mmol/L. The primary end-point was all-cause mortality. A 5-unit increase in the serum UCR during hospital stays was associated with an 8% increase in the hazard of all-cause death (HR = 1.08, 95% CI: 1.03–1.14, $p = 0.001$) after adjusting for potential confounders. In patients with a UCR > 40 at baseline, a > 10 mmol/L increase in serum sodium values within the first week of hospitalization was associated with higher odds of in-hospital death (OR = 2.93, 95% CI: 1.03–8.36, $p = 0.044$) compared to patients who experienced a < 10 mmol/L change. This was not observed in patients with a UCR < 40. Hypovolemia developing during hospital stays in COVID-19 patients with hyponatremia detected at hospital admission bears an adverse prognostic impact. Moreover, in hypovolemic patients, a > 10 mmol/L increase in serum sodium within the first week of hospital stays may further worsen the in-hospital prognosis.

Keywords: sodium; hyponatremia; urea-to-creatinine ratio; COVID-19; mortality; intensive care unit

1. Introduction

Hyponatremia is the most frequent electrolyte disorder in hospitalized patients and is associated with adverse outcomes [1,2]. Specifically, in patients with bacterial pneumonia, hyponatremia can be associated with increased mortality [3,4] and an increased risk of admission to the intensive care unit (ICU) [4].

Recently, the prognostic impact of hyponatremia has also been investigated in patients with COVID-19 hospitalized for interstitial pneumonia. Several pathophysiological and/or pharmacological mechanisms may explain hyponatremia in patients with COVID-19 and interstitial pneumonia. Inappropriate antidiuretic hormone (ADH) secretion is frequently involved. In fact, high circulating interleukin-6 (IL-6) levels may promote increased ADH secretion, as IL-6 can cross the blood–brain barrier and directly stimulate hormone release by supraoptic and paraventricular nuclei [5]. An inverse relationship between circulating levels of IL-6 and serum sodium concentration has been reported previously [6]. Moreover, increased ADH secretion may occur in COVID-19 patients due to hypovolemia, which can develop because of sodium loss during profuse diarrhea and vomiting. In addition, sodium loss during prolonged diuretic treatment with concomitant administration of hypotonic fluids (e.g., solutions for parenteral nutrition) in fluid-overloaded patients may represent another important cause of hyponatremia. Finally, because the entry of SARS-CoV-2 into the host cell via ACE2 disrupts the renin–angiotensin–aldosterone system (RAAS), creating an imbalance between ACE and ACE2 with an increased inflammatory response, we may speculate that this mechanism may also contribute to the development of hyponatremia in COVID-19 patients [7]. In this population, hyponatremic patients have been reported to have an increased risk of death in some [8–10] but not all [11,12] studies.

While hyponatremia can be associated with normal, decreased, or increased extracellular fluid volume [13], the clinical diagnosis of volume depletion is challenging, even upon expert judgment [14,15]. An elevated ($\geq$20) value of blood urea nitrogen (BUN)-to-serum-creatinine (sCr) (BUN/sCr) ratio has been proposed as a clinically useful proxy of hypovolemia independent of serum sodium concentration [16,17]. In fact, it is expected that a low effective arterial blood volume (EABV) will elicit a baroreceptor-mediated neurohormonal response, resulting in increased sodium and water reabsorption in the kidney proximal tubule and decreased tubular flow in the distal nephron, thus enhancing flow-dependent urea reabsorption in the collecting duct [18].

Indeed, an elevated BUN/sCr ratio value predicts adverse outcomes both in the general population [19] and in different clinical scenarios, including congestive heart failure [20,21], acute myocardial infarction [22,23], ischemic stroke [24–26], and subarachnoid hemorrhage [27].

In a recent study conducted in a cohort of Chinese patients hospitalized with COVID-19, an elevated BUN/sCr ratio value was identified as a potentially useful prognostic index [28]. Interestingly, Tzoulis et al. suggested that COVID-19 patients with hyponatremia and concomitant volume depletion, as judged based on a serum urea concentration value > 5 mmol/L, may be at a higher risk of death [11]. In Europe, as opposed to the US, urea is usually assayed in lieu of BUN. Based on the molecular weight expressed in daltons, serum urea concentration is approximately equivalent to half of the BUN value (i.e., 28/60 or 0.446) [29].

On these grounds, we decided to investigate whether an elevated serum urea-to-creatinine ratio (UCR), as a proxy of hypovolemia, is associated with in-hospital death or admission to the ICU in a cohort of noncritically ill patients hospitalized with COVID-19 and hyponatremia detected at the time of hospital admission. We also investigated whether a rapid increase in serum sodium concentration during hospital stays affects clinical outcomes in hypovolemic patients with different baseline UCRs.

2. Materials and Methods

2.1. Study Design

This observational, retrospective, multicenter study involved three large hospitals in Northern Italy. Adult ($\geq$18 years of age) patients diagnosed with COVID-19 and consecutively admitted to the three centers from January 2020 to May 2021 were included in the study. Clinical data were merged with the hospital lab database, and patients with at least one measurement of serum sodium, potassium, urea, and creatinine performed within 72 h since admission and with a serum sodium value below 135 mmol/L at the first measurement were included in the study. The patients lacking at least one valid measurement of serum sodium, potassium, urea, and creatinine within 72 h since admission were excluded.

Participants were followed up until the first occurrence of hospital discharge, transfer to another facility, or in-hospital death.

The study (STORM) was approved by the ethics committee of the coordinating center (San Gerardo Hospital, Monza) and by the IRB of each center and registered at ClinicalTrials.gov (accessed on 26 May 2023) (Identifier: NCT04670094, 15 December 2020).

2.2. Definition of Covariates

Study covariates included age, sex, history of comorbidities, drug treatments at admission, and blood chemistry parameters. We collected information on selected comorbidities, namely ischemic heart disease, heart failure, peripheral vascular disease, history of stroke, dementia, chronic obstructive pulmonary disease (COPD), liver failure, cancer, and diabetes mellitus. Charlson Comorbidity Index (CCI) was also computed.

Drug treatments at admission included angiotensin-converting enzyme inhibitors and angiotensin II receptor blockers classified as RAAS inhibitors, beta blockers, anticoagulants, and antiarrhythmic agents.

In addition to serum sodium, blood chemistry parameters included serum potassium, urea, and creatinine: hemoglobin, hematocrit, white blood cell count, and C-reactive protein.

Urea and creatinine measurements were used to compute UCR. Serum creatinine measurements were used to calculate the estimated glomerular filtration rate (eGFR) with the Chronic Kidney Disease Epidemiology Collaboration (CKD-EPI) equation [30]. Chronic kidney disease (CKD) was defined as eGFR < 60 mL/min/1.73 m^2.

2.3. Outcomes

The primary outcome was all-cause mortality. The secondary outcome was admission to ICU during hospital stays.

2.4. Statistical Analysis

The study population was subdivided into two subgroups based on UCR value at admission. Patients with admission UCR equal to or higher than 40 were regarded as being hypovolemic. The UCR value of 40 is equivalent to the value of BUN/sCr ratio of 20 proposed as a clinical proxy of hypovolemia (26,13,14).

Continuous data were described using medians and quartiles (first-third quartile Q1–Q3) and compared using the Kruskal–Wallis rank test, while categorical data were described using counts and percentages and compared using the chi-square (χ^2) test.

Estimated restricted cubic spline transformations were built using unadjusted logistic models on in-hospital mortality and admission to ICU to model the probability of death, as well as admission to ICU, by increasing level of admission UCR and placing five knots on the minimum, Q1, median, Q3, and maximum level of this ratio, respectively.

The Aalen–Johansen estimator was used to estimate the crude cumulative incidence of mortality and admission to ICU, accounting for discharge as a competing event, and the Gray test was used to test the null hypothesis of no difference in mortality and admission to ICU among the two groups according to admission UCR level.

Time-dependent Cox proportional hazards regression models were used to investigate the association between UCR and all-cause mortality, as well as admission to ICU. Urea-to-creatinine ratio during hospital stays was modeled as a time-varying covariate, and its association with outcomes was estimated for each 5-point increment. Potential confounders accounted for in the models were age, sex, CCI, treatment with diuretics or corticosteroids at any time during hospital stays, and serum potassium and eGFR at admission. We explored the impact of the time-varying serum UCR on in-hospital mortality patients treated with diuretics or corticosteroids at any time during hospital stays.

Furthermore, we also examined the prognostic role of changes in serum sodium values in hyponatremic patients when at least two serum sodium measurements were performed during the first 7 days of hospital stays. Increase in serum sodium values was categorized as lower or greater than 10 mmol/L. Logistic regression was applied separately in the two subgroups of hyponatremic patients classified according to UCR at admission, namely <40 and ≥40, to evaluate the prognostic impact of discrete changes in serum sodium within the first 7 days of hospital stays on in-hospital mortality.

Hazard ratios (HRs) or odds ratios (ORs) with 95% confidence intervals (CIs) were reported. SAS 9.4 was used for the statistical analyses, and the first-type error for tests was set at 0.05 (two-tailed).

3. Results

3.1. General Characteristics of Hyponatremic COVID-19 Patients

From an initial sample of 3470 patients admitted for COVID-19 between January 2020 and May 2021, we identified 258 patients who had at least one measurement of serum sodium, potassium, urea, and creatinine available within 72 h since hospital admission and had a serum sodium value below 135 mmol/L at the first measurement (Supplementary Figure S1). Of these, 231 patients (89.5%) had more than one measurement of urea and creatinine during their hospital stay, and 199 patients (77.1%) had more than one measurement of serum sodium within one week of hospitalization.

Overall, the median (1st–3rd quartile) patient age was 69 (59–78) years, with a majority of males (69.0%). Among comorbidities, diabetes (31.9%) and CKD (35.9%) had the highest relative frequencies, followed by ischemic heart disease (17.5%). Treatment with RAAS inhibitors and beta-adrenergic blockers had a prevalence of 42.9% and 34.3%, respectively. The median (1st–3rd quartile) value of the serum UCR was 40.6 (31.1–51.1) (Table 1, overall sample).

Table 1. Baseline characteristics of study population overall and within two strata defined according to categories of urea-to-creatinine ratio at admission. CKD, chronic kidney disease; COPD, chronic obstructive pulmonary disease; eGFR, estimated glomerular filtration rate; RAAS, renin–angiotensin–aldosterone system.

	Overall	Urea/Creatinine < 40	Urea/Creatinine ≥ 40	p	Missing (%)
n	258	126	132		
Male (n, %)	178 (69.0)	89 (70.6)	89 (67.4)	0.673	0
Age (years, median [Q1–Q3])	69 [59, 78]	65 [52, 75]	71 [65, 80]	<0.001	0
Hematocrit (%, median [Q1–Q3])	37.8 [34.0, 41.0]	38.2 [34.3, 41.5]	36.9 [34.0, 40.6]	0.432	2.7
Hemoglobin (g/dL, median [Q1–Q3])	12.8 [11.3, 13.9]	12.9 [11.3, 13.9]	12.5 [11.2, 14.0]	0.477	2.7
White blood cell count (10^3/μL, median [Q1–Q3])	6.38 [4.75, 10.10]	6.00 [4.45, 9.60]	7.00 [4.84, 10.44]	0.213	3.9
Urea (mg/dL, median [Q1–Q3])	41.5 [30.0, 63.8]	31.0 [24.0, 43.7]	52.0 [40.0, 78.7]	<0.001	0
Creatinine (mg/dL, median [Q1–Q3])	1.00 [0.82, 1.39]	1.00 [0.82, 1.33]	1.01 [0.82, 1.41]	0.879	0
Urea/Creatinine (median [Q1–Q3])	40.6 [31.1, 51.1]	31.0 [25.9, 34.8]	50.5 [44.5, 59.4]	-	0
Sodium (mmol/L, median [Q1–Q3])	133 [131, 134]	133 [131, 134]	133 [131, 134]	0.412	0.4
Potassium (mmol/L, median [Q1–Q3])	4.11 [3.76, 4.57]	4.02 [3.66, 4.38]	4.22 [3.92, 4.70]	0.002	0.4
C-reactive protein (mg/L, median [Q1–Q3])	84.6 [41.2, 133.0]	86.3 [46.5, 132.2]	81.4 [40.6, 133.0]	0.721	9.3

Table 1. Cont.

	Overall	Urea/Creatinine < 40	Urea/Creatinine ≥ 40	p	Missing (%)
Ischemic heart disease (n, %)	45 (17.5)	14 (11.2)	31 (23.5)	0.015	0.4
Heart failure (n, %)	14 (5.4)	5 (4.0)	9 (6.8)	0.472	0.4
Peripheral vascular disease (n, %)	24 (9.3)	7 (5.6)	17 (12.9)	0.073	0.4
History of stroke (n, %)	24 (9.3)	11 (8.8)	13 (9.8)	0.941	0.4
Dementia (n, %)	13 (5.1)	6 (4.8)	7 (5.3)	1	0.4
COPD (n, %)	26 (10.1)	4 (3.2)	22 (16.7)	0.001	0.4
Liver failure (n, %)	19 (7.4)	6 (4.8)	13 (9.8)	0.191	0.4
eGFR (mL/min/1.73 m^2, median [Q1–Q3])	69.7 [47.3, 87.8]	72.9 [51.6, 89.3]	67.1 [44.2, 84.5]	0.097	2.7
CKD (eGFR < 60 mL/min/1.73 m^2, n, %)	90 (35.9)	39 (31.5)	51 (40.2)	0.191	2.7
Cancer (n, %)	35 (13.8)	18 (14.5)	17 (13.1)	0.88	1.6
Diabetes mellitus (n, %)	82 (31.9)	33 (26.4)	49 (37.1)	0.087	0.4
Charlson Comorbidity Index (median [Q1–Q3])	2 [0, 3]	1 [0, 3]	2 [1, 3]	0.001	0
Systolic blood pressure (mmHg, median [Q1–Q3])	130 [120, 145]	130 [120, 147]	130 [120, 145]	0.78	2.7
Diastolic blood pressure (mmHg, median [Q1–Q3])	75 [67, 80]	75 [67, 80]	75 [67, 80]	0.89	2.7
Heart rate (bpm, median [Q1–Q3])	88 [75, 102]	87 [75, 100]	89 [75, 105]	0.259	33.7
RAAS inhibitors (n, %)	102 (42.9)	40 (33.9)	62 (51.7)	0.008	7.8
Beta blockers (n, %)	86 (34.3)	31 (25.4)	55 (42.6)	0.006	2.7
Anticoagulants (n, %)	28 (11.0)	12 (9.8)	16 (12.2)	0.671	1.6
Antiarrhythmics (n, %)	11 (4.3)	4 (3.3)	7 (5.4)	0.601	1.9

Thus, we divided our patient population into two subgroups based on a serum UCR value of 40 and regarded the patients with a UCR ≥ 40 as being hypovolemic.

3.2. General Characteristics of Hyponatremic COVID-19 Patients Partitioned Based on a UCR < or ≥40 at Baseline

Patients with a UCR ≥ 40 were older and had a higher CCI than those with a UCR < 40. Specifically, the former group had a higher prevalence of ischemic heart disease and COPD (Table 1). Serum potassium values were slightly but significantly ($p = 0.002$) higher in the patients with a UCR ≥ 40, while serum creatinine and eGFR were not different compared to the patients with a UCR < 40 ($p = 0.879$ and $p = 0.097$, respectively). The patients with a UCR ≥ 40 at admission were also more likely to be on treatment with RAAS inhibitors and with beta-adrenergic blockers (Table 1).

3.3. Relationship of Serum Urea-to-Creatinine Ratio at Admission and the Incidence of In-Hospital Death or Admission to Intensive Care Unit in Hyponatremic COVID-19 Patients

We observed 52 deaths in this cohort; the crude probability of in-hospital death as a function of the UCR at admission is depicted in Figure 1.

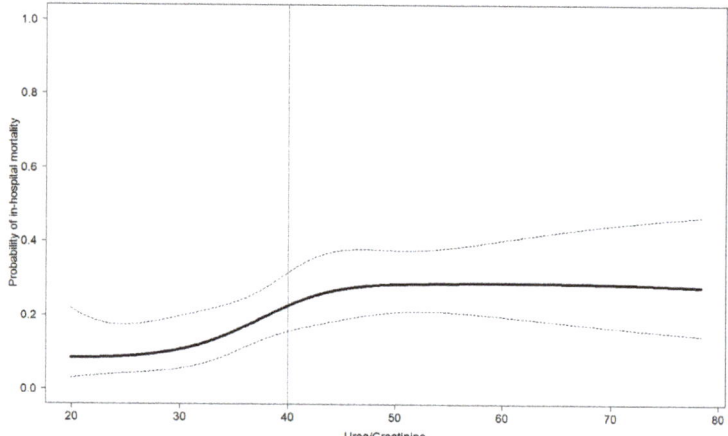

Figure 1. Estimated restricted cubic spline transformation of the probability of in-hospital mortality by values of the urea-to-creatinine ratio at admission. Estimate from unadjusted logistic model on in-hospital mortality. Restricted cubic spline with five knots on the minimum, first, second, and third quartile, and maximum value of the admission urea/creatinine ratio.

It can be seen that the probability of in-hospital death increased linearly with the UCR until a value of approximately 40, leveling off after this threshold. This threshold corresponded to the median value of the UCR distribution in the whole population of COVID-19 patients with hyponatremia at hospital admission (Table 1). The crude probability of admission to the ICU (37 patients) as a function of the UCR at admission is shown in Supplementary Figure S2. No specific trend was displayed in the probability of this outcome.

The crude cumulative incidence of in-hospital death was higher ($p = 0.011$) in patients with a UCR $\geq$ 40 at baseline than in those with a UCR < 40 (Figure 2, panel A). On the other hand, the unadjusted cumulative incidence of ICU admission was similar ($p = 0.516$) in the two subgroups (Figure 2, panel B).

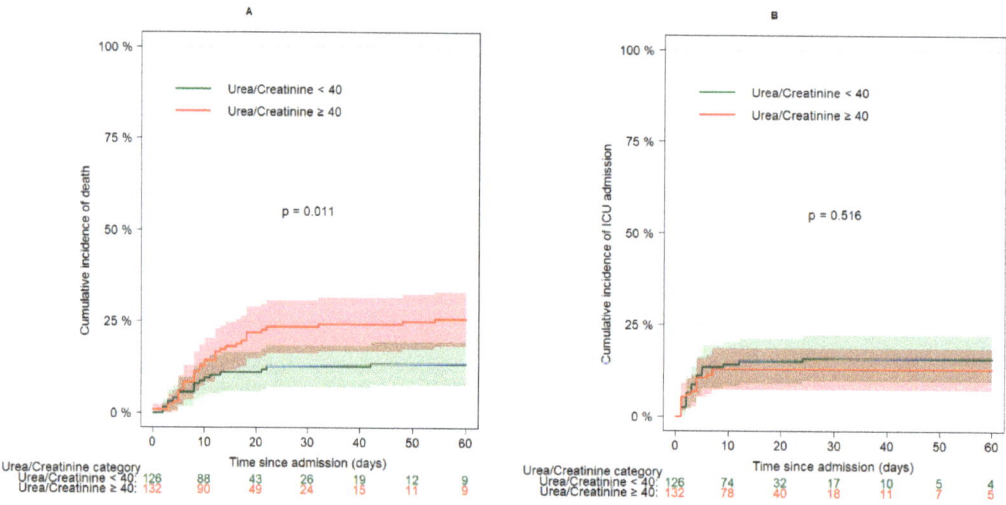

Figure 2. Cumulative incidence of death (panel **A**) and ICU admission (panel **B**) by categories of urea-to-creatinine ratio at admission.

3.4. Relationship between Changes in the Urea/Creatinine Ratio and Outcomes in Hyponatremic COVID-19 Patients

We examined the prognostic impact of the UCR during hospital stays by modeling this index as a time-varying covariate. We observed that every 5-unit increase in the UCR was associated with an 8% increase in the hazard of all-cause death (HR = 1.08, 95% CI: 1.03–1.14, $p = 0.001$) after adjusting for potential confounders, including treatment with diuretics or corticosteroids at any time during hospital stays (Table 2, Model C). When these latter variables were not considered, the regressors' results were very similar (Models A and B).

Table 2. Multivariable Cox regression models on mortality by time-varying urea-to-creatinine ratio. CI, confidence interval; eGFR, estimated glomerular filtration rate; HR, hazard ratio.

Parameter	Model A (n = 258, Deaths = 52)		Model B (n = 255, Deaths = 52)		Model C (n = 247, Deaths = 49)	
	HR (95% CI)	p Value	HR (95% CI)	p Value	HR (95% CI)	p Value
5-point increment of urea/creatinine	1.06 (1.02–1.12)	0.0093	1.07 (1.02–1.12)	0.0082	1.08 (1.03–1.14)	0.0011
Age (years)	1.04 (1.01–1.07)	0.0109	1.04 (1.01–1.07)	0.0131	1.03 (1.01–1.06)	0.0187
Male (yes vs. no)	1.40 (0.75–2.62)	0.2913	1.41 (0.75–2.63)	0.2884	1.68 (0.87–3.23)	0.1220
Charlson Comorbidity Index	1.46 (1.24–1.71)	<0.001	1.46 (1.23–1.74)	<0.001	1.18 (0.95–1.46)	0.1471
Diuretic during hospitalization (yes vs. no)			0.97 (0.52–1.80)	0.9246	1.12 (0.59–2.12)	0.7368
Corticosteroid during hospitalization (yes vs. no)			0.90 (0.51–1.59)	0.7216	0.53 (0.28–1.01)	0.0519
Potassium at admission (mmol/L)					1.61 (1.04–2.48)	0.0346
eGFR at admission (mL/min/1.73 m^2)					0.97 (0.96–0.99)	0.0007

We also detected a 6% increase in the hazard of ICU admission associated with a 5-unit increase in the UCR, which, however, did not reach statistical significance (HR = 1.06, 95% CI: 0.99–1.12, $p = 0.085$) in the fully adjusted model (Table 3, Model C).

Patients with a baseline UCR ≥ 40 were more likely to undergo diuretic treatment during hospital stays than those who had a UCR < 40 (41/132, 31.3% vs. 21/126, 16.9%; $p = 0.012$). Similarly, the former were also more likely than the latter to undergo treatment with corticosteroids at any time during hospital stays (84/132, 64.1% vs. 55/126, 44.4%; $p = 0.002$). We explored the impact of a time-varying UCR on in-hospital mortality in hyponatremic patients who were or were not treated with diuretics and with corticosteroids (Supplementary Tables S1 and S2) during hospital stays. We found that in patients who underwent diuretic treatment (Supplementary Table S1, Model A), a 5-unit increase in the UCR was associated with a 21% (HR = 1.21, 95% CI: 1.08–1.36, $p = 0.001$) greater hazard of all-cause death after adjusting for potential confounders. This did not hold true in the patients who were not treated with diuretics (Supplementary Table S1, Model B, HR = 1.05, 95% CI: 0.99–1.12, $p = 0.095$). In patients treated with corticosteroids (Supplementary Table S2, Model A), a 5-unit increase in the UCR was associated with a 12% (HR = 1.12, 95% CI: 1.05–1.19, $p = 0.001$) greater hazard of all-cause death after adjusting for potential confounders. This did not hold true in the patients who were not treated with corticosteroids (Supplementary Table S2, Model B, HR = 1.05 95% CI: 0.98–1.13, $p = 0.179$).

Table 3. Multivariable Cox regression models on ICU admission by time-varying urea-to-creatinine ratio. CI, confidence interval; eGFR, estimated glomerular filtration rate; HR, hazard ratio.

Parameter	Model A (n = 258, ICU = 37)		Model B (n = 255, ICU = 37)		Model C (n = 247, ICU = 37)	
	HR (95% CI)	p Value	HR (95% CI)	p Value	HR (95% CI)	p Value
5-point increment of urea/creatinine	1.04 (0.98–1.11)	0.1843	1.06 (0.99–1.12)	0.0664	1.06 (0.99–1.12)	0.0849
Age (years)	0.97 (0.94–0.99)	0.0112	0.96 (0.94–0.99)	0.0051	0.97 (0.94–0.99)	0.0108
Male (yes vs. no)	2.29 (0.95–5.51)	0.0652	2.28 (0.95–5.49)	0.0657	2.19 (0.90–5.36)	0.0833
Charlson Comorbidity Index	0.96 (0.76–1.21)	0.7272	0.96 (0.76–1.22)	0.7586	1.07 (0.81–1.41)	0.6273
Diuretic during hospitalization (yes vs. no)			0.93 (0.38–2.27)	0.8754	0.97 (0.39–2.38)	0.9382
Corticosteroid during hospitalization (yes vs. no)			0.63 (0.32–1.23)	0.1746	0.73 (0.36–1.48)	0.3814
Potassium at admission (mmol/L)					0.66 (0.36–1.22)	0.1848
eGFR at admission (mL/min/1.73 m^2)					1.01 (0.99–1.03)	0.3601

3.5. Prognostic Role of Changes in Serum Sodium Values in Hyponatremic Patients Partitioned Based on a UCR < or ≥40 at Baseline

Among the 199 (77.1%) hyponatremic patients with at least two measurements of sodium during the first 7 days from admission, 17.6% experienced an increase in serum sodium values equal to or greater than 10 mmol/L within 1 week of their hospital stay. The incidence of a serum sodium change of ≥10 mmol/L was higher in the subgroup of patients with a UCR ≥ 40 compared to the subgroup with a UCR < 40 at admission (22/107, 20.6% vs. 13/92, 14.1%, Figure 3).

We, therefore, examined the prognostic impact of this increase (≥10 mmol/L) in serum sodium on in-hospital mortality in the two subgroups of hyponatremic patients with a UCR ≥ 40 or <40 at admission. In the subgroup of patients with a UCR ≥ 40 (Table 4, Model B), those with a variation ≥ 10 mmol/L of serum sodium had higher odds of in-hospital death (OR = 2.93, 95% CI: 1.03–8.36, p = 0.0443) compared to the patients who experienced a < 10 mmol/L change in serum sodium; this was not observed in patients with a UCR < 40 (Table 4, Model A).

Table 4. Multivariable logistic regression models on mortality by maximum variation of sodium within 7 days after admission, stratified by value of the urea-to-creatinine ratio at admission (only the patients with at least two measurements of sodium within 7 days after admission were included in the analysis). CI, confidence interval; OR, odds ratio.

	Urea/Creatinine < 40		Urea/Creatinine ≥ 40	
	Model A (n = 92, Deaths = 13)		Model B (n = 107, Deaths = 30)	
Parameter	OR (95% CI)	p Value	OR (95% CI)	p Value
ΔNa ≥ 10 mmol/L vs. ΔNa < 10 mmol/L	0.22 (0.01–3.37)	0.2766	2.93 (1.03–8.36)	0.0443
Age (years)	1.05 (0.99–1.12)	0.1241	1.04 (0.99–1.09)	0.1144
Male (yes vs. no)	4.57 (0.77–27.1)	0.0936	0.79 (0.28–2.19)	0.6474
Charlson Comorbidity Index	1.79 (1.09–2.92)	0.0201	1.32 (1.02–1.71)	0.0335

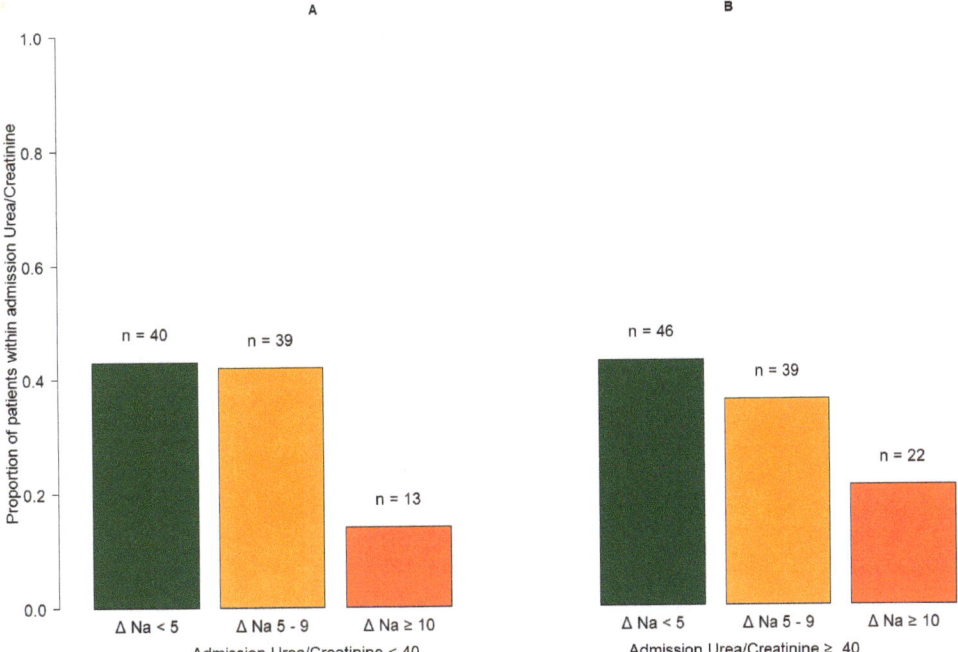

Figure 3. Proportion of patients' maximum variation of sodium (ΔNa, mmol/L) within 7 days after admission in patients with baseline urea-to-creatinine ratio <40 (panel **A**, n = 92) and ≥40 (panel **B**, n = 107). Only patients with at least two measurements of sodium within 7 days after admission were included in the analysis.

4. Discussion

The main result of this study is that hyponatremic patients who developed hypovolemia during hospitalization for COVID-19 experienced an increase in the hazard of in-hospital death. Moreover, in hyponatremic patients with hypovolemia already present at admission, as evidenced by a UCR value ≥ 40 at baseline, a ≥10 mmol/L increase in serum sodium values within the first week of hospitalization was associated with a nearly three-fold increase in the odds of in-hospital death compared with patients with a UCR value < 40 at baseline.

The UCR has been used as an index of a contracted effective circulating volume and/or neurohormonal activation in several areas of clinical research, including ischemic stroke [24,26], heart failure [20,21], acute myocardial infarction [22,23], and subarachnoid hemorrhage [27]. In these pathological conditions, an elevated UCR value has also been reported as a predictor of poor outcomes.

Hyponatremia is a common finding in hospitalized patients, including those with COVID-19-associated pneumonia [8–12]. However, the reported prognostic impact of hyponatremia in this patient population, especially with respect to the risk of death, varies across published studies. Moreover, it is unclear whether a different state of extracellular volume repletion may affect the association of hyponatremia with clinical outcomes. Indeed, Tzoulis et al. [11] observed that serum urea values above 5 mmol/L, as a proxy of volume depletion, may be associated with higher mortality in hyponatremic COVID-19 patients. Moreover, Liu et al. [28] reported that a high BUN/Cr ratio value may be used as a prognostic tool in these patients, although those investigators did not stratify their population based on serum sodium values. Thus, our results extend the previous findings by Tzoulis et al. [11] and ourselves [12], suggesting that the condition of hypovolemia detected at admission in hyponatremic COVID-19 patients portends an adverse prognosis.

Diuretic treatment can induce neurohumoral activation due to volume depletion [18,31], thus increasing the UCR value. Indeed, a diuretic-induced increase in the UCR, associated with poor outcomes, was also observed in different patient populations, including patients with ischemic stroke [25,26] and congestive heart failure. In the latter population, excessive hemoconcentration, expressed by a large increase in the BUN/Cr ratio value in patients treated with high-dose loop diuretics, was associated with increased mortality [20,32]. Furthermore, in patients with acute decompensated heart failure, the combination of hyponatremia (i.e., serum sodium values < 136 mmol/L) and elevated BUN values (i.e., >21 mg/dL) at discharge was associated with a higher hazard of death compared with hyponatremia alone or elevated BUN alone [33]. These findings support the role of excessive neurohormonal activation in predicting adverse prognosis. In our population, approximately one third of all hyponatremic patients who developed hypovolemia were treated with diuretics during their hospital stays. Therefore, we examined the association of a time-varying UCR with outcomes by adjusting for diuretic treatment administered at any time during hospital stays. Moreover, we also performed a stratified analysis of hyponatremic patients who were or were not treated with diuretics and found that increasing values of the UCR remained independently associated with an increased hazard of death in the former but not in the latter. Thus, we hypothesize that in our cohort of patients admitted with COVID-19 and hyponatremia at baseline, the adverse prognostic impact of the UCR increasing during hospital stays could have been related to neurohormonal hyperactivation secondary to worsening volume depletion, particularly in those submitted to diuretic treatment.

Hypovolemic patients with symptomatic hyponatremia, especially those treated with thiazides, are more prone to a rapid and greater increase in serum sodium concentration due to rapid volume expansion during treatment with hypertonic saline compared to normovolemic patients, conceivably due to the appropriate suppression of vasopressin secretion [34]. The overcorrection of serum sodium values may also be induced by infusions of isotonic saline solution in hypovolemic patients with hyponatremia [8]. In hyponatremic patients, the overcorrection of serum sodium values may be associated with severe brain damage and poor prognosis [35]. In our cohort of hyponatremic COVID-19 patients, we observed that the incidence of a change in serum sodium equal to or greater than 10 mmol/L within 1 week of hospital stays was higher in the subgroup of those who were hypovolemic (i.e., who had a UCR $\geq$ 40) at the time of the hospital admission compared to the subgroup who were not hypovolemic. Moreover, in hypovolemic patients, a $\geq$10 mmol/L increase in serum sodium within one week since admission was associated with higher odds of in-hospital death compared with nonhypovolemic patients experiencing a comparable change in serum sodium values. Our results are in line with those of Tzoulis et al. [11], who observed the highest mortality rate in COVID-19 patients experiencing a $\geq$8 mmol/L increase in serum sodium values in the first 5 days of hospital stays. We observed a $\geq$10 mmol/L increase in serum sodium in a relatively large fraction (35/199, 17.6%) of our hyponatremic patients, in whom at least two measurements of serum sodium were performed within one week since admission. Indeed, in patients admitted for COVID-19, hypovolemia could develop due to vomiting, diarrhea, or diuretic treatment. While we did not have information on the type and amount of fluids administered to our patients during hospital stays, we speculate that in a fraction of these patients, volume replenishment could have induced a diuresis-driven overcorrection of serum sodium values, which could have impacted overall survival.

The main strength of this study is that it was conducted on a representative sample of COVID-19 patients who had hyponatremia at hospital admission, from whom several measurements of serum urea, creatinine, and sodium values were collected during hospital stays. This allowed us to model the UCR as a time-varying variable and to explore the relative impact of worsening hypovolemia and serum sodium changes on clinical outcomes.

Moreover, we collected information on treatment with diuretics and corticosteroids during hospital stays, which allowed us to analyze the interaction of the UCR with these treatments and perform a subgroup analysis in the patients who did or did not receive diuretics during hospitalization.

Several limitations of our study must also be acknowledged. Firstly, while the UCR may be regarded as an index of contracted effective circulating volume [16–18], it is also affected by protein intake, gastrointestinal bleeding, muscle mass, and accelerated catabolism, especially in critically ill patients [36]. However, the patients enrolled in our study were not critically ill at baseline, nor did an increasing UCR predict admission to the ICU. Treatment with glucocorticoids may also increase the UCR by promoting protein breakdown [37]. However, although a greater fraction of the patients with a UCR value ≥ 40 received treatment with glucocorticoids compared to the patients who maintained a UCR < 40, we did not detect a significant interaction between the UCR value and corticosteroid treatment while analyzing the association of the time-varying UCR with in-hospital mortality. Secondly, we did not collect information on changes in the acid-base status; thus, we could not explore whether a putative increase in plasma bicarbonate concentration may have paralleled the increase in the UCR value, thus reinforcing the interpretation of a UCR ≥ 40 as an index of hypovolemia in hyponatremic patients, especially in those who received diuretics during hospital stays. However, patients with diarrhea-induced volume depletion usually develop metabolic acidosis rather than metabolic alkalosis. Hence, the impact of hypovolemia on changes in the acid-base status may be confounded by different clinical situations and may limit the clinical usefulness of those changes in the assessment of effective circulating volume. Thirdly, we had no information on urine output and fluid administration during hospital stays; thus, we could not analyze the impact of fluid balance on the changes in the UCR value and serum sodium. However, we observed that a greater fraction of hyponatremic patients who developed a UCR value ≥ 40 received diuretics during hospitalization compared with those in whom the UCR remained < 40, which suggests that diuretics may have contributed to fluid losses and may have favored a greater increase in serum sodium in the former. Finally, as this was an observational study, we cannot infer a cause–effect relationship of the changes in the UCR and serum sodium with patient outcomes. Notwithstanding adjustments for comorbidity burden, kidney function at baseline, and treatment with diuretics or corticosteroids during hospitalization in all analyses, residual confounding is possible, and our results must be considered merely hypothesis-generating.

5. Conclusions

Our results suggest that hypovolemia occurring during hospital stays in noncritically ill COVID-19 patients with hyponatremia detected at hospital admission may have an adverse prognostic impact. Moreover, in hypovolemic patients with hyponatremia, a ≥ 10 mmol/L increase in serum sodium may further worsen in-hospital survival.

Our findings reinforce and extend the existing data in the literature suggesting that hypovolemia developing in COVID-19 hospitalized patients with hyponatremia is associated with unfavorable outcomes. These findings may not necessarily be valid only in COVID-19 patients, as previous research indicates that an increasing UCR bears prognostic information in different patient populations. Thus, we suggest that clinicians should monitor the UCR in hospitalized patients with hyponatremia to detect those at the highest risk and take appropriate action to reverse hypovolemia using judicious volume expansion. However, while restoring an adequate effective circulating volume, great caution should be exerted to avoid a rapid and/or excessive increase in serum sodium concentration.

Supplementary Materials: The following are available online at https://www.mdpi.com/article/10.3390/biomedicines11061555/s1, Figure S1: Flowchart of patient selection, Figure S2: Estimated restricted cubic spline transformation of the probability of admission to ICU by admission urea-to-creatinine ratio. Estimate from unadjusted logistic model on admission to ICU. Restricted cubic spline with five knots on the minimum, first, second, and third quartile and maximum value of the admission urea-to-creatinine ratio. Table S1: Multivariable Cox regression models on mortality by time-varying urea-to-creatinine ratio, stratified by treatment with diuretics during the hospital stay. Table S2: Multivariable Cox regression models on mortality by time-varying urea/creatinine ratio, stratified by treatment with corticosteroids during the hospital stay.

Author Contributions: Conceptualization, G.R. and S.G.; methodology, P.R. and G.O.; formal analysis, P.R. and G.O.; investigation G.L., G.M., A.M., and C.G., data curation, M.A.; writing—original draft preparation, G.R. and S.G.; writing—review and editing, G.R. and S.G.; supervision, M.G.V.; funding acquisition, M.G.V. All authors have read and agreed to the published version of the manuscript.

Funding: The research was partially supported by the Italian Ministry of Education, University, and Research (MGV, 2017-NAZ-446/PRIN 0178S4EK9). The research was partially supported by the Italian Ministry of Health.

Institutional Review Board Statement: The study was conducted according to the guidelines of the declaration of Helsinki and was approved by the Ethics Committee of the coordinating center (San Gerardo Hospital, Monza) and by the IRB of each center and registered at ClinicalTrials.gov (Identifier: NCT04670094, 15 December 2020).

Informed Consent Statement: Where possible, informed consent was obtained from all subjects involved in the study. Otherwise, the study was conducted under authorizations guaranteed by Article 89 of the GDPR EU Regulation 2016/679, which guarantees the processing for purposes of public interest, scientific or historical or statistical purposes of health data. In addition, this is a retrospective study.

Data Availability Statement: Please contact the corresponding author regarding data requests.

Conflicts of Interest: The authors declare no conflict of interest.

References

1. Schrier, R.W.; Sharma, S.; Shchekochikhin, D. Hyponatraemia: More than Just a Marker of Disease Severity? *Nat. Rev. Nephrol.* **2013**, *9*, 37–50. [CrossRef]
2. Wald, R.; Jaber, B.L.; Price, L.L.; Upadhyay, A.; Madias, N.E. Impact of Hospital-Associated Hyponatremia on Selected Outcomes. *Arch. Intern. Med.* **2010**, *170*, 294–302. [CrossRef] [PubMed]
3. Müller, M.; Schefold, J.C.; Guignard, V.; Exadaktylos, A.K.; Pfortmueller, C.A. Hyponatraemia Is Independently Associated with In-Hospital Mortality in Patients with Pneumonia. *Eur. J. Intern. Med.* **2018**, *54*, 46–52. [CrossRef] [PubMed]
4. Zilberberg, M.D.; Exuzides, A.; Spalding, J.; Foreman, A.; Jones, A.G.; Colby, C.; Shorr, A.F. Hyponatremia and Hospital Outcomes among Patients with Pneumonia: A Retrospective Cohort Study. *BMC Pulm. Med.* **2008**, *8*, 16. [CrossRef] [PubMed]
5. Palin, K.; Moreau, M.L.; Sauvant, J.; Orcel, H.; Nadjar, A.; Duvoid-Guillou, A.; Dudit, J.; Rabié, A.; Moos, F. Interleukin-6 Activates Arginine Vasopressin Neurons in the Supraoptic Nucleus during Immune Challenge in Rats. *Am. J. Physiol. Endocrinol. Metab.* **2009**, *296*, E1289–E1299. [CrossRef]
6. Atila, C.; Monnerat, S.; Bingisser, R.; Siegemund, M.; Lampart, M.; Rueegg, M.; Zellweger, N.; Osswald, S.; Rentsch, K.; Christ-Crain, M.; et al. Inverse Relationship between IL-6 and Sodium Levels in Patients with COVID-19 and Other Respiratory Tract Infections: Data from the COVIVA Study. *Endocr. Connect.* **2022**, *11*, e220171. [CrossRef]
7. Govender, N.; Khaliq, O.; Moodley, J.; Naicker, T. Unravelling the Mechanistic Role of ACE2 and TMPRSS2 in Hypertension: A Risk Factor for COVID-19. *Curr. Hypertens. Rev.* **2022**, *18*, 130–137. [CrossRef]
8. Ruiz-Sánchez, J.G.; Núñez-Gil, I.J.; Cuesta, M.; Rubio, M.A.; Maroun-Eid, C.; Arroyo-Espliguero, R.; Romero, R.; Becerra-Muñoz, V.M.; Uribarri, A.; Feltes, G.; et al. Prognostic Impact of Hyponatremia and Hypernatremia in COVID-19 Pneumonia. A HOPE-COVID-19 (Health Outcome Predictive Evaluation for COVID-19) Registry Analysis. *Front. Endocrinol.* **2020**, *11*, 599255. [CrossRef]
9. Hirsch, J.S.; Uppal, N.N.; Sharma, P.; Khanin, Y.; Shah, H.H.; Malieckal, D.A.; Bellucci, A.; Sachdeva, M.; Rondon-Berrios, H.; Jhaveri, K.D.; et al. Prevalence and Outcomes of Hyponatremia and Hypernatremia in Patients Hospitalized with COVID-19. *Nephrol. Dial. Transpl.* **2021**, *36*, 1135–1138. [CrossRef]
10. Frontera, J.A.; Valdes, E.; Huang, J.; Lewis, A.; Lord, A.S.; Zhou, T.; Kahn, D.E.; Melmed, K.; Czeisler, B.M.; Yaghi, S.; et al. Prevalence and Impact of Hyponatremia in Patients With Coronavirus Disease 2019 in New York City. *Crit. Care Med.* **2020**, *48*, e1211–e1217. [CrossRef]

11. Tzoulis, P.; Waung, J.A.; Bagkeris, E.; Hussein, Z.; Biddanda, A.; Cousins, J.; Dewsnip, A.; Falayi, K.; McCaughran, W.; Mullins, C.; et al. Dysnatremia Is a Predictor for Morbidity and Mortality in Hospitalized Patients with COVID-19. *J. Clin. Endocrinol. Metab.* **2021**, *106*, 1637–1648. [CrossRef] [PubMed]
12. Genovesi, S.; Regolisti, G.; Rebora, P.; Occhino, G.; Belli, M.; Molon, G.; Citerio, G.; Beltrame, A.; Maloberti, A.; Generali, E.; et al. Negative Prognostic Impact of Electrolyte Disorders in Patients Hospitalized for Covid-19 in a Large Multicenter Study. *J. Nephrol.* **2022**, *36*, 621–626. [CrossRef] [PubMed]
13. Bhasin-Chhabra, B.; Veitla, V.; Weinberg, S.; Koratala, A. Demystifying Hyponatremia: A Clinical Guide to Evaluation and Management. *Nutr. Clin. Pr.* **2022**, *37*, 1023–1032. [CrossRef] [PubMed]
14. McGee, S.; Abernethy, W.B.; Simel, D.L. The Rational Clinical Examination. Is This Patient Hypovolemic? *JAMA* **1999**, *281*, 1022–1029. [CrossRef] [PubMed]
15. Fortes, M.B.; Owen, J.A.; Raymond-Barker, P.; Bishop, C.; Elghenzai, S.; Oliver, S.J.; Walsh, N.P. Is This Elderly Patient Dehydrated? Diagnostic Accuracy of Hydration Assessment Using Physical Signs, Urine, and Saliva Markers. *J. Am. Med. Dir. Assoc.* **2015**, *16*, 221–228. [CrossRef]
16. Stookey, J.D.; Pieper, C.F.; Cohen, H.J. Is the Prevalence of Dehydration among Community-Dwelling Older Adults Really Low? Informing Current Debate over the Fluid Recommendation for Adults Aged 70+years. *Public Health Nutr.* **2005**, *8*, 1275–1285. [CrossRef]
17. Liamis, G.; Tsimihodimos, V.; Doumas, M.; Spyrou, A.; Bairaktari, E.; Elisaf, M. Clinical and Laboratory Characteristics of Hypernatraemia in an Internal Medicine Clinic. *Nephrol. Dial. Transpl.* **2008**, *23*, 136–143. [CrossRef]
18. Schrier, R.W. Blood Urea Nitrogen and Serum Creatinine: Not Married in Heart Failure. *Circ. Heart Fail.* **2008**, *1*, 2–5. [CrossRef]
19. Shen, S.; Yan, X.; Xu, B. The Blood Urea Nitrogen/Creatinine (BUN/Cre) Ratio Was U-Shaped Associated with All-Cause Mortality in General Population. *Ren. Fail.* **2022**, *44*, 184–190. [CrossRef]
20. Sujino, Y.; Nakano, S.; Tanno, J.; Shiraishi, Y.; Goda, A.; Mizuno, A.; Nagatomo, Y.; Kohno, T.; Muramatsu, T.; Nishimura, S.; et al. Clinical Implications of the Blood Urea Nitrogen/Creatinine Ratio in Heart Failure and Their Association with Haemoconcentration. *ESC Heart Fail.* **2019**, *6*, 1274–1282. [CrossRef]
21. Zhen, Z.; Liang, W.; Tan, W.; Dong, B.; Wu, Y.; Liu, C.; Xue, R. Prognostic Significance of Blood Urea Nitrogen/Creatinine Ratio in Chronic HFpEF. *Eur. J. Clin. Investig.* **2022**, *52*, e13761. [CrossRef] [PubMed]
22. Aronson, D.; Hammerman, H.; Beyar, R.; Yalonetsky, S.; Kapeliovich, M.; Markiewicz, W.; Goldberg, A. Serum Blood Urea Nitrogen and Long-Term Mortality in Acute ST-Elevation Myocardial Infarction. *Int. J. Cardiol.* **2008**, *127*, 380–385. [CrossRef] [PubMed]
23. Huang, S.; Guo, N.; Duan, X.; Zhou, Q.; Zhang, Z.; Luo, L.; Ge, L. Association between the Blood Urea Nitrogen to Creatinine Ratio and In-hospital Mortality among Patients with Acute Myocardial Infarction: A Retrospective Cohort Study. *Exp. Med.* **2023**, *25*, 36. [CrossRef]
24. Schrock, J.W.; Glasenapp, M.; Drogell, K. Elevated Blood Urea Nitrogen/Creatinine Ratio Is Associated with Poor Outcome in Patients with Ischemic Stroke. *Clin. Neurol. Neurosurg.* **2012**, *114*, 881–884. [CrossRef]
25. Rowat, A.; Graham, C.; Dennis, M. Dehydration in Hospital-Admitted Stroke Patients: Detection, Frequency, and Association. *Stroke* **2012**, *43*, 857–859. [CrossRef] [PubMed]
26. Renner, C.J.; Kasner, S.E.; Bath, P.M.; Bahouth, M.N. VISTA Acute Steering Committee [Link] Stroke Outcome Related to Initial Volume Status and Diuretic Use. *J. Am. Heart Assoc.* **2022**, *11*, e026903. [CrossRef]
27. Chen, Z.; Wang, J.; Yang, H.; Li, H.; Chen, R.; Yu, J. Relationship between the Blood Urea Nitrogen to Creatinine Ratio and In-Hospital Mortality in Non-Traumatic Subarachnoid Hemorrhage Patients: Based on Propensity Score Matching Method. *J. Clin. Med.* **2022**, *11*, 7031. [CrossRef]
28. Liu, Q.; Wang, Y.; Zhao, X.; Wang, L.; Liu, F.; Wang, T.; Ye, D.; Lv, Y. Diagnostic Performance of a Blood Urea Nitrogen to Creatinine Ratio-Based Nomogram for Predicting In-Hospital Mortality in COVID-19 Patients. *Risk. Manag. Health Policy* **2021**, *14*, 117–128. [CrossRef]
29. Hosten, A.O. BUN and Creatinine. In *Clinical Methods: The History, Physical, and Laboratory Examinations*; Walker, H.K., Hall, W.D., Hurst, J.W., Eds.; Butterworths: Boston, NJ, USA, 1990; ISBN 978-0-409-90077-4.
30. Levey, A.S.; Stevens, L.A.; Schmid, C.H.; Zhang, Y.L.; Castro, A.F.; Feldman, H.I.; Kusek, J.W.; Eggers, P.; Van Lente, F.; Greene, T.; et al. A New Equation to Estimate Glomerular Filtration Rate. *Ann. Intern. Med.* **2009**, *150*, 604–612. [CrossRef]
31. Lindenfeld, J.; Schrier, R.W. Blood Urea Nitrogen. *J. Am. Coll. Cardiol.* **2011**, *58*, 383–385. [CrossRef]
32. Testani, J.M.; Cappola, T.P.; Brensinger, C.M.; Shannon, R.P.; Kimmel, S.E. Interaction Between Loop Diuretic-Associated Mortality and Blood Urea Nitrogen Concentration in Chronic Heart Failure. *J. Am. Coll. Cardiol.* **2011**, *58*, 375–382. [CrossRef]
33. Kajimoto, K.; Minami, Y.; Sato, N.; Takano, T. Investigators of the Acute Decompensated Heart Failure Syndromes (ATTEND) registry Serum Sodium Concentration, Blood Urea Nitrogen, and Outcomes in Patients Hospitalized for Acute Decompensated Heart Failure. *Int. J. Cardiol.* **2016**, *222*, 195–201. [CrossRef] [PubMed]
34. Mohmand, H.K.; Issa, D.; Ahmad, Z.; Cappuccio, J.D.; Kouides, R.W.; Sterns, R.H. Hypertonic Saline for Hyponatremia: Risk of Inadvertent Overcorrection. *Clin. J. Am. Soc. Nephrol.* **2007**, *2*, 1110–1117. [CrossRef] [PubMed]
35. Sterns, R.H.; Nigwekar, S.U.; Hix, J.K. The Treatment of Hyponatremia. *Semin. Nephrol.* **2009**, *29*, 282–299. [CrossRef] [PubMed]

36. Haines, R.W.; Fowler, A.J.; Wan, Y.I.; Flower, L.; Heyland, D.K.; Day, A.; Pearse, R.M.; Prowle, J.R.; Puthucheary, Z. Catabolism in Critical Illness: A Reanalysis of the REducing Deaths Due to OXidative Stress (REDOXS) Trial*. *Crit. Care Med.* **2022**, *50*, 1072–1082. [CrossRef]
37. Chapela, S.P.; Simancas-Racines, D.; Montalvan, M.; Frias-Toral, E.; Simancas-Racines, A.; Muscogiuri, G.; Barrea, L.; Sarno, G.; Martínez, P.I.; Reberendo, M.J.; et al. Signals for Muscular Protein Turnover and Insulin Resistance in Critically Ill Patients: A Narrative Review. *Nutrients* **2023**, *15*, 1071. [CrossRef]

Disclaimer/Publisher's Note: The statements, opinions and data contained in all publications are solely those of the individual author(s) and contributor(s) and not of MDPI and/or the editor(s). MDPI and/or the editor(s) disclaim responsibility for any injury to people or property resulting from any ideas, methods, instructions or products referred to in the content.

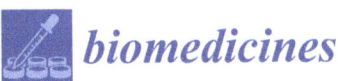

Article

Clinical and Personal Predictors of Helmet-CPAP Use and Failure in Patients Firstly Admitted to Regular Medical Wards with COVID-19-Related Acute Respiratory Distress Syndrome (hCPAP-f Study)

Francesco Cei [1,*,†], Ludia Chiarugi [1], Simona Brancati [1], Silvia Dolenti [1], Maria Silvia Montini [1], Matteo Rosselli [1], Mario Filippelli [1], Chiara Ciacci [1], Irene Sellerio [1], Marco Maria Gucci [1], Giulia Vannini [1], Rinaldo Lavecchia [1], Loredana Staglianò [1], Daniele di Stefano [1], Tiziana Gurrera [1], Mario Romagnoli [2], Valentina Francolini [2], Francesca Dainelli [2], Grazia Panigada [3], Giancarlo Landini [4], Gianluigi Mazzoccoli [5,*,†] and Roberto Tarquini [1,†]

1 Division of Internal Medicine I, San Giuseppe Hospital, 50053 Empoli, Italy
2 Division of Internal Medicine II, San Giuseppe Hospital, 50053 Empoli, Italy
3 Division of Internal Medicine, SS Cosma and Damiano Hospital, 51017 Pescia, Italy
4 Division of Internal Medicine, Santa Maria Nuova Hospital, 50100 Firenze, Italy
5 Division of Internal Medicine, Fondazione IRCCS Casa Sollievo della Sofferenza, 71013 San Giovanni Rotondo, Italy
* Correspondence: francesco.cei@uslcentro.toscana.it (F.C.); g.mazzoccoli@operapadrepio.it (G.M.)
† These authors contributed equally to this work.

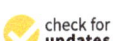

Citation: Cei, F.; Chiarugi, L.; Brancati, S.; Dolenti, S.; Montini, M.S.; Rosselli, M.; Filippelli, M.; Ciacci, C.; Sellerio, I.; Gucci, M.M.; et al. Clinical and Personal Predictors of Helmet-CPAP Use and Failure in Patients Firstly Admitted to Regular Medical Wards with COVID-19-Related Acute Respiratory Distress Syndrome (hCPAP-f Study). *Biomedicines* **2023**, *11*, 207. https://doi.org/10.3390/biomedicines11010207

Academic Editors: Elena Cecilia Rosca, Amalia Cornea and Toshihiro Kita

Received: 11 November 2022
Revised: 22 December 2022
Accepted: 11 January 2023
Published: 13 January 2023

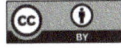

Copyright: © 2023 by the authors. Licensee MDPI, Basel, Switzerland. This article is an open access article distributed under the terms and conditions of the Creative Commons Attribution (CC BY) license (https://creativecommons.org/licenses/by/4.0/).

Abstract: Acute Respiratory Distress Syndrome (ARDS) caused by COVID-19 is substantially different from ARDS caused by other diseases and its treatment is dissimilar and challenging. As many studies showed conflicting results regarding the use of Non-invasive ventilation in COVID-19-associated ARDS, no unquestionable indications by operational guidelines were reported. The aim of this study was to estimate the use and success rate of Helmet (h) Continuous Positive Airway Pressure (CPAP) in COVID-19-associated ARDS in medical regular wards patients and describe the predictive risk factors for its use and failure. In our monocentric retrospective observational study, we included patients admitted for COVID-19 in medical regular wards. hCPAP was delivered when supplemental conventional or high-flow nasal oxygen failed to achieve respiratory targets. The primary outcomes were hCPAP use and failure rate (including the need to use Bilevel (BL) PAP or oro-tracheal intubation (OTI) and death during ventilation). The secondary outcome was the rate of in-hospital death and OTI. We computed a score derived from the factors independently associated with hCPAP failure. Out of 701 patients admitted with COVID-19 symptoms, 295 were diagnosed with ARDS caused by COVID-19 and treated with hCPAP. Factors associated with the need for hCPAP use were the PaO_2/FiO_2 ratio < 270, IL-6 serum levels over 46 pg/mL, AST > 33 U/L, and LDH > 570 U/L; age > 78 years and neuropsychiatric conditions were associated with lower use of hCPAP. Failure of hCPAP occurred in 125 patients and was associated with male sex, polypharmacotherapy (at least three medications), platelet count < 180 × 10^9/L, and PaO_2/FiO_2 ratio < 240. The computed hCPAP-f Score, ranging from 0 to 11.5 points, had an AUC of 0.74 in predicting hCPAP failure (significantly superior to Call Score), and 0.73 for the secondary outcome (non-inferior to IL-6 serum levels). In conclusion, hCPAP was widely used in patients with COVID-19 symptoms admitted to medical regular wards and developing ARDS, with a low OTI rate. A score computed combining male sex, multi-pharmacotherapy, low platelet count, and low PaO_2/FiO_2 was able to predict hCPAP failure in hospitalized patients with ARDS caused by COVID-19.

Keywords: hCPAP; non-invasive ventilation; COVID-19; SARS-CoV-2; ARDS; prognosis

1. Introduction

Since the first wave of the Severe Acute Respiratory Syndrome Coronavirus 2 (SARS-CoV-2) pandemic, the main cause for hospitalization and the need for intensive care was the systematic development of Acute Respiratory Distress Syndrome (ARDS), with the need for oro-tracheal intubation (OTI) and high mortality [1,2].

Many differences were described between classical ARDS and Coronavirus Disease 19 (COVID-19)-associated ARDS. In particular, COVID-19 patients manifested severe hypoxemia, confirmed by arterial blood gases (ABG) analysis, without correspondent signs of respiratory distress; often, they did not feel dyspnea, so the term "happy hypoxemia" was widely used [3,4].

In fact, in the initial phases of COVID-19 pneumonia, the most common mechanisms of hypoxia were the alteration of the ventilation/perfusion matching, due to lung edema, alteration in lung perfusion regulation, and microthrombi formation in the lung [5–7], with the preservation of lung mechanics [8]; however, in late phases, lung mechanics often deteriorated in COVID-19 pneumonia. Differentiation into three phenotypes was proposed to individualize treatment: (1) Ground-glass opacities with good perfusion; (2) inhomogeneous atelectasis; and (3) a patchy ARDS-like pattern. Phenotype 1 required low positive end-expiratory pressure (PEEP) ventilation, while phenotype 2 needed higher PEEP values and phenotype 3 usually received OTI [9].

Categorical clinical practice guidelines are lacking, hence significant treatment variability was reported [10]. Widespread use of early intubation compared to noninvasive ventilation (NIV) was described; however, since the first wave, a progressive increase in steroid treatment and NIV was reported, with a reduction in mortality [11]. Many studies tried to find a difference between supplemental high-flow nasal cannula (HFNC) oxygen and NIV, with diversified results. The HENIVOT study failed to find a difference in the median number of days free of respiratory support within 28 days in patients with COVID-19 and moderate to severe hypoxemic respiratory [12]. The HELMET-COVID study did not find a statistically significant difference in 28-day all-cause mortality between helmet NIV and usual respiratory support (including conventional oxygen therapy, HFNC, and nose or/and face mask NIV) in adults with acute hypoxemic respiratory failure related to COVID-19 [13].

Our study aimed to estimate the use and success rate of helmet continuous positive airway pressure (hCPAP) and evaluate the factors associated with its delivery and failure in patients first admitted to a regular medical ward and developing COVID-19-related ARDS. We also aimed to derive a predictive score (hCPAP-f Score) to identify patients at admission at high risk for hCPAP failure in the context of ARDS caused by COVID-19.

2. Methods

2.1. Patients and Data Collection

We performed a monocentric retrospective observational study. We evaluated the charts of patients first admitted to general medicine wards (Division of Internal Medicine I and II of the San Giuseppe Hospital, Empoli, Italy) for COVID-19 symptoms between 6 March and 30 May 2020 and between 1 October 2020 and 15 March 2021. All admitted patients exhibited epidemiological, clinical, laboratory, and radiologic findings suggesting COVID-19. Diagnosis of SARS-CoV-2 infection was confirmed by a real-time polymerase chain reaction (RT-PCR) assay or a second-generation antigenic test performed on specimens collected by nasopharyngeal swab.

We included COVID-19 patients aged 18 years or older admitted to the emergency department for symptomatic SARS-CoV-2 infection (fever, cough, dyspnea, nausea and vomiting, diarrhea, thoracic pain, asthenia, myalgias, pharyngodynia, and loss of smell and taste).

We excluded patients first admitted to the Intensive Care Unit (ICU) and those admitted for other medical or surgical conditions with concomitant asymptomatic SARS-CoV-2 infection.

For all enrolled patients, we reported personal data including age, gender, comorbidities, day of symptoms onset, home treatments, and length of stay (LOS). Comorbidity definitions and home treatment specifications are reported in the Supplementary Materials (File S1: Specifications and definition).

Clinical data, recorded at admission, included mean arterial blood pressure, the Glasgow Coma Scale (GCS), body temperature, cardiac frequency, peripheral oxygen saturation (SpO_2), the ratio of oxygen saturation to the fraction of inspired oxygen [SpO_2/FiO_2 (S/F)], and the ratio of partial pressure of oxygen to the fraction of inspired oxygen [PaO_2/FiO_2 (P/F)].

Laboratory data, recorded at admission, included complete blood count (CBC); prothrombin time (PT) expressed as the international normalized ratio (INR); activated partial thromboplastin time (aPTT); D-dimer value; fibrinogen; transaminases; total bilirubin; lactate dehydrogenase (LDH); C-reactive protein (CRP); procalcitonin (PCT); interleukin-6 (Il-6); brain natriuretic peptide (BNP); arterial partial pressure of oxygen (PaO_2) and carbon dioxide ($PaCO_2$); and PaO_2/FiO_2 ratio (P/F).

Radiology findings acquired by computer tomography (CT) or conventional radiology scans included the presence of interstitial pneumonia.

ARDS was defined by the Berlin Criteria [14] evaluated at admission; criteria were as follows: Beginning of the symptoms in the last seven days or worsening in the last seven days; the presence of bilateral opacities confirmed by conventional radiology or CT; respiratory distress not supportively explained by cardiac failure or fluid overload; and a PaO_2/FiO_2 (P/F) ratio below 300. The severity of the disease was also evaluated with the CALL Score [15].

hCPAP was delivered as first-line noninvasive respiratory support in patients in whom conventional supplemental oxygen therapy delivered via a simple mask, a Venturi mask (VM), or a non-rebreather mask failed to achieve and maintain respiratory targets. In particular, hCPAP was delivered in pure hypoxemic respiratory failure when oxygen supply with VM at 50% FiO_2 failed to maintain the target SpO_2 (94–98%) and respiratory rate (RR < 24 acts per minute). We present the stepwise approach to oxygen and ventilatory support in Figure 1.

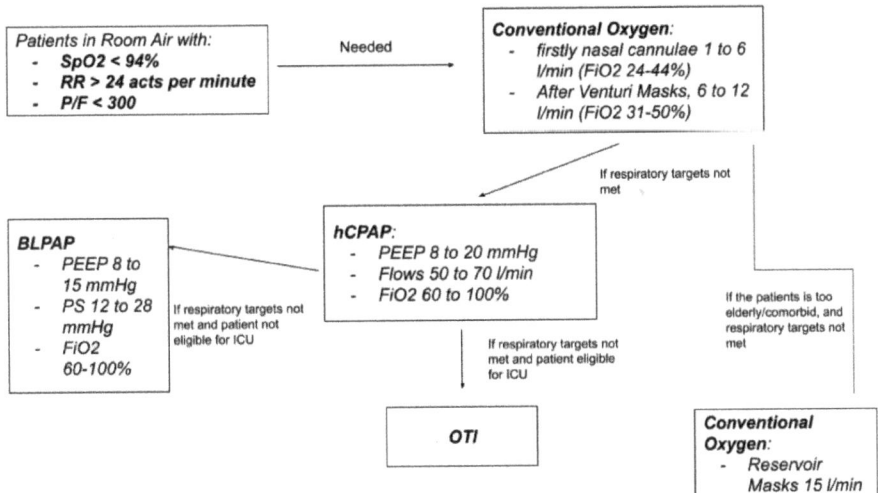

Figure 1. Stepwise approach to oxygen and ventilatory support for patients with COVID-19-related respiratory failure.

We delivered hCPAP using helmets that did not require a dedicated ventilator. These helmets convey high-flow medical gases in a closed space to generate the positive end-expiratory pressure (PEEP), required for alveolar recruitment.

High flows were generated by two systems:

- Flow-meters using both high-pressure oxygen and high-pressure medical air, with a target flow of 60 L/min at the beginning and a FiO_2 of 60%, obtained by mixing the flows of air and pure oxygen; both air and pure oxygen could generate a flow of 60 L/min, with the theoretical possibility of attaining 100% FiO_2;
- Flow meters using Venturi systems to generate the high flow; these systems convey oxygen in two ways with a maximum of 30 or 60 L/min to a strict canal in a Venturi valve; the high flow generates a low-pressure area, which recruits room air at high flows; this mix could generate an initial FiO2 of 60%, and upon closing the Venturi valve, we obtain a FiO_2 of 100%.

hCPAP was set to deliver 50 to 70 L/min flow and at least 8 mmHg PEEP (titrated to 20 mmHg) for almost 12 h per day, divided into 3 cycles (morning, afternoon, and night) alternated to HFNC (using the first type of flow meters and set with at least the same FiO_2 and flow) or non-rebreathing reservoir masks or Venturi masks (set with at least the same FiO_2).

BiLevel positive airway pressure (BLPAP) was delivered as first-line respiratory support only when respiratory acidosis occurred.

When hCPAP failed to maintain the respiratory targets (SpO_2 94–98% and a RR < 24 acts per minute) despite titrating FiO_2 to 80–100% and PEEP to 15–20 mmHg, we could consider two ways to increase the respiratory support:

- If the patient, evaluated by a trained intensivist, was considered recruitable for ICU, OTI was performed.
- If the patient, after collegial evaluation by the intensivist and the internist, was considered to have a scarce brief-term prognosis, was very elderly, and had multiple comorbidities, a trial for BLPAP was considered.

BLPAP was also delivered in the case of the appearance of moderate respiratory acidosis (pH 7.25–7.30). We usually started with pressure support of 12 mmHg (titratable to 26–28 mmHg) and PEEP of 8 mmHg (titratable to 15 mmHg), with at least the same FiO_2 as in hCPAP.

Technical details of the devices used for hCPAP and BLPAP delivery in regular medical wards are reported in the Supplementary Materials.

BLPAP delivery and ICU admission decisions involved collaboration between internists and intensivists, but the decision to intubate the patient pertained to the intensivists.

We calculated the number of days from admission and from symptom onset to the beginning of hCPAP.

For patients who received hCPAP, we reported data on in-hospital pharmacological therapy, particularly the use of steroids (dexamethasone 8 mg or equivalent), venous thromboembolism prophylaxis (enoxaparin 4000 UI or equivalent), tocilizumab (intravenously 8 mg per kilogram of actual body weight, up to a maximum of 800 mg, in two infusions, 12 h apart, or subcutaneously at 162 mg administered in two simultaneous doses, one in each thigh, up to 324 mg in total), and antibiotics (beta-lactams, glycopeptides, aminoglycosides, tetracyclines, quinolones, and oxazolidinones).

The primary outcomes were hCPAP delivery and failure rates. hCPAP failure was a combined endpoint including the need for BLPAP or OTI as a rescue respiratory support technique and mortality during ventilation. The secondary outcome was the combination of intra-hospital death and the need for OTI.

We retrospectively collected patients' data by reviewing paper and digital medical records (ARGOS version 4.2422820 and GALILEO version 1.5.3.14.2787 by Dedalus Italy S.p.A., via di Collodi 6/C, 50141 Florence, Italy). A structured web-based data collection form was developed for the retrospective chart review and for collecting clinical and personal data.

Data were collected by the physician staff of the Division of Internal Medicine I and II of the San Giuseppe Hospital, Empoli, Italy. Retrospective chart review studies relying on previously collected data may be wronged by biases due to the study operations, data collection, data entry, and data quality declaration causing a loss of information or approximation. To minimize this possibility, the first author comprehensively and carefully revised data collection, while also verifying the sources in the case of missing data, to curtail errors and biases. Data were analyzed after anonymization.

We included all the patients who met the inclusion criteria during the period described above. Regarding power and sample size calculation, designed for an observational study, the sample size was calculated considering differences between groups (hCPAP success and hCPAP failure); we considered a probable rate of hCPAP failure of approximately one-third [12,13] (ratio 2:1). Considering alpha 0.05 and power 0.90, and a Cohen's effect size d of 0.4, we calculated a necessary sample size of at least 254 patients (169 with hCPAP success and 85 with hCPAP failure).

The study was carried out and is reported according to the Strengthening the Reporting of Observational studies in Epidemiology (STROBE) guidelines for observational studies [16].

The local Ethical Committee approved the study (BIGCOVID, No. 2161 date 6 September 2021). Patients gave their written informed consent to participate. Only data collection from clinical records was allowed for patients unable to give their consent or those deceased. The study was conducted according to the Declaration of Helsinki for experiments involving humans.

2.2. Statistical Analysis

Continuous variables were reported as means and their 95th percentile confidence intervals (CIs) if normally distributed, and as medians and interquartile ranges (IQRs) if non-normally distributed. The D'Agostino–Pearson test of normality was used to test the normal distribution. Categorical variables were reported as absolute counts and percentages.

Differences in continuous variables between groups were tested with the t-test in normally distributed variables, with the Mann–Whitney test in non-normally distributed variables. Differences over time were tested with a paired-sample t-test or Wilcoxon test.

Categorical variables were tested with the Chi-square (χ^2) probability distribution test and the Chi-square (χ^2) test for trends (Cochran–Armitage test for trends).

We calculated Odds Ratios (ORs) and their 95th percentile CIs in univariate and multivariate logistic regression models. Only variables that resulted in being significantly different in the univariate analysis were included in the multivariate analysis. For continuous variables that resulted as statistically significant in the univariate analysis, we calculated ORs at values associated with the best of their sensitivity and specificity according to Youden's J statistic (Youden index) for the primary outcomes [17] (see also Supplementary Materials).

We performed a retrospective database analysis, with some clinical and laboratory data eventually being corrupted, deleted, and/or made unreadable at random. We reported data and univariate analysis for all the variables included in the study. Listwise deletion of missing values was performed, and to maintain the power of the analysis, variables with a loss of data of over 10% were not included in the multivariate analysis, even if significantly altered in the univariate analysis.

We derivated a score (hCPAP-f Score) using the variables that resulted as independently associated with hCPAP failure; for categorical values, points were directly obtained by the OR in the regression models; for continuous variables, we estimated the ORs for each quartile of distribution to obtain correspondent points. An OR in the range between 0.5 and 1.5 was considered 0 (not influent).

We tested the ability of the derived score to predict hCPAP failure by calculating the area under the curve (AUC) of the receiver operating characteristic (ROC) curves and tested the non-inferiority with both the Call Score and IL-6 serum levels. We estimated both sensitivity and specificity. We also tested the score for the secondary outcomes.

For all analyses, a *p*-value below 0.05 was considered statistically significant.

All the statistical analyses were performed using MedCalc statistical software (MedCalc Software, Acacialaan 22, 8400 Ostend, Belgium). The sample size was calculated with G*Power (The G*Power Team, Heinrich-Heine-Universität Düsseldorf, Universitätsstr. 1 40225 Düsseldorf, Germany).

3. Results

A total of 764 patients were admitted in the regular medical wards for COVID-19 respiratory symptoms, 63 (8.2%) were excluded for hospitalization due to other acute medical or surgical conditions, and 463 (66%) were admitted with clinical characteristics of ARDS, with a severe increase in the risk of OTI and death (OR 8.9, CI 4.8–16, $p < 0.001$). The overall rate of death and OTI was 23.5% (165), in-hospital mortality was 20.3% (142), and 36.6% (52) were in the non-ventilated group. The median length of stay in the hospital was 11 days (7–17) (Figure 2).

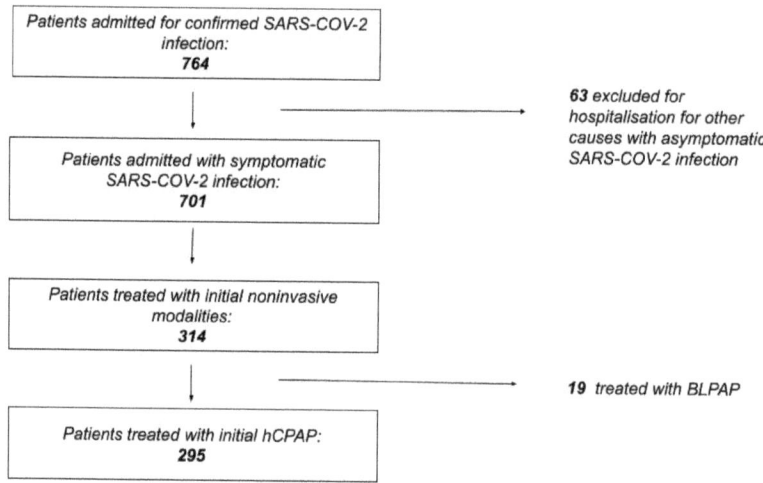

Figure 2. Flow diagram rendering the process of patient selection.

Noninvasive mechanical ventilatory support was needed in 314 patients (44.8% of the patients included in the analysis and 67.8% of patients with COVID-19-related ARDS). Furthermore, 19 patients (6.1%) needed BLPAP ab initio and 295 patients started a trial of hCPAP. Moreover, 86 patients (12.3%) were transferred to ICU, and OTI was needed in 46 patients (6.5%).

Of the patients treated with hCPAP, only three patients did not meet all of Berlin's criteria for ARDS, for higher values of P/F at admission; however, they met Berlin's criteria for ARDS during hospitalization. No patient without ARDS was treated with both BLPAP and OTI.

The median number of days from admission to the beginning of hCPAP was 2 (1–3), and between symptoms onset and the beginning of hCPAP, it was 7 (5–9). The median duration of noninvasive ventilation was 6 days (2–10) and the median length of stay in hospital for ventilated patients was 15 (11–24, $p < 0.001$). Supplemental HFNC oxygen alternated with hCPAP was delivered to 203 patients (68.8%).

Among the patients who needed noninvasive ventilation, 290 (92%) received steroids, 283 (90%) thromboprophylaxis (however, the other patients continued oral anticoagulation), 204 (64.9%) antibiotics, and 56 (17.8%) tocilizumab.

Differences between patients who needed hCPAP and those treated with conventional oxygen supplementation are reported in Table 1. Pre-existing factors associated with an increased risk of the need for hCPAP were the following: Young age, male sex, the presence of chronic kidney disease (CKD), active neoplasia, and severe obesity; lower applications of hCPAP were found to be associated with neuropsychiatric disorders, a serious risk factor for nonadherence and poor compliance. These patients also showed higher hemoglobin values, neutrophils count, INR, transaminases, fibrinogen, LDH, inflammatory markers, and Call Score values, in addition to lower P/F.

Table 1. Differences between patients treated with hCPAP and conventional oxygen therapy.

Variables	hCPAP	Conventional Oxygen	Younden Index	p-Value
Age (years)	69 (61–78)	73 (58–84)	<78	0.006
Male Sex n(%)	189/295 (64%)	177/386 (45.9%)		0.01
Hypertension	142/295 (48.1%)	188/384 (48.9%)		0.93
Cardiovascular disease	80/295 (27.1%)	117/384 (30%)		0.14
Respiratory diseases	44/295 (14.9%)	60/384 (15.6%)		0.10
Chronic kidney disease	35/295 (11.8%)	68/386 (17.6%)		0.04
Active cancer	26/295 (8.8%)	28/386 (7.3%)		0.047
Severe obesity	42/295 (14.2%)	34/384 (8.9%)		0.004
Neuropsychiatric disorders	34/295 (11.5%)	99/386 (25.6%)		<0.001
Diabetes	50/295 (16.9%)	81/384 (21%)		0.08
Polytherapy at home	137/295 (46.4%)	183/384 (47.7%)		0.62
Haemoglobin (g/dL)	14 (13–15)	13 (12–15)	>13	<0.001
Platelets (10^9/L)	207 (157–260)	204 (163–259)		0.98
Neutrophils (units/L)	5900 (4550–8600)	4900 (3370–7650)	>4700	<0.001
Lymphocytes (units/L)	800 (570–1100)	860 (600–1200)		0.30
International Normalized Ratio (INR)	1.2 (1.1–1.3)	1.1 (1.0–1.2)	>1.1	0.026
D-dimer (µg/mL)	847 (523–1550)	900 (530–1500)		0.95
Fibrinogen (mg/dL)	770 (640–880)	680 (570–790)		<0.001
Aspartate aminotransferase (U/L)	39 (31–54)	31 (24–46)	>33	<0.001
Alanine aminotransferase (U/L)	31 (19–51)	24 (16–39)		<0.001
Lactate dehydrogenase (U/L)	620 (480–760)	470 (380–600)	>570	<0.001
Total Bilirubin (mg/dL)	0.6 (0.5–0.8)	0.6 (0.5–0.8)		0.125
C-reactive protein (mg/dL)	8.3 (4–13)	4.8 (2–11)	>4.6	<0.001
Procalcitonin (ng/mL)	0.12 (0.07–0.3)	0.09 (0.05–0.22)	>0.1	<0.001
Interleukin-6 (pg/mL)	58 (31–100)	34 (14–66)	>46	<0.001
Horowitz Index	230 (130–275)	260 (180–310)	<270	0.006
Brain natriuretic peptide (pg/mL)	64 (35–140)	79 (34–190)		0.31
Call score	12 (10–13)	11 (9–12)	>9	<0.001

Independent factors associated with the need for hCPAP confirmed by multivariate analysis (Table 2, Figure 3) were the following: P/F < 270 (OR 3.1, 1.9–4.9), IL-6 serum levels > 46 pg/mL (OR 2, 1.3–3.2), AST > 33 U/L (OR 1.7, 1.1–2.8), and LDH > 570 U/L (OR 1.75, 1.1–2.8). Moreover, a reduction in the administration of hCPAP was found in patients 78 years old and older (OR 0.38, 0.23–0.64) and in those with neuropsychiatric disorders (OR 0.43, 0.23–0.78).

hCPAP failure occurred in 125 patients (42.4%), of them, 102 required OTI or died (34.5%), and 47 (15.9%) died during hCPAP without the advancement of respiratory support. In 25 patients, a trial of BLPAP was performed, and 11 (44%) died during BLPAP. After OTI, 23 (50%) patients died. Patients initially treated with BLPAP showed high rates of OTI and death (13.68%).

Patients with hCPAP failure were elderly, male, and affected by hypertension, cardiovascular diseases, respiratory diseases, CKD, active cancer, and neuropsychiatric disorders, polytherapy at home (at least three medications), and were treated with antibiotics during hospitalization. They also showed lower values of platelet count, fibrinogen, and P/F and higher values of total bilirubin, C-reactive protein, D-dimer, procalcitonin, interleukin-6, and serum creatinine. Details are shown in Table 3.

Table 2. Multivariate analysis of the factors associated with increased risk for need of hCPAP.

Variables	OR (CI)	p-Value
Age > 78 years	0.38 (0.23–0.64)	<0.001
Male sex	1.14 (0.72–1.81)	0.561
Cronic kidney disease	0.95 (0.49–1.86)	0.874
Active cancer	1.84 (0.91–3.73)	0.088
Severe obesity	1.57 (0.84–2.9)	0.153
Neuropsychiatric disorders	0.43 (0.23–0.78)	0.006
Hemoglobin > 13 g/dL	1.5 (0.91–2.46)	0.113
Neutrophils > 4000 units/L	1.02 (0.71–1.44)	0.933
INR > 1.1	1.06 (0.76–1.47)	0.72
Aspartate aminotransferase U/L	1.72 (1.08–2.74)	0.022
Lactate dehydrogenase (U/L)	1.75 (1.09–2.82)	0.021
C-reactive protein > 5 mg/dL	1.18 (0.71–1.96)	0.527
Procalcitonin > 0.1 ng/mL	1.06 (0.64–1.74)	0.829
Interleukin-6 > 46 pg/mL	2.04 (1.28–3.24)	0.003
Horowitz index < 270	3.11 (1.95–4.95)	<0.001

Table 3. Differences between patients with the success and failure of hCPAP. Younden indexes for hCPAP failure are also reported.

Variables	hCPAP Success	hCPAP Failure	Younden Index	p-Value
Age (years)	66 (57–73)	73 (63–83)	70	<0.001
Male Sex	98/170	94/125		0.002
Hypertension	74/170	17/125		0.037
Cardiovascular disease	38/170	44/125		0.021
Respiratory diseases	21/170	26/125		0.05
Chronic kidney disease	11/170	22/125		0.002
Active cancer	10/170	18/125		0.048
Severe obesity	26/170	16/125		0.53
Neuropsychiatric disorders	15/170	20/125		0.044
Diabetes	31/170	22/125		0.057
Polytherapy at home	62/170	77/125		<0.001
Haemoglobin (g/dL)	14 (13–15)	14 (13–15)		0.37
Platelets (10^9/L)	220 (180–280)	174 (135–237)	<180	<0.001
Neutrophils (units/L)	6000 (4400–8500)	6000 (4400–8500)		0.59
Lymphocytes (units/L)	860 (600–1200)	780 (510–1040)		0.051
International Normalized Ratio (INR)	1.2 (1.1–1.3)	1.2 (1.1–1.3)		0.46
D-dimer (µg/mL)	730 (470–1280)	1070 (630–1900)	>1160	0.001
Fibrinogen (mg/dL)	800 (660–890)	720 (600–850)		0.001
Aspartate aminotransferase (U/L)	39 (25–60)	39 (25–60)		0.2
Alanine aminotransferase (U/L)	31 (20–53)	31 (20–53)		0.44
Lactate dehydrogenase (U/L)	620 (470–780)	620 (470–780)		0.11
Total Bilirubin (mg/dL)	0.6 (0.5–0.7)	0.7 (0.5–0.9)		0.027
C-reactive protein (mg/dL)	7.4 (3.7–13)	9.4 (5–14)	>7	0.013
Procalcitonin (ng/mL)	0.09 (0.06–0.2)	0.2 (0.1–0.43)	>0.1	<0.001
Interleukin-6 (pg/mL)	48 (24–84)	75 (40–130)	>63	<0.01
Creatinine (mg/dL)	0.87 (0.78–1.05)	1.07 (0.86–1.5)	>1.1	<0.001
Horowitz Index	250 (170–290)	190 (26–250)	<240	0.001
Brain natriuretic peptide (pg/mL)	58 (34–127)	75 (34–180)		0.16
Call Score	11 (9–13)	12 (10–13)	>10	0.002
Days from hospital admission to hCPAP delivery	2 (1–3)	1 (1–3)		0.58
Days from symptom onset to hCPAP delivery	8 (5–10)	7 (5–9)		0.083
Days of ventilation	8 (6–10)	7 (3–13)		0.233
Therapy with tocilizumab	25/170	26/125		0.10
Therapy with antibiotics	94/170	98/125		0.048

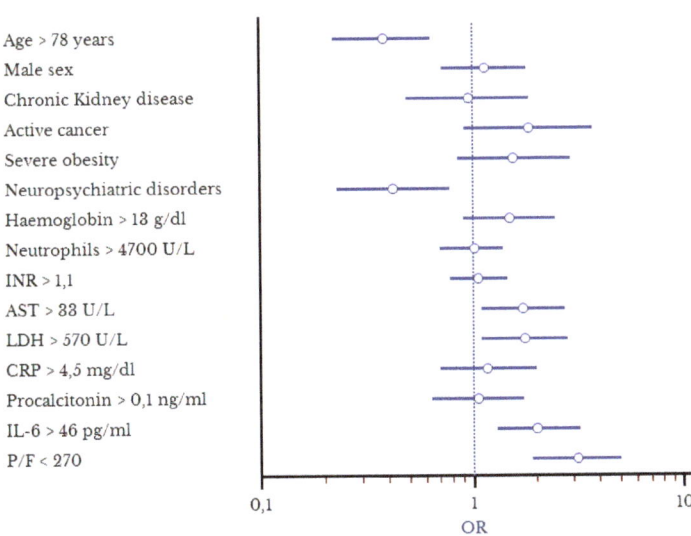

Figure 3. Forest Plot of the factors associated with increased risk of hCPAP delivery.

Multivariate regression models confirmed the following independent factors were associated with hCPAP failure: Male sex (OR 2.2, 1.1–4.8), polytherapy at home (at least three medications) (OR 2.4, 1.1–5.1), platelet count < 180 × 10^9/L (OR 3.2, 1.6–6.2), and P/F < 240 (OR 2, 1.04–4), as detailed in Table 4 and Figure 4.

Table 4. Multivariate analysis for factors associated with hCPAP failure.

Variables	Odds Ratio (OR)	p-Value
Age > 70 years	1.86 (0.96–3.62)	0.066
Male sex	2.24 (1.12–4.78)	0.023
Hypertension	0.71 (0.35–1.44)	0.345
Cardiovascular diseases	1.01 (0.44–2.36)	0.973
Respiratory diseases	0.75 (0.31–1.81)	0.525
Cronic kidney disease	1.48 (0.44–4.98)	0.524
Active cancer	2.04 (0.75–5.5)	0.161
Neuropsychiatric disorders	1.26 (0.47–3.35)	0.646
Polytherapy at home	2.4 (1.09–5.13)	0.03
Platelet count < 180 × 10^9/L	3.17 (1.58–6.34)	<0.001
D-dimer > 1160 µg/mL	1 (0.49–2.0)	0.979
C-reactive protein > 10 mg/dL	1 (0.5–2.01)	0.993
Interleukin-6 > 63 pg/mL	1.74 (0.89–2.45)	0.106
Procalcitonin > 0.1 ng/mL	1.47 (0.73–2.96)	0.281
Creatinine > 1.1 mg/dL	1.19 (0.53–2.67)	0.669
Horowitz index < 240	2.04 (1.04–3.99)	0.037
Therapy with antibiotics	1.47 (0.7–3.1)	0.31

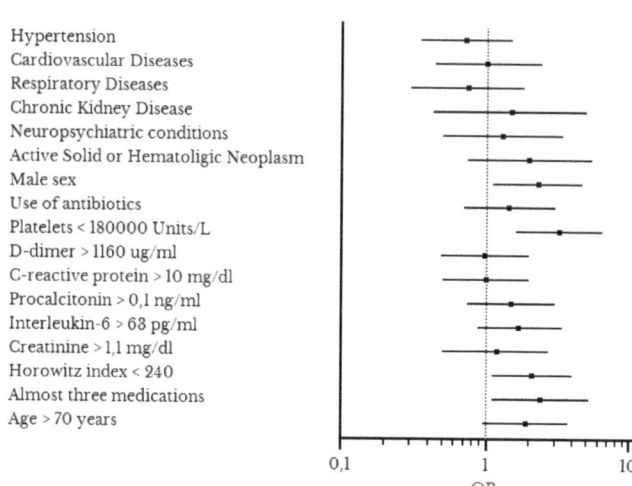

Figure 4. Forest plot rendering factors associated with hCPAP failure.

In Table 5, the derived hCPAP-f Score is presented, ranging from a minimum value of 0 to a maximum value of 11.5 (see Section 2).

Table 5. Odds Ratios (OR) and points used to compute the hCPAP-f score.

Variable	OR	Score Points
Male Sex	2.2	2
Polytherapy at home	2.4	2.5
P/F		
<84	3.1	3
84–240	2.2	2
241–300	1.2	0
>300	0.7	0
Platelet count ($\times 10^9$/L)		
<160	3.9	4
160–205	2	2
206–260	1.3	0
>260	0.85	0

In the group of patients forced to undergo hCPAP-f, the median hCPAP-f score value was 4.5 (2.5–6.5) and was higher in patients with hCPAP failure (6.5, 4–8.5) with respect to patients with hCPAP success (4, 2–5, $p < 0.001$). The hCPAP-f Score showed an AUC of 0.74 (0.69–0.79) and Younden's value > 4.5, $p < 0.001$) with a sensitivity of 63% and a specificity of 74%. As shown in Figure 5, the hCPAP-f Score appeared superior to the Call Score in predicting hCPAP failure (AUC of Call Score 0.6, 0.53–0.66, $p < 0.001$).

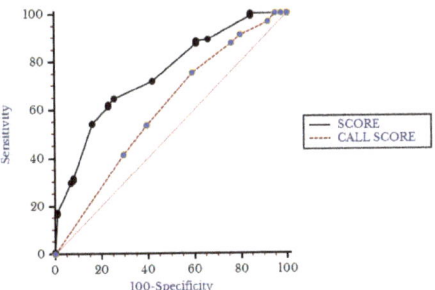

Figure 5. Comparison between Score and Call score for primary outcome.

In the overall group of patients, the median hCPAP-f score value was also 4.5 (2.5–6.5), with higher values for patients who died or needed OTI (6.5, 4–8.5) with respect to other patients (4, 2–5, $p < 0.001$). The hCPAP-f score retained its predictive value for the secondary outcome (AUC 0.73, 0.69–0.76, Younden's value > 4.5, $p < 0.001$, sensitivity 64% and specificity 72%) and appeared superior to the Call Score (AUC 0.67, 0.63–0.71, $p = 0.037$) and non-inferior to Interleukin-6 (0.72, 0.68–0.76, $p = 0.58$, Figure 6).

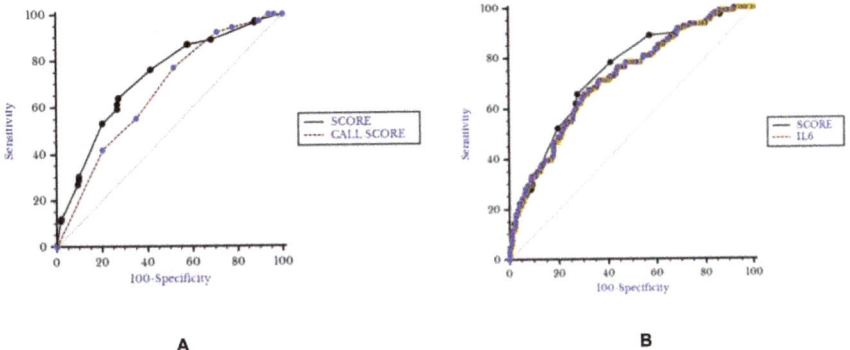

Figure 6. Comparison between Score and Call Score (**A**) and Interleukin-6 (**B**) for secondary outcome.

4. Discussion

During the SARS-CoV-2 pandemic, the prevalence of COVID-19-related ARDS in hospitalized patients varied substantially over time and geographical areas, and data in the scientific literature are heterogeneous. A report from the New York City area showed a prevalence of respiratory insufficiency of almost 27.8% and the need for intensive care of 14.2% with a high rate of OTI (12.2%) [18]. A register-based study of both the first and the second waves (March–December 2020) in Poland showed a very low prevalence of ARDS (3.6%) [19], while a higher percentage (32%) was found in Ethiopia during the second and third waves (September 2020–June 2021) [20]. In an early report from the Milan metropolitan area (February–March 2020), a very high prevalence (68%) of ARDS was found in hospitalized patients for COVID-19 [21]. A global literature survey reported an overall 26% prevalence of ARDS in hospitalized patients for COVID-19 [1]. Most of the studies included patients first admitted to both ordinary hospital and intensive-care beds. The heterogeneity of the prevalence of ARDS in the committed studies could be explained by many reasons, including the definition of ARDS used, the different rates of hospitalization in many countries, the inclusion of all patients with a positive RT-PCR or antigenic test (even those hospitalized for other reasons rather than symptomatic COVID-19), and the impact of virus variants.

In our experience, prior to the institution of mass vaccination programs, patients hospitalized for symptomatic COVID-19 had a high rate of ARDS after admission to medical regular wards (66%), with a median P/F of 242 (95–300) and a very significant increase in risk for adverse events (OR 8.9 for OTI and death). These could, in part, be explained by the ministerial recommendations for general practitioners to hospitalize patients with severe COVID-19 symptoms, particularly low oxygen desaturation index, dyspnea, and persistent fever. Moreover, inpatient transfers to the ICU were substantially low (12.5%) considering the disease severity detailed in Table 1.

The optimal respiratory support for COVID-19-related ARDS is not clearly defined. Experiences with early intubation lead to high mortality rates [2]. A choice between noninvasive modalities, including HFNC, CPAP, and BLPAP, was hazardous for the scarce data and the lack of indications from international guidelines. In Anglo-Saxon countries, an initial preference for HFNC was proposed [18,22]; this indication was based on data on undifferentiated acute hypoxemic respiratory failure, which showed no differences between conventional respiratory support, NIV, and HFNC in OTI rates, with a small advantage regarding 90-day survival for HFNC [23,24].

In our study, we reported data derived from our large experience in using hCPAP, frequently associated with HFNC, as a synergic oxygen delivery support technique. We report similar death and OTI rates to those reported by the recent Recovery-Rs prospective trial (34.3% in our study and 36.3% in the Recovery-Rs trial) [25].

Factors associated with an increased need for hCPAP were low P/F, increased interleukin-6 serum levels, increased AST values, and high LDH values. Our results are in agreement with those reported in a small study (97 patients) showing that fever > 37.5 °C, LDH value > 250 UI, and D-dimer over 1000 µg/mL were associated with the requirement for NIV [26]. In another small study considering all the noninvasive respiratory support techniques, only hypertension was found to be associated with an increased need for NIV [27].

In our study, transaminases, especially AST, were associated with an increased risk of death and OTI; AST is considered a marker of systemic disease, while ALT is considered a more liver-specific marker [28]. Increased LDH levels are also considered a marker of cell death/lisys and multi-organ failure due to cytokine storm, and it was associated with the severity of COVID-19 disease and the risk of death [29]. Interleukin-6 is a highly studied marker of immune activation in COVID-19, and its association with adverse outcomes (including the need for transfer to the ICU and death) was analyzed in systematic reviews [30]. The combination of these parameters, including low P/F, seemed to indicate that patients with unwarranted production of pro-inflammatory cytokines (cytokine storm) leading to ARDS and widespread tissue damage resulting in multi-organ failure are at increased risk of needing hCPAP delivery.

Despite being generally well tolerated, in our study, a reduction in the delivery of hCPAP was demonstrated in the elderly and in patients affected by neuropsychiatric disorders. However, as the decision to apply hCPAP was in the hands of the attending physicians, a very poor performance status, high dependency, and altered mentation could lead to more conservative and/or conventional approaches to oxygen therapy, using nasal prongs, cannula, or masks. Moreover, the benefit of ventilation in those patients could be questionable. In fact, the use of CPAP in the very elderly with acute hypoxemia due to heart failure did not lead to an increase in the survival of hospitalized patients [31], and the use of HFNC in very elderly patients with COVID-19 was associated with a high mortality rate (63.6%) [32].

Factors associated with hCPAP failure were male sex, polytherapy (the use of at least three medications at home), platelet count below 180×10^9/L, and P/F < 240.

Male sex is associated with an increased risk of death and OTI in COVID-19 and other coronavirus syndromes, due to a different pattern of the immune response, considering that females had higher CD8+ and CD4+ lymphocyte counts, and stronger immunoglobulin response [33]. This was also confirmed by our study population, in which males had higher values of IL-6 with respect to females ($p < 0.001$). Furthermore, males were more frequently affected by almost one comorbidity, particularly hypertension and cardiovascular disease ($p = 0.03$) even if they were slightly younger (median age 70 vs. 73 years, $p = 0.045$). No differences were found in the risk of developing ARDS ($p = 0.6$).

No single comorbidity showed a significant association with hCPAP failure, while the use of multiple medications at home was associated with an increased risk of hCPAP failure, envisaging polytherapy as a marker of the patient's frailty. Furthermore, the use of some medications (i.e., acetylsalicylic acid, digoxin, folic acid, mirtazapine, linagliptin, enalapril, atorvastatin, and allopurinol) was found associated with an increased risk of death [34]. COVID-19 can lead to thrombocytopenia via many mechanisms, including direct and direct platelet destruction, microthrombi formation, and reduced hematopoiesis induced by cytokine storm and low platelet count was also found associated with adverse events [35]. A very low P/F could suggest the need for more invasive treatments instead of hCPAP to resolve the hypoxemic respiratory failure. Furthermore, in an Italian cohort of COVID-19 patients hospitalized in 2020, the severity of ARDS (stratified as mild, moderate, and severe according to P/F value) was found to correlate with the risk of NIV failure (when considering both hCPAP and BLPAP) [36].

We derived a four-factor, 11.5-point score (hCPAP-f) showing good reliability in predicting hCPAP failure in COVID-19 patients. The hCPAP-f score was superior to the Call Score, first derived to detect the clinical deterioration of COVID-19 patients [15] and non-inferior for the secondary outcome in the overall COVID-19 patient population. It also resulted in being non-inferior to interleukin-6 serum levels, which we evaluated as a prognostic factor [37], to predict the secondary outcome in the overall COVID-19 patient population.

Varied results are found in the scientific literature regarding NIV failure prediction, and only the HACOR score was associated with CPAP failure, with an AUC of 0.74 [38]. However, in this observational study, many personal and laboratory factors analyzed in our study were not tested. A large multicenter study found low P/F, low platelet count, and high C-reactive protein to reliably predict NIV failure [39]. However, these two studies did not differ systematically between hCPAP and BLPAP, and both studies did not include the need for BiPAP in the outcomes as a rescue technique for patients who experienced hCPAP failure. Moreover, we also derived a new score to help physicians in rapidly stratifying high-risk patients for ICU transfer and selection for more aggressive respiratory support strategies (BLPAP, OTI).

Our study has some limitations, primarily related to its monocentric retrospective observational design, while the strengths are related to the real-world setting, the large sample size, and the great number of variables analyzed. Our derived score needs external validation for application in clinical practice.

5. Conclusions

Defining optimal respiratory support in COVID-19-related ARDS is challenging; nonetheless, NIV is realistically valuable to decrease the need for invasive mechanical ventilation, while the specific role of HFNC remains uncertain. As a first-line therapy, CPAP plus HFNC and additional interventions may be a useful option according to the patient's condition and compliance [40].

In our clinical setting, hCPAP was largely used to treat COVID-19-related ARDS, leading to a low rate of OTI. Factors associated with the need for hCPAP were high AST, LDH, and IL-6 serum levels, as well as low P/F; older age and neuropsychiatric disorders led to a reduction in its use. Failure of hCPAP was associated with male sex, polytherapy with the use of at least three medications at home, low platelet count, and very low P/F. A feasible and reliable four-variable early score was derived, with good reliability in predicting both hCPAP failure and the combination of OTI and death in patients hospitalized for symptomatic COVID-19. The hCPAP-f score could be used at the time of hospital admission for the initial stratification of high-risk COVID-19 patients to assess the need for the selection of more aggressive respiratory support and/or early transfer to the ICU.

Supplementary Materials: The following supporting information can be downloaded at: https://www.mdpi.com/article/10.3390/biomedicines11010207/s1, File S1: Specifications and definitions.

Author Contributions: F.C. and R.T. conceived the article and wrote the paper; G.M. reviewed the scientific literature, supervised the statistical analysis, and wrote the paper; F.C. and R.T. created the database, performed the statistical analysis, and reviewed data collection; L.C., S.B., S.D., M.S.M., M.R. (Matteo Rosselli), M.F., C.C., I.S., M.M.G., G.V., R.L., L.S., D.d.S., T.G., M.R. (Mario Romagnoli), V.F., F.D. and G.P. collected the data; F.C., G.L. and R.T. administered and supervised the whole project. All authors approved the final version of the manuscript and agreed to the published version of the manuscript. F.C., G.M. and R.T. take the responsibility for the integrity of the work as a whole.

Funding: APCs were funded by the "5 × 1000" voluntary contribution and by a grant from the Italian Ministry of Health (RC2022–2024) to G.M.

Institutional Review Board Statement: BIGCOVID, No. 2161 date 6 September 2021; promoter Azienda Usl Toscana Centro, first researcher G.L.

Informed Consent Statement: Written informed consent was obtained from all study participants or their legal representatives.

Data Availability Statement: The data that support the findings of this study are available upon request from the first author, F.C. The data are not publicly available due to containing information that could compromise the privacy of research participants.

Acknowledgments: We thank all the patients who voluntarily consented to participate in the study.

Conflicts of Interest: The author declares that there are no conflict of interest with respect to the authorship and/or publication of this article.

References

1. Tzotzos, S.J.; Fischer, B.; Fischer, H.; Zeitlinger, M. Incidence of ARDS and outcomes in hospitalized patients with COVID-19: A global literature survey. *Crit. Care* **2020**, *24*, 516. [CrossRef] [PubMed]
2. Grasselli, G.; Zangrillo, A.; Zanella, A.; Antonelli, M.; Cabrini, L.; Castelli, A.; Cereda, D.; Coluccello, A.; Foti, G.; Fumagalli, R.; et al. COVID-19 Lombardy ICU Network. Baseline Characteristics and Outcomes of 1591 Patients Infected With SARS-CoV-2 Admitted to ICUs of the Lombardy Region, Italy. *JAMA* **2020**, *323*, 1574–1581. [CrossRef] [PubMed]
3. Tobin, M.J.; Laghi, F.; Jubran, A. Why COVID-19 Silent Hypoxemia Is Baffling to Physicians. *Am. J. Respir. Crit. Care Med.* **2020**, *202*, 356–360. [CrossRef] [PubMed]
4. Wilkerson, R.G.; Adler, J.D.; Shah, N.G.; Brown, R. Silent hypoxia: A harbinger of clinical deterioration in patients with COVID-19. *Am. J. Emerg. Med.* **2020**, *38*, 2243.e5–2243.e6. [CrossRef]
5. Komorowski, M.; Aberegg, S.K. Using applied lung physiology to understand COVID-19 patterns. *Br. J. Anaesth.* **2020**, *125*, 250–253. [CrossRef]
6. Lang, M.; Som, A.; Mendoza, D.P.; Flores, E.J.; Reid, N.; Carey, D.; Li, M.D.; Witkin, A.; Rodriguez-Lopez, J.M.; Shepard, J.O.; et al. Hypoxaemia related to COVID-19: Vascular and perfusion abnormalities on dual-energy CT. *Lancet Infect. Dis.* **2020**, *20*, 1365–1366. [CrossRef]
7. Dhont, S.; Derom, E.; Van Braeckel, E.; Depuydt, P.; Lambrecht, B.N. The pathophysiology of 'happy' hypoxemia in COVID-19. *Respir. Res.* **2020**, *21*, 198. [CrossRef] [PubMed]
8. Gattinoni, L.; Coppola, S.; Cressoni, M.; Busana, M.; Rossi, S.; Chiumello, D. COVID-19 Does Not Lead to a "Typical" Acute Respiratory Distress Syndrome. *Am. J. Respir. Crit. Care Med.* **2020**, *201*, 1299–1300. [CrossRef]
9. Robba, C.; Battaglini, D.; Ball, L.; Patroniti, N.; Loconte, M.; Brunetti, I.; Vena, A.; Giacobbe, D.R.; Bassetti, M.; Rocco, P.R.M.; et al. Distinct phenotypes require distinct respiratory management strategies in severe COVID-19. *Respir. Physiol. Neurobiol.* **2020**, *279*, 103455. [CrossRef]
10. Azoulay, E.; de Waele, J.; Ferrer, R.; Staudinger, T.; Borkowska, M.; Povoa, P.; Iliopoulou, K.; Artigas, A.; Schaller, S.J.; Shankar-Hari, M.; et al. International variation in the management of severe COVID-19 patients. *Crit. Care* **2020**, *24*, 486. [CrossRef]
11. Docherty, A.B.; Mulholland, R.H.; Lone, N.I.; Cheyne, C.P.; De Angelis, D.; Diaz-Ordaz, K.; Donegan, C.; Drake, T.M.; Dunning, J.; Funk, S.; et al. ISARIC4C Investigators. Changes in in-hospital mortality in the first wave of COVID-19: A multicentre prospective observational cohort study using the WHO Clinical Characterisation Protocol UK. *Lancet Respir. Med.* **2021**, *9*, 773–785. [CrossRef] [PubMed]
12. Grieco, D.L.; Menga, L.S.; Cesarano, M.; Rosà, T.; Spadaro, S.; Bitondo, M.M.; Montomoli, J.; Falò, G.; Tonetti, T.; Cutuli, S.L.; et al. Effect of Helmet Noninvasive Ventilation vs High-Flow Nasal Oxygen on Days Free of Respiratory Support in Patients With

COVID-19 and Moderate to Severe Hypoxemic Respiratory Failure: The HENIVOT Randomized Clinical Trial. *JAMA* **2021**, *325*, 1731–1743. [CrossRef] [PubMed]
13. Arabi, Y.M.; Aldekhyl, S.; Al Qahtani, S.; Al-Dorzi, H.M.; Abdukahil, S.A.; Al Harbi, M.K.; Al Qasim, E.; Kharaba, A.; Albrahim, T.; Alshahrani, M.S.; et al. Effect of Helmet Noninvasive Ventilation vs Usual Respiratory Support on Mortality Among Patients with Acute Hypoxemic Respiratory Failure Due to COVID-19: The HELMET-COVID Randomized Clinical Trial. *JAMA* **2022**, *328*, 1063–1072. [CrossRef]
14. ARDS Definition Task Force; Ranieri, V.M.; Rubenfeld, G.D.; Thompson, B.T.; Ferguson, N.D.; Caldwell, E.; Fan, E.; Camporota, L.; Slutsky, A.S. Acute respiratory distress syndrome: The Berlin Definition. *JAMA* **2012**, *307*, 2526. [CrossRef]
15. Ji, D.; Zhang, D.; Xu, J.; Chen, Z.; Yang, T.; Zhao, P.; Chen, G.; Cheng, G.; Wang, Y.; Bi, J.; et al. Prediction for Progression Risk in Patients With COVID-19 Pneumonia: The CALL Score. *Clin. Infect. Dis.* **2020**, *71*, 1393–1399. [CrossRef] [PubMed]
16. Von Elm, E.; Altman, D.G.; Egger, M.; Pocock, S.J.; Gøtzsche, P.C.; Vandenbroucke, J.P. STROBE initiative. The Strengthening the Reporting of Observational Studies in Epidemiology (STROBE) statement: Guidelines for reporting observational studies. *Prev. Med.* **2007**, *45*, 247–251. [CrossRef] [PubMed]
17. Ruopp, M.D.; Perkins, N.J.; Whitcomb, B.W.; Schisterman, E.F. Youden Index and optimal cut-point estimated from observations affected by a lower limit of detection. *Biom. Z.* **2008**, *50*, 419–430. [CrossRef]
18. The Northwell COVID-19 Research Consortium; Richardson, S.; Hirsch, J.S.; Narasimhan, M.; Crawford, J.M.; McGinn, T.; Davidson, K.W.; Barnaby, D.P.; Becker, L.B.; Chelico, J.D.; et al. Presenting Characteristics, Comorbidities, and Outcomes Among 5700 Patients Hospitalized With COVID-19 in the New York City Area. *JAMA* **2020**, *323*, 2052–2059. [CrossRef]
19. Gujski, M.; Jankowski, M.; Rabczenko, D.; Goryński, P.; Juszczyk, G. The Prevalence of Acute Respiratory Distress Syndrome (ARDS) and Outcomes in Hospitalized Patients with COVID-19-A Study Based on Data from the Polish National Hospital Register. *Viruses* **2022**, *14*, 76. [CrossRef]
20. Tolossa, T.; Merdassa Atomssa, E.; Fetensa, G.; Bayisa, L.; Ayala, D.; Turi, E.; Wakuma, B.; Mulisa, D.; Seyoum, D.; Getahun, A.; et al. Acute respiratory distress syndrome among patients with severe COVID-19 admitted to treatment center of Wollega University Referral Hospital, Western Ethiopia. *PLoS ONE* **2022**, *17*, e0267835. [CrossRef]
21. Ciceri, F.; Castagna, A.; Rovere-Querini, P.; De Cobelli, F.; Ruggeri, A.; Galli, L.; Conte, C.; De Lorenzo, R.; Poli, A.; Ambrosio, A.; et al. Early predictors of clinical outcomes of COVID-19 outbreak in Milan, Italy. *Clin. Immunol.* **2020**, *217*, 108509. [CrossRef] [PubMed]
22. COVID-19 Treatment Guidelines Panel. Coronavirus Disease 2019 (COVID-19) Treatment Guidelines. National Institutes of Health. Available online: https://www.covid19treatmentguidelines.nih.gov/ (accessed on 7 August 2022).
23. Alhazzani, W.; Evans, L.; Alshamsi, F.; Møller, M.H.; Ostermann, M.; Prescott, H.C.; Arabi, Y.M.; Loeb, M.; Ng Gong, M.; Fan, E.; et al. Rhodes, Andrew Surviving Sepsis Campaign Guidelines on the Management of Adults With Coronavirus Disease 2019 (COVID-19) in the ICU: First Update. *Crit. Care Med.* **2021**, *49*, e219–e234. [CrossRef] [PubMed]
24. Frat, J.P.; Thille, A.W.; Mercat, A.; Girault, C.; Ragot, S.; Perbet, S.; Prat, G.; Boulain, T.; Morawiec, E.; Cottereau, A.; et al. REVA Network. High-flow oxygen through nasal cannula in acute hypoxemic respiratory failure. *N. Engl. J. Med.* **2015**, *372*, 2185–2196. [CrossRef] [PubMed]
25. Perkins, G.D.; Ji, C.; Connolly, B.A.; Couper, K.; Lall, R.; Baillie, J.K.; Bradley, J.M.; Dark, P.; Dave, C.; De Soyza, A.; et al. Effect of Noninvasive Respiratory Strategies on Intubation or Mortality Among Patients With Acute Hypoxemic Respiratory Failure and COVID-19: The RECOVERY-RS Randomized Clinical Trial. *JAMA* **2022**, *327*, 546–558. [CrossRef]
26. Suardi, L.R.; Pallotto, C.; Esperti, S.; Tazzioli, E.; Baragli, F.; Salomoni, E.; Botta, A.; Covani Frigieri, F.; Pazzi, M.; Stera, C.; et al. Risk factors for non-invasive/invasive ventilatory support in patients with COVID-19 pneumonia: A retrospective study within a multidisciplinary approach. *Int. J. Infect. Dis.* **2020**, *100*, 258–263. [CrossRef]
27. Brusasco, C.; Corradi, F.; Di Domenico, A.; Raggi, F.; Timossi, G.; Santori, G.; Brusasco, V.; Galliera CPAP-COVID-19 Study Group. Collaborators of the Galliera CPAP-COVID-19 study group are. Continuous positive airway pressure in COVID-19 patients with moderate-to-severe respiratory failure. *Eur. Respir. J.* **2021**, *57*, 2002524. [CrossRef]
28. Wagner, J.; Garcia-Rodriguez, V.; Yu, A.; Dutra, B.; Larson, S.; Cash, B.; DuPont, A.; Farooq, A. Elevated transaminases and hypoalbuminemia in Covid-19 are prognostic factors for disease severity. *Sci. Rep.* **2021**, *11*, 10308. [CrossRef]
29. Henry, B.M.; Aggarwal, G.; Wong, J.; Benoit, S.; Vikse, J.; Plebani, M.; Lippi, G. Lactate dehydrogenase levels predict coronavirus disease 2019 (COVID-19) severity and mortality: A pooled analysis. *Am. J. Emerg. Med.* **2020**, *38*, 1722–1726. [CrossRef]
30. Coomes, E.A.; Haghbayan, H. Interleukin-6 in COVID-19: A systematic review and meta-analysis. *Rev. Med. Virol.* **2020**, *30*, 1–9. [CrossRef]
31. L'Her, E.; Duquesne, F.; Girou, E.; de Rosiere, X.D.; Le Conte, P.; Renault, S.; Allamy, J.P.; Boles, J.M. Noninvasive continuous positive airway pressure in elderly cardiogenic pulmonary edema patients. *Intensive Care Med.* **2004**, *30*, 882–888. [CrossRef]
32. Lagier, J.C.; Amrane, S.; Mailhe, M.; Gainnier, M.; Arlotto, S.; Gentile, S.; Raoult, D. High-flow oxygen therapy in elderly patients infected with SARS-CoV2 with a contraindication for transfer to an intensive care unit: A preliminary report. *Int. J. Infect. Dis.* **2021**, *108*, 1–3. [CrossRef] [PubMed]
33. Peckham, H.; de Gruijter, N.M.; Raine, C.; Radziszewska, A.; Ciurtin, C.; Wedderburn, L.R.; Rosser, E.C.; Webb, K.; Deakin, C.T. Male sex identified by global COVID-19 meta-analysis as a risk factor for death and ITU admission. *Nat. Commun.* **2020**, *11*, 6317. [CrossRef] [PubMed]

34. Monserrat Villatoro, J.; Mejía-Abril, G.; Díaz García, L.; Zubiaur, P.; Jiménez González, M.; Fernandez Jimenez, G.; Cancio, I.; Arribas, J.R.; Suarez Fernández, C.; Mingorance, J.; et al. A Case-Control of Patients with COVID-19 to Explore the Association of Previous Hospitalisation Use of Medication on the Mortality of COVID-19 Disease: A Propensity Score Matching Analysis. *Pharmaceuticals* **2022**, *15*, 78. [CrossRef] [PubMed]
35. Yang, X.; Yang, Q.; Wang, Y.; Wu, Y.; Xu, J.; Yu, Y.; Shang, Y. Thrombocytopenia and its association with mortality in patients with COVID-19. *J. Thromb. Haemost.* **2020**, *18*, 1469–1472. [CrossRef]
36. Tetaj, N.; Piselli, P.; Zito, S.; De Angelis, G.; Marini, M.C.; Rubino, D.; Gaviano, I.; Antonica, M.V.; Agostini, E.; Porcelli, C.; et al. Timing and Outcomes of Noninvasive Ventilation in 307 ARDS COVID-19 Patients: An Observational Study in an Italian Third Level COVID-19 Hospital. *Medicina* **2022**, *58*, 1104. [CrossRef] [PubMed]
37. Grifoni, E.; Valoriani, A.; Cei, F.; Lamanna, R.; Gelli, A.M.G.; Ciambotti, B.; Vannucchi, V.; Moroni, F.; Pelagatti, L.; Tarquini, R.; et al. Interleukin-6 as prognosticator in patients with COVID-19. *J. Infect.* **2020**, *81*, 452–482. [CrossRef]
38. Santus, P.; Pini, S.; Amati, F.; Saad, M.; Gatti, M.; Mondoni, M.; Tursi, F.; Rizzi, M.; Chiumello, D.A.; Monzani, V.; et al. Predictors of Helmet CPAP Failure in COVID-19 Pneumonia: A Prospective, Multicenter, and Observational Cohort Study. *Can. Respir. J. 2022*, **2022**, 1499690. [CrossRef]
39. Bellani, G.; Grasselli, G.; Cecconi, M.; Antolini, L.; Borelli, M.; De Giacomi, F.; Bosio, G.; Latronico, N.; Filippini, M.; Gemma, M.; et al. Noninvasive Ventilatory Support of Patients with COVID-19 outside the Intensive Care Units (WARd-COVID). *Ann. Am. Thorac. Soc.* **2021**, *18*, 1020–1026. [CrossRef]
40. Zampieri, F.G.; Ferreira, J.C. Defining Optimal Respiratory Support for Patients with COVID-19. *JAMA* **2022**, *327*, 531–533. [CrossRef]

Disclaimer/Publisher's Note: The statements, opinions and data contained in all publications are solely those of the individual author(s) and contributor(s) and not of MDPI and/or the editor(s). MDPI and/or the editor(s) disclaim responsibility for any injury to people or property resulting from any ideas, methods, instructions or products referred to in the content.

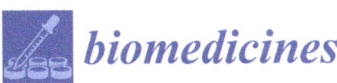

Case Report

COVID-19 Related Myocarditis and Myositis in a Patient with Undiagnosed Antisynthetase Syndrome

Daniel Duda-Seiman [1], Nilima Rajpal Kundnani [2,*], Daniela Dugaci [3], Dana Emilia Man [1], Dana Velimirovici [1] and Simona Ruxanda Dragan [1]

1. Department of Cardiology, "Victor Babes" University of Medicine and Pharmacy, 300041 Timisoara, Romania
2. Department of Functional Sciences, Physiology, Center of Immuno-Physiology and Biotechnologies (CIFBIOTEH), "Victor Babes" University of Medicine & Pharmacy, 300041 Timisoara, Romania
3. Institute of Cardiovascular Diseases, 300310 Timisoara, Romania
* Correspondence: knilima@umft.ro

Abstract: Background: The clinical presentation of SARS-CoV-2 varies from patient to patient. The most common findings noted were respiratory tract infections, of different severity grades. In some cases, multi-organ damage was noted. Due to its high potential for causing severe systemic inflammation such as myositis and myocarditis, patients should be properly investigated, which carries high chances of SARS-CoV-2 being easily missed if not investigated on time and which can result in more fatal outcomes. Case report: We present a case of COVID-19 infection in a non-vaccinated male patient, who presented to our clinic with no symptoms of respiratory involvement but with severe muscle aches. Cardiac markers and procalcitonin levels were high, and concentric hypertrophy of the left ventricle, severe hypokinesia of the interventricular septum and of the antero-lateral wall, hypokinesia of the inferior and posterior wall and an ejection fraction of the left ventricle being around 34% was noted. Coronary angiography showed no lesions. Corticosteroids and antibiotics were instituted which showed improvement. A possible link to an autoimmune process was suspected, due to the presence of anti-PL-7 antibody, suggesting an antisynthetase syndrome. Conclusion: Each and every patient should be thoroughly investigated, and presently little is known in regards to this virus. Studies focusing on possible relationships between the COVID-19 and autoimmune disease can help to potentially generate better outcomes.

Keywords: myocarditis; COVID-19; myositis; autoimmune diseases

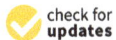

Citation: Duda-Seiman, D.; Kundnani, N.R.; Dugaci, D.; Man, D.E.; Velimirovici, D.; Dragan, S.R. COVID-19 Related Myocarditis and Myositis in a Patient with Undiagnosed Antisynthetase Syndrome. *Biomedicines* 2023, 11, 95. https://doi.org/10.3390/biomedicines11010095

Academic Editor: Elena Cecilia Rosca

Received: 14 December 2022
Revised: 27 December 2022
Accepted: 28 December 2022
Published: 30 December 2022

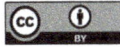

Copyright: © 2022 by the authors. Licensee MDPI, Basel, Switzerland. This article is an open access article distributed under the terms and conditions of the Creative Commons Attribution (CC BY) license (https://creativecommons.org/licenses/by/4.0/).

1. Introduction

COVID-19 was declared a global pandemic after the first case was detected in 2019, which led to a massive spread worldwide, infecting and affecting lives of millions of people with very high mortality rates [1–3]. Healthcare system around the globe were not prepared to fight this unprecedented situation, especially because very little was known about it, and no vaccinations or medications to prevent it were on hand. Many changes were instituted to separate entry and exit of the infected cases in most hospitals. WHO guidelines were issued to stop the spread of this devastating virus [3,4]. Surgical interventions were done only on an emergency basis, and elective surgeries were postponed [5]. The clinical presentation varied widely depending on different strains of the virus [6,7]. Few patients were found to be asymptomatic, while some had serious respiratory symptoms, to the extent that oxygen therapy was mandatory, while some developed multi-organ failure [7]. The vaccination programs were implemented as soon as they were approved by the WHO to minimize the spread. The use of pharmacological and non-pharmacological measures were evaluated and implemented on a large scale to combat the pandemic [8].

Angiotensin-converting enzyme 2 (ACE2) is crucial in cardiovascular neurohumoral regulation. The increased binding affinity of the SARS-CoV-2 virus to ACE2 receptors modifies the ACE2 signaling pathways, leading to acute myocardial injuries [9]. The cytokine release syndrome is the prerogative of severe forms of COVID-19. This extreme inflammatory response with high levels of cytokines determines systemic injuries, including endothelial and myocardial ones, as well as acute respiratory distress syndrome and various end-organ damage. Viral myocarditis might appear as a result of a direct myocardium infection [10]. From 8–62% of COVID-19 hospitalized patients show increased levels of cardiac troponins, as a consequence of acute cardiac injury. If echocardiographic changes are present, there is an increased risk of in-hospital mortality, which, fortunately, did not happen in our case. Common echocardiographic abnormalities are: left ventricular wall motion changes, global left ventricular systolic dysfunction, right ventricular dysfunction, pericardial effusion, and diastolic dysfunction [11]. There is a large clinical variety of presentations of COVID-19 myocarditis: from mild symptoms (fatigue, dyspnea), to severe situations with hemodynamic instability. Recent literature illustrates the possibility of variable evolution of the subject with myocardial injury in the context of SARS-CoV-2 infection. Patients with no or mild cardiac symptoms at the onset might develop acute heart failure and cardiogenic shock [12]. The Antisynthetase Syndrome (ASS) is a rare condition belonging to the Idiopathic Inflammatory Myopathies (IMS), which is quite difficult to diagnose. Its clinical presentation is heterogenous, with interstitial lung disease and/or inflammatory myositis, and with positive antisynthetase antibodies [13].

Here we present a non-vaccinated, infected COVID-19 male, who developed serious cardiac complications.

2. Case Details

A 62-year-old male patient, known to have primary hypertension and type 2 diabetes mellitus, presented with a brutal onset of loss of consciousness, muscle pain in the upper limbs accompanied by increased movement impairment. In the emergency department a rapid antigen test for SARS-CoV-2 was performed which was found to be positive. The patient had not been vaccinated against SARS-CoV-2. Clinical assessment showed no significant changes: BMI = 32.41 kg/m^2; BP = 140/85 mmHg; HR = 95 bpm with normal rhythmic heart beats; SpO$_2$ = 97% (room air); no fever; no pulmonary rales. Initial lab values showed increased inflammation (CRP = 59.5 mg/L), increased values of cardiac enzymes (hsTnI = 8248 ng/L) and possible sepsis (procalcitonin = 68.03 ng/L). The ECG showed no acute ischemic changes. A CT angiography of the pulmonary arteries was performed with the following result: cardiomegaly with contrast refluxed into the hepatic veins, pulmonary arteries with dimensions at the upper limits for normal values, homogeneously opacified, without acute pulmonary lesions. Considering these data, the patient underwent a standard cardiac ultrasound examination revealing concentric hypertrophy of the left ventricle, severe hypokinesia of the interventricular septum, of the anterior and antero-lateral wall, and hypokinesia of the inferior and posterior wall with an estimated ejection fraction of the left ventricle to be approximately 34% (Figure 1); global strain was −7.7% (Figure 2); systolic pressure in the pulmonary artery was 50 mmHg. Approximately 2 h after admission, the dynamics of myocardial necrosis was entertained, enzymes registered an increasing trend (hsTnI = 9755 ng/mL; CK = 51432 U/L; CK-MB = 189 U/L). As a result of the accumulated data, an acute coronary syndrome without ST segment elevation was suspected. The patient underwent coronary angiography using the right radial artery approach, in which the coronary arteries revealed no significant angiographic lesions. Figures 3 and 4 show the dynamics of hsTnI, CK and CK-MB.

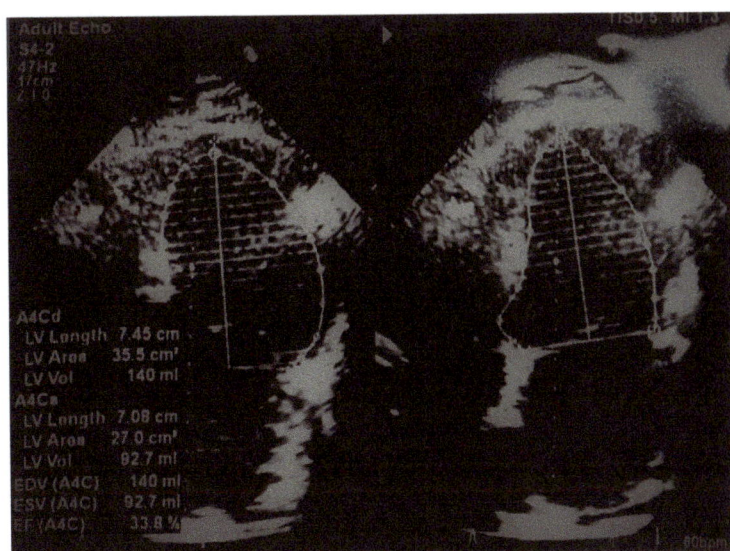

Figure 1. Apical 4-chambers (A4C) echocardiography: moderately decreased left ventricular ejection fraction (LV, left ventricle; EDV, end-diastolic volume; ESV, end-systolic volume; EF, ejection fraction).

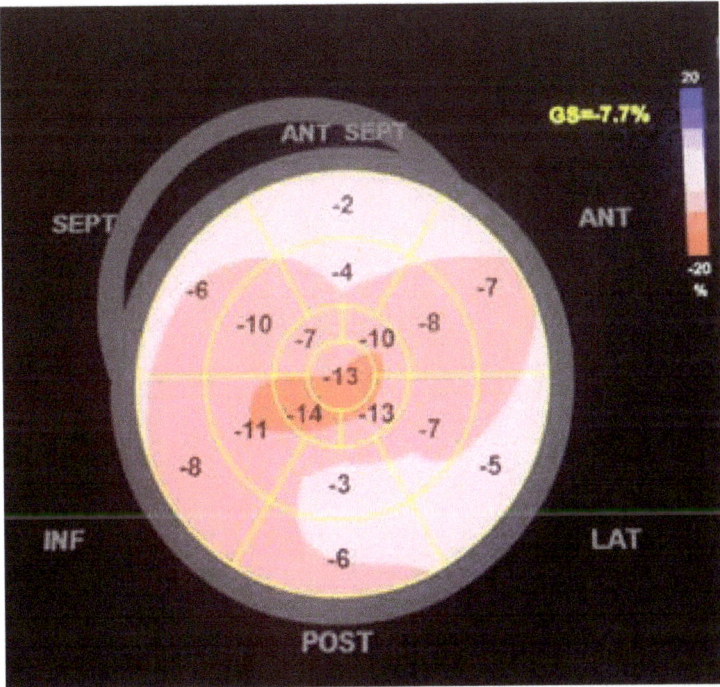

Figure 2. Global strain (GS) of the left ventricle: polar map with the regional values and the GS value calculated from the 17 segments of the left ventricle, which is significantly impaired (ANT, anterior; ANT SEPT, anteroseptal; GS, global strain; INF, inferior; LAT, lateral; POST, posterior; SEPT, septal).

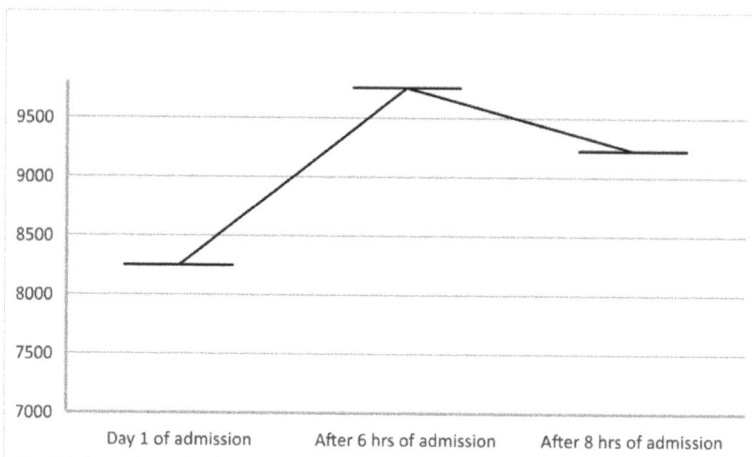

Figure 3. hsTnI (high sensitive I troponin) behavior during hospitalization.

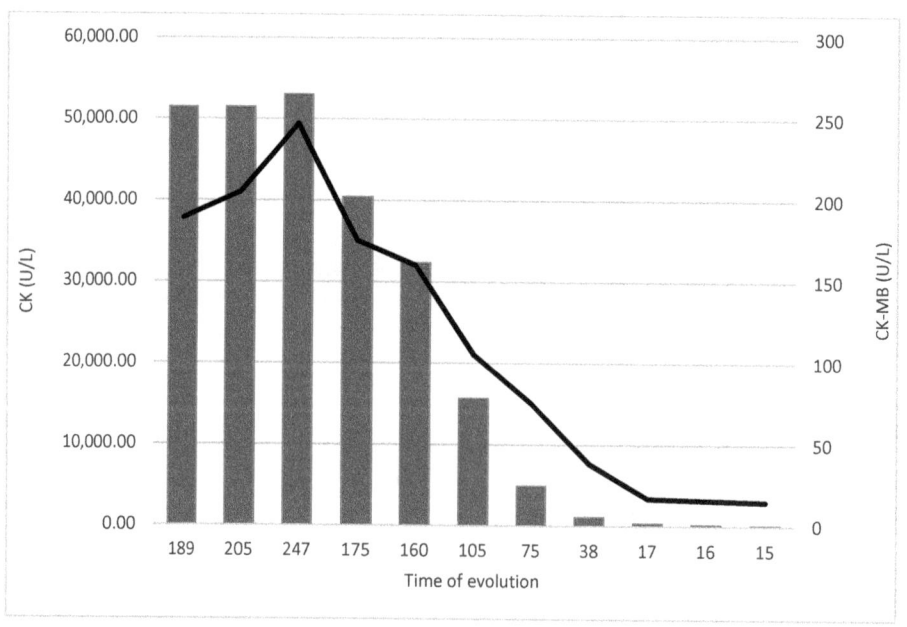

Figure 4. CK and CK-MB behavior during hospitalization. (CK, creatine phosphokinase; CK-MB, muscle-brain creatine phosphokinase isoenzyme).

Considering possible sepsis of unknown origin, antibiotics were initiated with ceftriaxone. A sputum culture was positive for Klebsiella pneumoniae spp pneumoniae, and ceftriaxone was continued according to the antibiogram. Blood cultures taken consecutively were negative. During day 3, a thorax CT scan was performed, which showed fine areas of ground glass arranged peripherally and classified as minimal lung damage (Figure 5) and small bilateral areas of pleurisy with a maximum thickness of 10 mm in the right costo-phrenic recess. Methylprednisolone was given, with progressive decreasing of the dose over time. Standard medication for heart failure with a reduced ejection fraction was given [14]. The serum level of interleukin-6 was 2.32 pg/mL, which was considered to be normal [15]. The evolution was favorable: cardiac enzymes, inflammatory markers and procalcitonin continued to decrease and eventually were normalized. Kidney function was preserved. The muscle pain in the upper limbs subsided, with full recovery of functionality. Patient tested negative for SARS-CoV-2 infection on day 14 (RT-PCR).

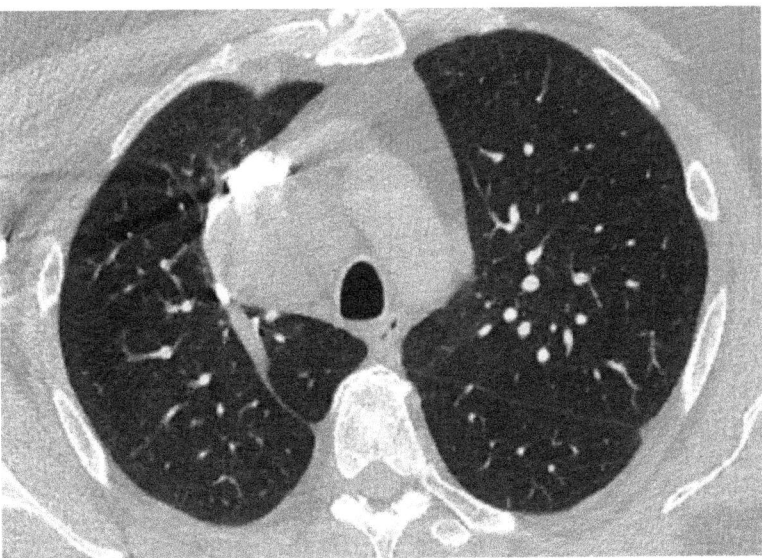

Figure 5. Native chest computer-tomography in the context of confirmed SARS-CoV-2 infection: fine areas of ground glass arranged peripherally classified as minimal lung damage.

Corroborating the clinical, paraclinical and biological context, the panel of IgG antibodies specific for myositis was observed, with a positive result for anti-PL-7 antibodies. We consider that the episode of myocarditis and extensive myositis was clinically triggered by the SARS-CoV-2 infection, possibly linked to his autoimmune status, which was unknown to the patient.

3. Discussion

This is a case of a patient diagnosed with COVID-19, not vaccinated against SARS-CoV-2 infection, with no respiratory symptoms, but with the presence of an inflammatory syndrome with skeletal and myocardial muscle damage. Intriguingly, symptomatology due to myocarditis and heart failure was lacking and a bacterial pulmonary superinfection did not produce classic clinical symptoms such as dyspnea, cough or fever. Laboratory assessment documented sepsis. Cytokine storm was not documented and specific biologic therapy was not considered.

As previously described [16], COVID-19 may be associated with an extreme inflammatory response of both skeletal muscles and the myocardium, with respiratory symptoms being poorly expressed or even absent. We considered that the muscle damage in this case was due to SARS-CoV-2 infection, previously reported by Pawar et al., who observed similar findings in their case study [17]. Myositis and myocarditis were reported, but post vaccination, which in our case, could not be correlated as our patient was unvaccinated [18]. Given its severity, we also considered investigating the potential of an underlying autoimmune condition for myositis for which the anti-PL-7 antibodies were positive. Of course, a muscular biopsy would have been necessary to further document the findings, but the patient refused. Myalgia and muscular weakness can be found quite frequently in COVID-19 patients (11–50%) [19], but an association with a connective tissue disorder is rare. It has been found that patients positive for anti-PL-7 or anti-PL-12 antibodies may develop a severe form of interstitial lung disease with myositis not being a frequent association [13]. More evidence is evolving, illustrating the fact that SARS-CoV-2 may induce different myopathies, while anti-PL-7 positive patients may clinically express dermatomyositis, during the course of a COVID-19 infection [20]. In the case of patients with known and therapy-controlled ASS, healing for COVID-19 infection was achieved if they were asymptomatic for acute COVID-19 and had at least one negative SARS-CoV-2 polymerase chain reaction test. Long-term evolution after COVID-19 in unvaccinated patients with ASS may be characterized by a worsening of the underlying condition (pulmonary hypertension, myocarditis) [21]. Momin and Nagori [22] presented the case of a female patient with family exposure to COVID-19 infection and vaccinated with the second dose of a mRNA vaccine. She developed symptoms (body ache/pain, dyspnea and leg swelling), but testing for SARS-CoV-2 infection was negative. Thorax computer tomography was suggestive for COVID-19. Laboratory findings were consistent for ASS. As in our case, ASS might be revealed by exposure to SARS-CoV-2 infection, corticosteroids being the treatment of choice for clinical and biological improvement.

Myositis-specific autoantibodies and myositis-associated autoantibodies should be determined in COVID-19 patients who present with clinical myositis. Autoimmunity might be caused by molecular triggers, or by a potential mechanism which primes an underlying predisposition, or by the COVID-19 induced immune dysfunction [23].

Cortico-therapy is beneficial by decreasing rhabdomyolysis and the inflammatory syndrome, consistent with literature data [13,16,19,20]. The COVID-19 pandemic led to increased diagnosis of anti-synthetase syndromes [24], which needs more investigation into the link between SARS-CoV-2 infections and autoimmune diseases.

4. Conclusions

Since the nature and clinical pattern is unclear and differs from patient to patient, physicians should leave no stone unturned while dealing with a COVID-19 positive patient. A thorough investigation is a must even in the absence of classical symptoms. More extensive studies are still required to better understand the link between the virus and different pathologies, especially in patients suffering from autoimmune diseases.

Author Contributions: D.D.-S. and N.R.K.: drafting and revising the manuscript, data curation, D.D.-S.: investigation and visualization. D.D. and D.E.M.: data collection and analysis, D.V. and S.R.D.: conceptualization and supervision. All authors have read and agreed to the published version of the manuscript.

Funding: This research received no external funding.

Institutional Review Board Statement: Not applicable.

Informed Consent Statement: Written informed consent was signed by the patient at the time of admission in the hospital, as a part of routine protocol. That his results will be used for research purposes respecting confidentiality norms.

Data Availability Statement: Data will be provided upon written request.

Conflicts of Interest: The authors declare no conflict of interest.

References

1. Tsai, S.C.; Lu, C.C.; Bau, D.T.; Chiu, Y.J.; Yen, Y.T.; Hsu, Y.M.; Fu, C.W.; Kuo, S.C.; Lo, Y.S.; Chiu, H.Y.; et al. Approaches towards fighting the COVID-19 pandemic (Review). *Int. J. Mol. Med.* **2021**, *47*, 3–22. [CrossRef] [PubMed]
2. Sreepadmanabh, M.; Sahu, A.K.; Chande, A. COVID-19, Advances in diagnostic tools, treatment strategies, and vaccine development. *J. Biosci.* **2020**, *45*, 148. [CrossRef] [PubMed]
3. Umakanthan, S.; Sahu, P.; Ranade, A.V.; Bukelo, M.M.; Rao, J.S.; Abrahao-Machado, L.F.; Dahal, S.; Kumar, H.; Kv, D. Origin, transmission, diagnosis and management of coronavirus disease 2019 (COVID-19). *Postgrad. Med. J.* **2020**, *96*, 753–758. [PubMed]
4. Muralidar, S.; Ambi, S.V.; Sekaran, S.; Krishnan, U.M. The emergence of COVID-19 as a global pandemic: Understanding the epidemiology, immune response and potential therapeutic targets of SARS-CoV-2. *Biochimie* **2020**, *179*, 85–100. [CrossRef]

5. Tunescu, M.; Christodorescu, R.; Sharma, A.; Barsac, C.R.; Rogobete, A.F.; Crisan, D.C.; Popovici, S.E.; Kundnani, N.R.; Sandesc, D.; Bedreag, O. The preoperative evaluation of post-COVID-19 patients scheduled for elective surgery-What is important not to miss! *Eur. Rev. Med. Pharmacol. Sci.* **2021**, *25*, 7607–7615.
6. Mocanu, V.; Bhagwani, D.; Sharma, A.; Borza, C.; Rosca, C.I.; Stelian, M.; Bhagwani, S.; Haidar, L.; Kshtriya, L.; Kundnani, N.R.; et al. COVID-19 and the Human Eye: Conjunctivitis, a Lone COVID-19 Finding-A Case-Control Study. *Med. Princ. Pract.* **2022**, *31*, 66–73. [CrossRef]
7. Parasher, A. COVID-19, Current understanding of its Pathophysiology, Clinical presentation and Treatment. *Postgrad. Med. J.* **2021**, *97*, 312–320. [CrossRef]
8. Horga, N.G.; Cirnatu, D.; Kundnani, N.R.; Ciurariu, E.; Parvu, S.; Ignea, A.L.; Borza, C.; Sharma, A.; Morariu, S. Evaluation of Non-Pharmacological Measures Implemented in the Management of the COVID-19 Pandemic in Romania. *Healthcare* **2022**, *10*, 1756. [CrossRef]
9. Soumya, R.S.; Unni, T.G.; Raghu, K.G. Impact of COVID-19 on the Cardiovascular System: A Review of Available Reports. *Cardiovasc. Drugs Ther.* **2021**, *35*, 411–425. [CrossRef]
10. Basu-Ray, I.; Almaddah, N.K.; Adeboye, A.; Soos, M.P. Cardiac Manifestations of Coronavirus (COVID-19). In *Treasure Island*; StatPearls Publishing LLC: Tampa, FL, USA, 2022.
11. Chung, M.K.; Zidar, D.A.; Bristow, M.R.; Cameron, S.J.; Chan, T.; Harding, C.V., 3rd; Kwon, D.H.; Singh, T.; Tilton, J.C.; Tsai, E.J.; et al. COVID-19 and Cardiovascular Disease: From Bench to Bedside. *Circ. Res.* **2021**, *128*, 1214–1236. [CrossRef]
12. Siripanthong, B.; Asatryan, B.; Hanff, T.C.; Chatha, S.R.; Khanji, M.Y.; Ricci, F.; Muser, D.; Ferrari, V.A.; Nazarian, S.; Santangeli, P.; et al. The Pathogenesis and Long-Term Consequences of COVID-19 Cardiac Injury. *JACC Basic Transl. Sci.* **2022**, *7*, 294–308. [CrossRef]
13. Blake, T.; Noureldin, B. Anti-PL-7 antisynthetase syndrome presenting as COVID-19. *Rheumatology* **2021**, *60*, e252–e254. [CrossRef]
14. McDonagh, T.A.; Metra, M.; Adamo, M.; Gardner, R.S.; Baumbach, A.; Böhm, M.; Burri, H.; Butler, J.; Čelutkienė, J.; Chioncel, O.; et al. 2021 ESC Guidelines for the diagnosis and treatment of acute and chronic heart failure: Developed by the Task Force for the diagnosis and treatment of acute and chronic heart failure of the European Society of Cardiology (ESC) With the special contribution of the Heart Failure Association (HFA) of the ESC. *Eur. Heart J.* **2021**, *42*, 3599–3726. [PubMed]
15. Zhang, J.; Hao, Y.; Ou, W.; Ming, F.; Liang, G.; Qian, Y.; Cai, Q.; Dong, S.; Hu, S.; Wang, W.; et al. Serum interleukin-6 is an indicator for severity in 901 patients with SARS-CoV-2 infection: A cohort study. *J. Transl. Med.* **2020**, *18*, 406. [CrossRef] [PubMed]
16. Shabbir, A.; Camm, C.F.; Elkington, A.; Tilling, L.; Stirrup, J.; Chan, A.; Bull, S. Myopericarditis and myositis in a patient with COVID-19, a case report. *Eur. Heart J. Case Rep.* **2020**, *4*, 1–6. [CrossRef] [PubMed]
17. Dushyant Pawar, K.P.; Nandini, N. A case of myocarditis and myositis following COVID19 vaccine. *J. Am. Coll. Cardiol.* **2022**, *79*, 2693. [CrossRef]
18. Durucan, I.; Guner, S.; Kilickiran Avci, B.; Unverengil, G.; Melikoglu, M.; Ugurlu, S. Post Covıd-19 Vaccınatıon Inflammatory Syndrome: A Case Report. *Mod. Rheumatol. Case Rep.* **2022**, *12*, rxac041. [CrossRef] [PubMed]
19. Beydon, M.; Chevalier, K.; Al Tabaa, O.; Hamroun, S.; Delettre, A.S.; Thomas, M.; Herrou, J.; Riviere, E.; Mariette, X. Myositis as a manifestation of SARS-CoV-2. *Ann. Rheum. Dis.* **2021**, *80*, e42. [CrossRef]
20. Shimizu, H.; Matsumoto, H.; Sasajima, T.; Suzuki, T.; Okubo, Y.; Fujita, Y.; Temmoku, J.; Yoshida, S.; Asano, T.; Ohira, H.; et al. New-onset dermatomyositis following COVID-19, A case report. *Front. Immunol.* **2022**, *13*, 1002329. [CrossRef]
21. Vertui, V.; Zanframundo, G.; Castañeda, S.; Biglia, A.; Palermo, B.L.; Cavazzana, I.; Meloni, F.; Cavagna, L. Clinical evolution of antisynthetase syndrome after SARS-CoV2 infection: A 6-month follow-up analysis. *Clin. Rheumatol.* **2022**, *41*, 2601–2604. [CrossRef]
22. Momin, E.; Nagori, M. Unusual case of anti-synthetase syndrome correlated with exposure to covid-19 infection or vaccine. *Chest* **2022**, *162*, A2165. [CrossRef]
23. Swartzman, I.; Gu, J.J.; Toner, Z.; Grover, R.; Suresh, L.; Ullman, L.E. Prevalence of Myositis-Specific Autoantibodies and Myositis-Associated Autoantibodies in COVID-19 Patients: A Pilot Study and Literature Review. *Cureus* **2022**, *14*, e29752. [CrossRef] [PubMed]
24. Phillips, B.; Martin, J.; Rhys-Dillon, C. Correction to: Increased incidence of anti synthetase syndrome during COVID-19 pandemic. *Rheumatology* **2022**, *61*, 3875. [CrossRef] [PubMed]

Disclaimer/Publisher's Note: The statements, opinions and data contained in all publications are solely those of the individual author(s) and contributor(s) and not of MDPI and/or the editor(s). MDPI and/or the editor(s) disclaim responsibility for any injury to people or property resulting from any ideas, methods, instructions or products referred to in the content.

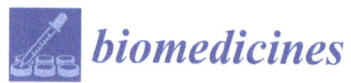

Article

Parosmia COVID-19 Related Treated by a Combination of Olfactory Training and Ultramicronized PEA-LUT: A Prospective Randomized Controlled Trial

Arianna Di Stadio [1,*,†], Elena Cantone [2,†], Pietro De Luca [3], Claudio Di Nola [2], Eva A. Massimilla [4], Giovanni Motta [4], Ignazio La Mantia [1] and Gaetano Motta [4]

[1] Department GF Ingrassia, Otolaryngology Unit, University of Catania, 95131 Catania, Italy
[2] Department of Otolaryngology, Federico II University, 80131 Naples, Italy
[3] Department of Otolaryngology, San-Giovanni Addolorata Hospital, 00100 Rome, Italy
[4] Department of Otolaryngology, Volvatellid University, 81055 Naples, Italy
* Correspondence: ariannadistadio@hotmail.com or arianna.distadio@unict.it
† These authors contributed equally to this work.

Abstract: During COVID-19 pandemic, clinicians have had to deal with an ever-increasing number of cases of olfactory disturbances after SARS-CoV-2 infections and in some people this problem persisted for long time after negativization from virus. This a prospective randomized controlled trial aims at evaluating the efficacy of ultramicronized palmitoylethanolamide (PEA) and Luteolin (LUT) (umPEA-LUT) and olfactory training (OT) compared to OT alone for the treatment of smell disorders in Italian post-COVID population. We included patients with smell loss and parosmia who were randomized and assigned to Group 1 (intervention group; daily treatment with umPEA-LUT oral supplement and OT) or Group 2 (control group; daily treatment with placebo and OT). All subjects were treated for 90 consecutive days. The Sniffin' Sticks identification test was used to assess the olfactory functions at the baseline (T0) and the end of the treatment (T1). Patients were queried regarding any perception of altered olfaction (parosmia) or aversive smell, such as cacosmia, gasoline-type smell, or otherwise at the same observational points. This study confirmed the efficacy of combination of umPEA-LUT and olfactory training as treatment of quantitative smell alteration COVID-19 related, but the efficacy of the supplement for parosmia was limited. UmpEA-LUT is useful for the treatment of brain neuro-inflammation (origin of quantity smell disorders) but has limited/no effect on peripheral damage (olfactory nerve, neuro-epithelium) that is responsible of quality disorders.

Keywords: smell loss; parosmia; qualitative smell disorders; treatment; PEA; olfactory training

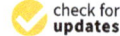

Citation: Di Stadio, A.; Cantone, E.; De Luca, P.; Di Nola, C.; Massimilla, E.A.; Motta, G.; La Mantia, I.; Motta, G. Parosmia COVID-19 Related Treated by a Combination of Olfactory Training and Ultramicronized PEA-LUT: A Prospective Randomized Controlled Trial. *Biomedicines* 2023, 11, 1109. https://doi.org/10.3390/biomedicines11041109

Academic Editors: Elena Cecilia Rosca and Amalia Cornea

Received: 5 March 2023
Revised: 29 March 2023
Accepted: 5 April 2023
Published: 6 April 2023

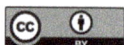

Copyright: © 2023 by the authors. Licensee MDPI, Basel, Switzerland. This article is an open access article distributed under the terms and conditions of the Creative Commons Attribution (CC BY) license (https://creativecommons.org/licenses/by/4.0/).

1. Introduction

Smell disorders are classically divided into two main categories, they can be quantitative and qualitative. Hyposmia and anosmia are quantitative disorders diagnosed and managed more easily than qualitative disorders namely parosmia and phantosmia, that are areas of research more open to interpretation. Unlike phantosmia, in which distorted smell detection occurs without any smell stimuli to trigger it, parosmia is a distortion of smell detection in the presence of smell stimuli. The two subtypes of parosmia are cacosmia, the detection of unpleasant smell and euosmia the detection of pleasant smell.

Although parosmia was an already known condition but with limited clinical interventions, it is only after the COVID pandemic that researchers have had to deal with an ever-increasing number of cases, thus contributing to an accumulation of knowledge and new approaches [1].

For instance, about 35% of people suffering from smell disorders are found to have parosmia, but the prevalence of smell disorders in COVID-19 infections are up to 75% and up to 45% for parosmia [2–5].

Generally, parosmia recovers in the first 1–2 months after the onset of symptoms but recent studies emphasize an improvement in parosmia even after 40 years of symptoms. [6]

The highly variable durations of parosmia explain why qualitative smell disorders require multiple approaches and treatments. This significant variation must induce clinicians to approach a therapeutic protocol even in cases of long-lasting parosmia. In addition, some patients could take up to 6 months to recover, so it is important to extend treatment duration [7,8].

Recent literature demonstrated that traditional treatment methods as olfactory training and steroids were rarely effective in the treatment of post-COVID parosmia highlighting the importance of finding new therapeutic approaches [9].

Because of the origin of parosmia and the absence of a treatment we speculated that a treatment by an anti-neuroinflammatory molecule could benefit. Di Stadio in 2022 [5] identified a high prevalence of parosmia in their patients affected by smell disorders COVID-19 related; the authors justified the presence of this symptom because of neuroinflammatory process in the olfactory bulbs [10,11]. The inflammation, in the authors opinion, negative impact on the recovery causing the persistence of the qualitative disorder [12].

Several authors showed the efficacy of umPEA-LUT to fight the inflammation caused by COVID-19 infection [13–15], as well as the ability of the molecule of inhibiting the penetration of the SARS-CoV-2 virus protecting people from the infection [16].

Different studies have shown the efficacy of combination between a supplement containing ultramicronized-palmytoiletanolamide and luteolin (umPEA-LUT) and olfactory training in ameliorating the quantitative smell alteration in patients who suffered from this persistent concern [17–19].

This randomized clinical trial aims at evaluating the efficacy of umPEA-LUT on the quality smell disorders in Italian post-COVID population suffering from parosmia following daily treatment with PEA-LUT and olfactory training compared to conventional therapy.

2. Materials and Methods

2.1. Study Population and Demographic Data

This prospective randomized controlled trial was conducted in a tertiary referral hospital of Naples from January 2022 to December 2022. A total of 130 people were included in this trial. The randomized controlled trials registration number is NCT04853836.

For patients' recruitment, we used both clinician communication and mass media. At the moment of recruitment, we assigned a number to the patient, and we elucidated that the study aim was to identify new methods for treating persistent loss of smell after COVID-19. We informed patients that after baseline assessment they would be re-checked after 90 days, with up to two possible intermediary olfactory assessments, as dictated by protocol. Patients were aware that their participation was voluntary and that they could leave the study at any time. To guarantee the blinding we divided the investigations in two; one physician, who did not know the assignation to the experimental group, performed the endoscopy to study the baseline condition (e.g., polyps or tumors), and another did olfactory testing using validated measures of threshold, discrimination, and identification scores. Self-report data on mental clouding/brain fog was also collected. The anonymized data were recorded on a protected Excel sheet [Google (Mountain View, CA, USA)].

Study participants were included or excluded based on the following criteria.

2.1.1. Inclusion Criteria

Inclusion criteria for outpatients were ages between 18 and 65 years, confirmed history of COVID-19 by positive nasopharyngeal swab for SARS-CoV-2), and anosmia/hyposmia identified by using the 16-pen version of the Sniffin' sticks psychophysical test (I score 0–16), olfactory impairment persisting ≥ 180 days (6 months) after sub-sequent negative

COVID-19 nasopharyngeal swab, acceptance to participate to the study by signature of written consent.

2.1.2. Exclusion Criteria

We identified specific exclusion criteria like history of smell and taste alterations, current or past alterations of memory or cognitive functions, current under chemotherapy or estaromatase, neuroinflammatory/neurodegenerative diseases in active phase, use of therapy able to alter smell and taste, active rhino-sinusitis including allergic and athropic rhinitis, previous chemo-radiotherapy in the head/neck, previous removal of tumor in nose or paranasal sinuses, recent history (<3 years) of stroke or moderate/severe head trauma, nasal septal deviation or turbinate hypertrophy, recent use of steroid nasal therapy within 30 days from the enrollment. The patients who were using drugs that could either independently reduce inflammation or interfere with PEA-LUT were excluded from the study.

2.2. Demographic Data Extraction

All this demographic information was collected for each patient included in the study: age, sex, time elapsed since negative COVID-19 test, prior treatment for olfactory disorders, presence of major disease, tobacco/alcohol use and medications. We designed a personal medical record to collect info about current and history of systemic diseases, including previous olfactory disorders or neuroinflammatory/neurodegenerative concerns, details about COVID as onset symptoms, swab results, treatments used, symptom persistence and COVID vaccine. The medical recorder also contained a section to annotate patient's self-perception of the smell alteration; we explained the differences and type of quantitative and qualitative smell alteration before asking for this specific info. After three from the beginning of the therapy the data of the patients who concluded the therapeutic scheme were extracted and analyzed by a statistician supervised by the study coordinator (ADS).

2.3. Experimental Groups

The consecutive patients enrolled in the study were assigned to 2 groups, as follows:

1. Intervention therapy (intervention group): Daily treatment with co-ultra-micronized PEA 700 mg and Luteolin 70 mg (umPEA-LUT) (Glialia ®, Epitech Group SpA, Milano, Italy) ultraPEA-LUT oral supplement and olfactory training. The oral supplement was prescribed as single dose to be assumed 5–10 min before breakfast in combination with daily olfactory training. The latter was done using four 100% organic essences of Lemon, Rose, Eucalyptus and Cloves three times a for 6 min each session; the olfactory stimulus consisted in smelling an odor for 4–6 s, then 40 s of relaxation, and then, new stimulation for 4–6 s with another odor. The short duration-stimulus was necessary to avoid "saturation" of the olfactory receptors [20]. This treatment was performed for 90 consecutive days.
2. Conventional therapy (control group): patients assigned to this group performed daily olfactory training exactly as previously described plus a placebo supplement therapy (multivitamin, vitamin D (400 UI), and/or alpha-lipoic acid (120 mg). The dosages used for vitamin D and of alpha-lipoic acid were selected based on an evidence-based literature review that showed these dosages did not have significant systemic anti-inflammatory, immunomodulatory, or antioxidant effects [13–15,18,19].

For ethical reason it was not possible to recruit patients and leave them without any treatment, creating in this way a "real" control group. By the way, because we included patients who were without treatment for at least 6 months; this could be supportive of the concept that without any treatment, neither OT nor supplement, there was no recovery and could justify this study design that compared traditional therapy (OT performed in control) and OT plus umPEA-LUT.

All patients performed their house-olfactory training (self-administered rehabilitation) after being adequately trained by the physician. Initially, the patients were trained in the hospital by face-to-face explanation on how to perform the sniffing exercise, practice performing the exercise. A written description on how to prepare the sniffing essence was given to each participants and for detailed instruction we provided a "YouTube" link (https://www.youtube.com/watch?v=Ri5YwM6EmWM; accessed on 1 January 2022). The video used was previously selected by the study coordinator and it was always the same for all patients.

To follow our participants and promote adherence to the study, members of clinic staff and physician regularly contacted people (1 contact each 15 days) by via phone calls, electronic communications, and office visits.

2.4. Nasal Endoscopy Assessment of Olfactory Dysfunction

A nasal endoscopy to exclude nasal conditions was always performed to identify conditions that could alter the olfactory functions or interfere with the treatment. In presence of conditions described in the exclusion criteria (for example nasal mass prior impaired smell, history of nasal/nasopharyngeal malignancy, history of radiation, or other anatomical abnormalities) the patients were excluded.

2.5. Assessment of Olfactory Dysfunction

The Sniffin' Sticks identification test was administered to assess olfactory function following a previously established protocol [16]. Briefly, clinicians used standard pen-like devices filled with odorants to score olfactory function and were blinded to the patients' experimental groups. During the odor identification task, participants were presented with 16 common odors. In multiple-choice format, participants were asked to select which of 4 odor labels matched the presented odor. Possible scores for odor identification ranged from 1–16. These scores were used classify olfactory function as anosmia (score <7), hyposmia (score from 7–14), or normosmia (score $\geq$14), and scores were then recorded for subsequent analysis.

2.6. Parosmia Evaluation

Patients after being educated about the quality alterations of the smell were asked about presence of parosmia (distorted perception of smell) or cacosmia (aversive smell like gasoline-type odor). This method, which modified the questionnaire used by Di Stadio et al. [11], was validate by De Luca et al. [19] on 100 patients.

2.7. Statistical Analysis

One-way ANOVA for repeated measures and Bonferroni-Holmes (BH) post-hoc tests were used to compare the results of the Sniffin' stick score at T0 and T1 between treatment and control groups. Chi-square (c) was used to compare nominal data represented by the changes or not of the parosmia after treatment considering both groups, and to evaluate the recovery based on the >3 points, <3 points, stable or worsening. Multi-linear regression analyses were performed to evaluate the effect of age, sex and TDI at T0 (x variables) on TDI at T1 (y variables).

Multi-linear regression including age, sex, smoke, TDI at T0 and TDI at T1 (x variables) and parosmia (y variable) were performed in each group to identify which of the parameters could affect the presence/absence of parosmia. p was considered significant < 0.05.

3. Results

A total of 130 patients were included in the study. Because the efficacy of combination between umPeaLut and olfactory training was known [12–15], the allocation of patients in the treatment was 4:2.7.

94 patients (49 women and 45 men, age average 36.7 ± 11.8) were assigned to the treatment group and 36 (21 women and 15 men, age average 50.5 ± 12.7) to the control group.

The patients in treatment group suffered from smell alteration for 8.8 ± 3.7 months average, patients in the control for 8.5 ± 2 months average.

Table 1 shows the demographic characteristics of the two groups including comorbidities and previous treatments performed for smell loss.

Table 1. Characteristic of patients of patients included in the study.

Variable	Group 1 (n = 94)	Group 2 (n = 36)
Mean age ± SD (range), yr	36.7 ± 11.8	50.5 ± 12.7
Gender—no (%)		
Female	49 (52%)	21 (58%)
Male	45 (48%)	15 (42%)
Smoking habits		
Smokers	14 (15%)	6 (16.6%)
Non-smokers	80 (85%)	18 (50%)
Comorbidities		
Hypertension	1 (1%)	2 (5%)
Thyroid Disorders	6 (6%)	2 (5.5%)
Allergy	5 (5%)	2 (5.5%)
Psychiatric disturbances	2 (2%)	6 (16%)
Time from symptoms onset (mean ± SD, range), months	8.8 ± 3.68 (3–15)	8.5 ± 1.97 (5–12)
Type of olfactory disfunction—no. (%)		
Anosmia	39 (41.5%)	8 (22%)
>Hyposmia alone	0 (0%)	14 (39%)
Parosmia/Cacosmia alone	7 (7.5%)	2 (5.5%)
Hyposmia ± Parosmia/Cacosmia	48 (51%)	14 (39%)
T0 Identification score (Sniffin' Sniff Test) (mean ± SD, range)	8.2 ± 2.7	9.6 ± 2.4
T1 Identification score (Sniffin' Sniff Test) (mean ± SD, range)	11.1 ± 2.2	10.1 ± 2.3

SD—standard deviation.

Most of the patients both in treatment (83) and in the control (33) did not perform brain MRI, however the ones who did, 11 in treatment and 6 in the control group did not show olfactory bulbs atrophy.

14 patients (14.9%) in the treatment group were smokers, 9 (27.2%) in control.

At the baseline (T0) 48 patients were anosmic and 46 hyposmic in the treatment group, while in the control group 12 were anosmic and 24 hyposmic.

The average Sniffin' score at the baseline (T0) was 8.2 ± 2.7 (CI95%: 2–15) in the patients assigned to the treatment group and 9.6 ± 2.4 (CI95%: 8–13) in the control. The difference between the two groups at the T0 was not statistically significant ($p > 0.05$).

The average Sniffin' score at T1 was 11.1 ± 2.2 in the treatment group and 10.1 ± 2.3 in the control.

In the treatment group, despite sex, age and TDI at T0 influenced the Sniffin' score at T1 ($p < 0.00001$), the only variable that had statistically significant impact on the final results was the Sniffing score at T0 ($p < 0.00001$).

In the control, despite sex, age and TDI at T0 affected the Sniffin' score at T1 ($p = 0.0009$), as well as observed in the treatment group, the only variable that had statistically significant impact on the Sniffin' score at T1 was the Sniffing score at T0 ($p = 0.009$).

We identified statistically significant differences comparing T0 and T1 in the treatment group (ANOVA: $p < 0.0001$; BH: $p < 0.01$), but not statistically significant difference comparing the Sniffin' score at T0 and T1 in the control (HB: $p > 0.05$). Statistically significant differences were observed between treatment and control (HB: $p < 0.05$) at T1(Figure 1).

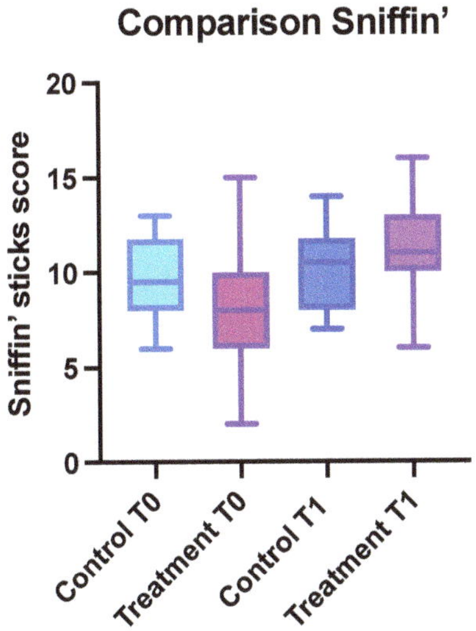

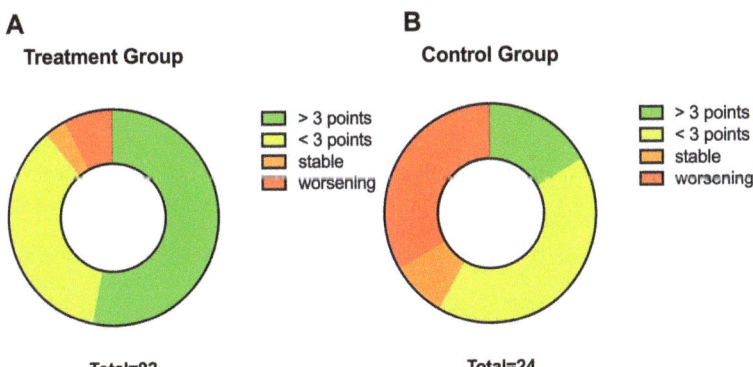

Figure 1. Comparison between the Sniffin' Score at T0 and T1 both in the treatment group and in control group. A statistically significant difference was observed T0 and T1 in the treatment group (ANOVA: $p < 0.0001$; BH: $p < 0.01$), and between treatment and control group at T1 (HB: $p < 0.05$) but not statistically significant difference comparing the Sniffin' score at T0 and T1 in the control (HB: $p > 0.05$).

49 patients (52.1%) in the treatment (average 11.4 ± 2.5, CI95%: 8–16) and 6 (18.2%) in the control (average 10.5 ± 0.7; CI95% 10–11) recovered more than 3 points at T1. 33 (35.1%) in the treatment (average 10.6 ± 1.7, CI95%: 8–13) and 15 (45.4%) in the control recovered less than 3 points. 3 patients (3.2%) in the treatment group did not change they score comparing T0 and T1 (average 12.6 ± 0.6, CI95%: 12–13), while in the control group three subjects (9.1%). Finally, we observed 7 patients (7.4%) in the treatment group that worsened their Sniffin' score comparing T0 and T1 (average 10.6 ± 2.5, CI95%: 6–14) and 12 (36.4%) in the control presented the same concern (average 8.5 ± 2.4, CI95%: 7–12). The differences between treatment and control in term of recovery were statistically significant (c: $p = 0.0008$) (Figure 2A,B).

Figure 2. This figure shows the comparative results in term of recovery between the treatment group and the control group. (**A**) the graph shows the results obtained in the treatment group; (**B**) the figure illustrates the results in the control group.

The totality of the patients in both groups had associated parosmia before the treatment. After treatment 58 patients (61.7%) in the treatment group and 21 (58.3%) in the control resolved the parosmia. The difference was not statistically significant (χ: $p = 0.3$) between treatment and control at T1 (Figure 3).

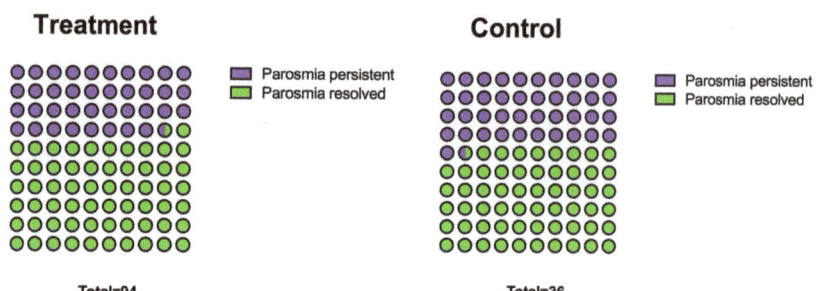

Figure 3. Comparison between the patients who recovered from parosmia in treatment group and in control group; the difference was not statistically significant (χ: $p = 0.3$).

The multilinear regression analysis showed that in the treatment group the score of the Sniffin' score at T1 were not correlated to the resolution of the parosmia ($p = 0.06$), while in the control this was related to the age ($p = 0.0007$) and the Sniffin'score at T0 ($p = 0.02$).

4. Discussion

This prospective randomized controlled trial confirmed the efficacy of combination between olfactory training and umPEA-LUT as treatment of quantitative post COVID smell disorders; the efficacy of the treatment on qualitative smell disorders should be deeply investigated because several co-factors other than the Sniffn'scores can impact on the persistence or resolution of parosmia after treatment.

Based on the hypothesis that quantitative smell disorders could be related to the inflammation in the olfactory bulbs, while qualitative disorders might be caused by the damage of neuro-epithelium [5] the absence of statistically significant difference regarding the recovery from parosmia that we observed was totally predictable. On the other hand, Di Stadio et al. speculated that the use of umPEA-LUT might help even in case of parosmia because the qualitative disorders might be also caused by an abnormal regeneration of the olfactory nerve; our study, despite preliminary because performed on a small sample of patients, seems confirming the hypothesis that neuro-epithelium is responsible of parosmia. UmPEA-LUT is a drug active on the central structures (olfactory bulbs) rather than on the peripheral ones (olfactory nerve and neuro-epithelium) [18] and this can explain why, despite an important effect on the recovery of the smell, the compound did not do the difference on the quality of odors perception between treatment and control groups.

In this study, patients in the treatment group started with worsen quantitative smell problems than control (respectively 8.2 ± 2.7 and 9.6 ± 2.4); however, despite that, the patients in the treatment group recovered as well as the ones in the control, but with more homogeneous scores (lower standard deviation than control). All subjects included were affected by olfactory disorders from 8.5 months at least (8.8 treatment and 8.5 control) so part of the recovery might be spontaneous; in fact, some authors reported recovery of olfactory functions by spontaneous recovery within two years [21] but the authors did not reported info about the SS. Moreover, in this study over 60% of patients did not recover fully olfactory capacities. Probably the concept of spontaneous recovery should be re-evaluated even considering that the treatment with umPEA-LUT and olfactory training allowed the return to normal olfactory function in over 60% of patients as previously showed [18].

This current study confirms the efficacy of the Di Stadio et al. protocol [14,15]; 80% patients treated with umPEA-LUT improved their SS in most of cases with gain over

3 points. On the contrary, in control less than 25% of patients recovered over 3 points and the likelihood of worsening was around 30%.

We noted that the only variable that affected the SS at T1 both in the control and treatment group with statistically significant impact was the score that patients had at the baseline (T0); this result confirms previous studies that did not identify an effect of the age and gender on the recovery of the olfactory function in young population (<60 ies) [2,3,18,20].

Anyway, although only SS at T1 was correlated (not statistically significant p) with the resolution of parosmia, no statistically significant differences for this finding were observed between treatment and control. In the latter the resolution of the qualitative disorder was correlated (with statistically significant p) with age and SS at T0. Because patients in control were younger than treatment and McWilliams et al. showed that in patients <40 spontaneously recovery of smell is likely [21], the improvement of parosmia in the control could be related to the young age rather than to the olfactory training. Additional study with the same design but with homogeneous ages among groups should be performed to understand if umPEA-LUT could really benefit the qualitative smell problems [21].

Although only few patients performed brain MRI both in the treatment and control group, in none of them we identified an atrophy of the olfactory bulbs. The atrophy of these structures was identified as negative prognostic factors in the recovery of normal olfactory functions [22]. Other authors showed that a change in the shape of the olfactory bulbs [23], without atrophy, could be observed in patients with post-COVID anosmia. The authors speculated that these changes could be related to the neuro-inflammation [23] and this could explain why, despite absence of atrophy, the patients in our sample suffered from anosmia. The use of umPEA-LUT, which reduces neuro-inflammation [13–15,18,19], improved the quantitative smell functions in our patients; additional study using 3T MRI and/or functional MRI focused on the olfactory bulbs could elucidate the mechanism of action of the supplement.

Overall, this study confirmed the efficacy of the combination of umPEA-LUT and olfactory training to recover quantitative olfactory functions, but additional study with age and sex stratification should be performed to understand the benefit of this treatment for qualitative disorders.

Our group is currently testing a new combination of supplements (umPEA-LUT and alpha-lipoic acid) to solve both quantitative and qualitative smell problems.

Limitations of the Study

The present study has some limitations. First, we only did odor identification, and the lack of a comprehensive battery of olfactory assessments incorporating thresholds and discrimination (complete TDI score) it is extremely important especially in patients with parosmia. Second, we used a previously published method for measuring parosmia, but this tool is not well-validated due to the limited published experience with COVID-19 parosmia, and it relies on subjective patient assessments. Third, the number of patients quite differed between the treatment group and the control group, and this disproportion could affect our results. Last, there is a significant difference between the mean age of the two groups, and this could be another confounding factor.

Despite these limitations, the prospective nature of the study, the presence of control group, the strengthens of the statistical analysis, and the promising results are the strengths of the present analysis.

5. Conclusions

This study confirmed the efficacy of combination of umPEA-LUT and olfactory training as treatment of quantitative smell alteration COVID-19 related. The results we obtained regarding the efficacy of the same treatment on parosmia are limited and their interpretation has been impacted by the difference in age average among the groups. In fact, control group included younger patients than treatment, who could have benefit by spontaneous recovery which is less likely in patients over 40 ies; this finding was confirmed by the identification of age and sniffing score at T0 as elements that impacted on the parosmia resolution. Additional studies comparing patients with same age are necessary to understand if umPEA-LUT might be helpful for the treatment of qualitative smell alterations.

Moreover, we are currently evaluating a combination between umPEA-LUT and alpha lipoic acid to understand if this combination of supplements associated with olfactory training can help to recovery full sense of smell.

Author Contributions: Conceptualization, A.D.S. and E.C.; methodology A.D.S.; validation, A.D.S., E.C., I.L.M., G.M. (Gaetano Motta); formal analysis, A.D.S., P.D.L.; investigation E.C., C.D.N., E.A.M., G.M. (Giovanni Motta); data curation, A.D.S.; writing—original draft preparation, A.D.S., E.C.; writing—review and editing, P.D.L., E.A.M., I.L.M.; Supervision E.C., A.D.S., I.L.M., G.M. (Gaetano Motta). All authors have read and agreed to the published version of the manuscript.

Funding: This research received no external funding.

Institutional Review Board Statement: The study was conducted in accordance with the Declaration of Helsinki, and approved by the Institutional Review Board of Federico II hospital (NA010122).

Informed Consent Statement: Informed consent was obtained from all subjects involved in the study.

Data Availability Statement: Data are available under request to the corresponding author.

Acknowledgments: Thanks to Thomas Hummel that supported us in the statistical analyses of the data.

Conflicts of Interest: The authors declare no conflict of interest.

References

1. Altundag, A. Parosmia and Phantosmia: Managing Quality Disorders. *Curr. Otorhinolaryngol. Rep.* **2023**, *11*, 19–26. [CrossRef]
2. Ohla, K.; Veldhuizen, M.G.; Green, T.; Hannum, M.E.; Bakke, A.J.; Moein, S.T.; Tognetti, A.; Postma, E.M.; Pellegrino, R.; Hwang, D.L.D.; et al. A follow-up on quantitative and qualitative olfactory dysfunction and other symptoms in patients recovering from COVID-19 smell loss. *Rhinol. J.* **2022**, *60*, 207–2017. [CrossRef]
3. Lechien, J.R.; Vaira, L.A.; Saussez, S. Prevalence and 24-month recovery of olfactory dysfunction in COVID-19 patients: A multicenter prospective study. *J. Intern. Med.* **2022**, *293*, 82–90. [CrossRef]
4. Pellegrino, R.; Mainland, J.D.; Kelly, C.E.; Parker, J.K.; Hummel, T. Prevalence and correlates of parosmia and phantosmia among smell disorders. *Chem. Senses* **2021**, *46*, bjab046. [CrossRef]
5. Di Stadio, A.; D'Ascanio, L.; La Mantia, I.; Ralli, M.; Brenner, M.J. Parosmia after COVID-19: Olfactory training, neuroinflammation and distortions of smell. *Eur. Rev. Med. Pharmacol. Sci.* **2022**, *26*, 1–3. [CrossRef]
6. Philpott, C.; Dixon, J.; Boak, D. Qualitative Olfactory Disorders: Patient Experiences and Self-Management. *Allergy Rhinol.* **2021**, *12*, 215265672110042. [CrossRef]
7. Altundag, A.; Cayonu, M.; Kayabasoglu, G.; Salihoglu, M.; Tekeli, H.; Saglam, O.; Hummel, T. Modified olfactory training in patients with postinfectious olfactory loss. *Laryngoscope* **2015**, *125*, 1763–1766. [CrossRef]
8. Altundag, A.; Yilmaz, E.; Kesimli, M.C. Modified Olfactory Training Is an Effective Treatment Method for COVID-19 Induced Parosmia. *Laryngoscope* **2022**, *132*, 1433–1438. [CrossRef]
9. Gary, J.B.; Gallagher, L.; Joseph, P.V.; Reed, D.; Gudis, D.A.; Overdevest, J.B. Qualitative Olfactory Dysfunction and COVID-19: An Evidence-Based Review with Recommendations for the Clinician. *Am. J. Rhinol. Allergy* **2023**, *37*, 95–101. [CrossRef]
10. Ralli, M.; Di Stadio, A.; Greco, A.; De Vincentiis, M.; Polimeni, A. Defining the burden of olfactory dysfunction in COVID-19 patients. *Eur. Rev. Med. Pharmacol. Sci.* **2020**, *24*, 3440–3441.
11. Di Stadio, A.; D'Ascanio, L.; De Luca, P.; Roccamatisi, D.; La Mantia, I.; Brenner, M.J. Hyperosmia after COVID-19: Hedonic perception or hypersensitivity? *Eur. Rev. Med. Pharmacol. Sci.* **2022**, *26*, 2196–2200.
12. Ferreli, F.; Gaino, F.; Russo, E.; Di Bari, M.; Rossi, V.; De Virgilio, A.; Di Stadio, A.; Spriano, G.; Mercante, G. Long-term olfactory dysfunction in COVID-19 patients: 18-month follow-up study. *Int. Forum Allergy Rhinol.* **2022**, *12*, 1078–1080. [CrossRef]
13. Noce, A.; Albanese, M.; Marrone, G.; Di Lauro, M.; Pietroboni Zaitseva, A.; Palazzetti, D.; Guerriero, C.; Paolino, A.; Pizzenti, G.; Di Daniele, F.; et al. Ultramicronized Palmitoylethanolamide (um-PEA): A New Possible Adjuvant Treatment in COVID-19 patients. *Pharmaceuticals* **2021**, *14*, 336. [CrossRef]
14. Albanese, M.; Marrone, G.; Paolino, A.; Di Lauro, M.; Di Daniele, F.; Chiaramonte, C.; D'Agostini, C.; Romani, A.; Cavaliere, A.; Guerriero, C.; et al. Effects of Ultramicronized Palmitoylethanolamide (um-PEA) in COVID-19 Early Stages: A Case–Control Study. *Pharmaceuticals* **2022**, *15*, 253. [CrossRef]
15. Roncati, L.; Lusenti, B.; Pellati, F.; Corsi, L. Micronized/ultramicronized palmitoylethanolamide (PEA) as natural neuroprotector against COVID-19 inflammation. *Prostaglandins Other Lipid Mediat.* **2021**, *154*, 106540. [CrossRef]

16. Fonnesu, R.; Thunuguntla, V.B.S.C.; Veeramachaneni, G.K.; Bondili, J.S.; La Rocca, V.; Filipponi, C.; Spezia, P.G.; Sidoti, M.; Plicanti, E.; Quaranta, P.; et al. Palmitoylethanolamide (PEA) Inhibits SARS-CoV-2 Entry by Interacting with S Protein and ACE-2 Receptor. *Viruses* **2022**, *14*, 1080. [CrossRef]
17. D'Ascanio, L.; Vitelli, F.; Cingolani, C.; Maranzano, M.; Brenner, M.J.; Di Stadio, A. Randomized clinical trial "olfactory dysfunction after COVID-19: Olfactory rehabilitation therapy vs. intervention treatment with Palmitoylethanolamide and Luteolin": Preliminary results. *Eur. Rev. Med. Pharmacol. Sci.* **2021**, *25*, 4156–4162.
18. Di Stadio, A.; D'Ascanio, L.; Vaira, L.A.; Cantone, E.; De Luca, P.; Cingolani, C.; Motta, G.; De Riu, G.; Vitelli, F.; Spriano, G.; et al. Ultramicronized Palmitoylethanolamide and Luteolin Supplement Combined with Olfactory Training to Treat Post-COVID-19 Olfactory Impairment: A Multi-Center Double-Blinded Randomized Placebo-Controlled Clinical Trial. *Curr. Neuropharmacol.* **2022**, *20*, 2001–2012. [CrossRef]
19. De Luca, P.; Camaioni, A.; Marra, P.; Salzano, G.; Carriere, G.; Ricciardi, L.; Pucci, R.; Montemurro, N.; Brenner, M.J.; Di Stadio, A. Effect of Ultra-Micronized Palmitoylethanolamide and Luteolin on Olfaction and Memory in Patients with Long COVID: Results of a Longitudinal Study. *Cells* **2022**, *11*, 2552. [CrossRef]
20. Oleszkiewicz, A.; Schriever, V.A.; Croy, I.; Hähner, A.; Hummel, T. Updated Sniffin' Sticks normative data based on an extended sample of 9139 subjects. *Eur. Arch. Oto Rhino Laryngol.* **2019**, *276*, 719–728. [CrossRef]
21. McWilliams, M.P.; Coelho, D.H.; Reiter, E.R.; Costanzo, R.M. Recovery from COVID-19 smell loss: Two-years of follow up. *Am. J. Otolaryngol.* **2022**, *43*, 103607. [CrossRef]
22. Aragão, M.; Leal, M.; Filho, O.C.; Fonseca, T.; Valença, M. Anosmia in COVID-19 Associated with Injury to the Olfactory Bulbs Evident on MRI. *Am. J. Neuroradiol.* **2020**, *41*, 1703–1706. [CrossRef]
23. Kandemirli, S.G.; Altundag, A.; Yildirim, D.; Sanli, D.E.T.; Saatci, O. Olfactory Bulb MRI and Paranasal Sinus CT Findings in Persistent COVID-19 Anosmia. *Acad. Radiol.* **2021**, *28*, 28–35. [CrossRef]

Disclaimer/Publisher's Note: The statements, opinions and data contained in all publications are solely those of the individual author(s) and contributor(s) and not of MDPI and/or the editor(s). MDPI and/or the editor(s) disclaim responsibility for any injury to people or property resulting from any ideas, methods, instructions or products referred to in the content.

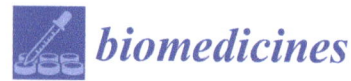

Systematic Review

Parsonage-Turner Syndrome Following SARS-CoV-2 Infection: A Systematic Review

Amalia Cornea [1,2], Irina Lata [2], Mihaela Simu [1,2] and Elena Cecilia Rosca [1,2,*]

1. Department of Neurology, Victor Babes University of Medicine and Pharmacy Timisoara, Eftimie Murgu Sq. no. 2, 300041 Timisoara, Romania
2. Department of Neurology, Clinical Emergency County Hospital Timisoara, Bd. Iosif Bulbuca no. 10, 300736 Timisoara, Romania
* Correspondence: roscacecilia@yahoo.com; Tel.: +40-746-173-794

Abstract: Parsonage-Turner syndrome (PTS) is an inflammatory disorder of the brachial plexus. Hypothesized underlying causes focus on immune-mediated processes, as more than half of patients present some antecedent event or possible predisposing condition, such as infection, vaccination, exercise, or surgery. Recently, PTS was reported following the severe acute respiratory syndrome coronavirus 2 (SARS-CoV-2) infection. We aimed to investigate data on PTS triggered by SARS-CoV-2 infection to provide an extensive perspective on this pathology and to reveal what other, more specific, research questions can be further addressed. In addition, we aimed to highlight research gaps requiring further attention. We systematically reviewed two databases (LitCOVID and the World Health Organization database on COVID-19) to January 2023. We found 26 cases of PTS in patients with previous SARS-CoV-2 infection. The clinical and paraclinical spectrum was heterogeneous, ranging from classical PTS to pure sensory neuropathy, extended neuropathy, spinal accessory nerve involvement, and diaphragmatic palsy. Also, two familial cases were reported. Among them, 93.8% of patients had severe pain, 80.8% were reported to present a motor deficit, and 53.8% of patients presented muscle wasting. Paresthesia was noted in 46.2% of PTS individuals and a sensory loss was reported in 34.6% of patients. The present systematic review highlights the necessity of having a high index of suspicion of PTS in patients with previous SARS-CoV-2 infection, as the clinical manifestations can be variable. Also, there is a need for a standardized approach to investigation and reporting on PTS. Future studies should aim for a comprehensive assessment of patients. Factors including the baseline characteristics of the patients, evolution, and treatments should be consistently assessed across studies. In addition, a thorough differential diagnosis should be employed.

Keywords: Parsonage-Turner syndrome; neuralgic amyotrophy; SARS-CoV-2; COVID-19; systematic review

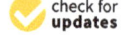

Citation: Cornea, A.; Lata, I.; Simu, M.; Rosca, E.C. Parsonage-Turner Syndrome Following SARS-CoV-2 Infection: A Systematic Review. *Biomedicines* **2023**, *11*, 837. https://doi.org/10.3390/biomedicines11030837

Academic Editor: Romina Salpini

Received: 21 February 2023
Revised: 7 March 2023
Accepted: 8 March 2023
Published: 9 March 2023

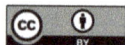

Copyright: © 2023 by the authors. Licensee MDPI, Basel, Switzerland. This article is an open access article distributed under the terms and conditions of the Creative Commons Attribution (CC BY) license (https://creativecommons.org/licenses/by/4.0/).

1. Introduction

Neuralgic amyotrophy, or Parsonage-Turner syndrome (PTS), is a peripheral nervous system disorder with two prominent features: severe pain and significant muscle atrophy. The symptoms primarily affect the forequarter region of the body, including the cranial, shoulder, upper limb, and ipsilateral chest wall. A precipitating antecedent event, or a trigger, can be recognized in most cases.

In the mid-1800, two separate disorders, serratus magnus paralysis and post-infectious paralysis, were initially described, indicating the muscle involved (serratus anterior) and that the syndrome followed an infection. Subsequently, two other entities were reported: serogenic neuropathy and vaccinogenic neuropathy, relating to their presumed triggers. Later, several other entities were identified and labeled with terms relevant to their location, pathology, or trigger. In 1948, Parsonage and Turner recognized the common characteristics of these conditions, concluding that they represented a single entity with various presentations [1]. They coined the term neuralgic amyotrophy based on recognizing these two major clinical features: severe pain and significant muscle wasting. Ultimately, a unifying clinical triad was identified: an antecedent event or trigger, sudden onset of intense forequarter region pain, and severe weakness and wasting of regional muscles. Nowadays, it is widely recognized that these disorders represent phenotypic variations of a single syndrome.

1.1. Epidemiology

Traditionally, PTS has been considered a rare disorder, with an annual incidence estimated at 1.64 cases per 100,000 population [2]. Nonetheless, the actual incidence is much higher, as the condition is underrecognized. A prospective study reported an incidence of 1 case per 1000 population [3]. PTS presents two major forms: sporadic and hereditary. The sporadic form is more frequent, affecting primarily young to middle-aged adults, with a mean age of onset of 40 years; the male-to-female ratio has been reported to be 2–2.3 [4]. The hereditary form has a mean age of onset of 25 years [4].

1.2. Clinical Presentation

Van Alfen and van Engelen presented one of the most comprehensive case series of PTS to date. They reported on 246 patients in a tertiary care setting [3], defining the typical clinical characteristics of PTS. In this series, PTS manifested with the primary onset of severe neuropathic pain, followed by patchy upper limb paresis, ranging from isolated anterior interosseous nerve palsy to severe bilateral paresis of both upper limbs. Nonetheless, despite significant variations in presentation, the triad comprising of (i) a recognized trigger, (ii) forequarter region pain, and (iii) forequarter region muscle weakness and wasting are distinctive, enabling easy diagnosis. Even if the triad is incomplete, PTS is typically identified based on the two most significant clinical features (severe pain, muscle weakness, and/or atrophy) that are almost invariably present. Although most patients report focal pain as the primary chief complaint, a focal sensory loss is rarely found; when present, it is usually minor. Accordingly, the neurologic examination abnormalities primarily involve the motor system [5].

The pain typically has a sudden onset; usually, it awakens the patient from sleep or is noted immediately upon awakening. The pain increases in intensity over several hours. Due to its severity, it leads the patient to seek medical attention promptly. The pain is exacerbated by movements of the shoulder or the upper extremity. Notably, it is not aggravated by head or neck movement, differentiating it from acute radiculopathies. After 1–2 weeks, the symptom resolves or is replaced by dull aching pain. Despite severe pain, cutaneous sensory axon involvement producing numbness is rare [6].

Forequarter motor deficit and muscle wasting follow the pain. The symptoms are generally identified when the pain subsides and the patient starts to use the affected limb. The weakness is sometimes not initially noted; muscle atrophy is the identified feature. Muscle wasting usually appears within a few weeks of the PTS onset. Rarely, weakness and atrophy might be absent.

1.3. Etiology and Pathophysiology

Triggering events are reported to be associated with at least 50% of PTS cases. The most common is an upper respiratory infection or influenza-like illness. Bacterial infections that may trigger PTS include pneumonia, malaria, typhus, diphtheria, rheumatic fever, borreliosis, dysentery, sepsis, rickettsia coroni, and bartonella henselae (cat claw). Among viruses, influenza, cytomegalovirus, herpes virus, varicella-zoster virus, parvovirus B19, Epstein-Barr, coxsackie, Echo 13/30 virus, smallpox, poliomyelitis, and hepatitis B were reported to trigger PTS [7]. Furthermore, approximately 10% of PTS patients were found to have a concomitant hepatitis E virus infection in the acute phase, thereby explaining previous reports of elevated liver enzymes in some [3]. Other triggers include immunizations and vaccinations, medical or surgical procedures, childbirth, unaccustomed physical activity, and trauma, including the minor trauma associated with falling (without apparent injury) and intravenous procedures (intravenous therapy, intravenous contrast, or intravenous blood withdrawal) [7]. In addition, PTS has been reported after administering some medications, including nivolumab [8] and botulinum toxin [9].

These triggers are considered to activate the immune system in susceptible individuals. The latency between the trigger and PTS is generally reported to range from several hours up to 4 to 6 weeks. Nonetheless, in about two-thirds of patients, the pain starts during the first week [6].

Most triggering factors indicate an underlying autoimmune process with selected peripheral nerve inflammation. Furthermore, pathological studies from nerve biopsies in acute PTS report the presence of lymphocytic inflammatory infiltrates in the affected nerves. The initial inflammation causes intraneural edema. The swollen fascicles are less flexible, and the motion of a nearby articulation induces kinking. Repetitive kinking and rotation of the nerves can lead to constriction and fascicular entwinement. Many patients report intense physical activity of the upper body before the onset of PTS [3]; this indicates that mechanical stress to the nerves plays a predisposing role [3]. Repeated microtrauma to the brachial plexus nerves of the plexus might determine an increase in the permeability of the blood-nerve barrier, opening the endoneurial space to immune factors and enabling the autoimmune process [10].

The sudden onset, monophasic course of PTS, association with preceding infection, serum sickness, vaccinations, and use of immunomodulating agents all support immune-mediated pathology. In addition, this hypothesis is supported by the involvement of both immune mechanisms, humoral and cellular, the existence of focal chronic inflammatory infiltrates, edema, and onion bulb appearance. The endoneurial and epineurial vessels are surrounded by mononuclear inflammatory infiltrates without features of necrotizing vasculitis. Furthermore, the PTS patients were reported to present altered lymphocyte subsets (decreased CD3 levels and increased CD4/CD8 ratios due to decreased CD8 levels), antiganglioside and anti-peripheral nerve myelin antibodies, and terminal complement activation products [11–14]. Oligoclonal bands were reported in the cerebrospinal fluid (CSF) [11,12,14]. Moreover, triggers of PTS, such as an upper respiratory infection, also represent triggers for other autoimmune diseases, including acute and chronic inflammatory demyelinating polyradiculoneuropathy [6].

The hereditary form of PTS has been described in approximately 200 families worldwide [15]. This form accounts for about 10–19% of PTS cases [4]. The patients present similar clinical features with the sporadic form, including antecedent triggers, intense pain, muscle weakness, and atrophy. Differences between the hereditary and sporadic forms include the age of onset, the frequency of recurrences, and some morphological features [6]. For example, although hereditary and sporadic forms are generally present in the third and fourth decades, and both forms may present in the first decade, children are more frequently affected by the hereditary form.

The hereditary form of PTS transmits in an autosomal dominant manner. Researchers found that approximately 55% of gene mutations in North American families affect the SEPT9 gene on chromosome 17 q and show high penetrance of 80–90% [10,16,17]. The genetic abnormality in the other 45% of these families is unknown, suggesting that hereditary PTS is a genetically heterogeneous syndrome.

Electrodiagnostic research indicates that the primary pathophysiology associated with both forms of PTS comprises axon disruption with Wallerian degeneration. Following Wallerian degeneration, conduction failure occurs as action potentials can no longer propagate along the axon. In contrast to focal myelin disruption, which remains focal, focal axon disruption presents with distant effects. Clinically, early muscle wasting and long recovery periods are also consistent with these findings. However, rarely (less than 1% of cases), PTS patients with sporadic forms might present focal demyelination [6].

1.4. Diagnostic Workup

Laboratory investigations have only a limited diagnostic value. They may aid in identifying specific infections associated with the onset of PTS and are used primarily for some differential diagnoses [10].

Electrodiagnostic investigations are widely used, supporting the diagnosis of PTS. Needle electromyography (EMG) is an invasive but valuable tool to detect muscle denervation. However, denervation may take up to four weeks to be fully apparent in EMG, and early measurements can thus be of limited value [18]. Nerve conduction studies (NCS) indicate the site of the lesion [5]. Nonetheless, in the subacute stages, after some reinnervation has appeared, the parameters of affected nerves may be normal, limiting the sensitivity of this diagnostic tool [10].

Furthermore, conduction slowing or blockage may be technically challenging to detect in some specific nerves due to their anatomical location. Sensory abnormalities are absent on NCS in 80% of clinically affected nerves [19]. Therefore, a normal NCS does not exclude a PTS diagnosis.

There is no differential diagnosis when a patient presents a PTS with paralysis of a long thoracic nerve and a left suprascapular nerve simultaneously. Otherwise, the main differential diagnoses include cervical root and shoulder joint disorders [9]. In patients with mononeuropathies, an entrapment neuropathy associated with a fibrous arcade, synovial cyst, or lipoma may cause the symptoms. Depending on clinical and additional investigations, meningoradiculitis, neoplastic plexopathy, or vasculitis could be considered. If the patient presents no pain, the differential diagnosis includes chronic idiopathic demyelinating polyneuropathy, multifocal motor neuropathy, Lewis Sumner syndrome, hereditary neuropathy with liability to pressure palsy, and facio-scapulo-humeral myopathy [7].

Recently, PTS was reported following the severe acute respiratory syndrome coronavirus 2 (SARS-CoV-2) infection. Our objective is to provide a comprehensive report on existing literature by investigating data on PTS triggered by SARS-CoV-2 infection, provide an extensive perspective on this pathology, and reveal what other, more specific, research questions can be further addressed. In addition, we aim to highlight research gaps requiring further attention. Therefore, we aim to evaluate the clinical, laboratory, neurophysiological, and neuroimaging features of PTS in patients with Coronavirus disease 2019 (COVID-19) and explore possible links in this pathology.

2. Materials and Methods

This systematic review was performed following the guidelines of the Preferred Reporting Items for Systematic reviews and Meta-Analyses extension for Scoping Reviews (PRISMA-ScR) [20–23] (see Supplemental Materials S1) and the current recommendations on the synthesis of case reports and case series [24].

The research questions were defined based on the Population, Concept, and Context (PCC) of the review, as recommended by the Joanna Briggs Institute [20]:

- Is there a relationship between SARS-CoV-2 infections and the apparition of PTS?
- If yes, what are the clinical features?
- What do we know about laboratory, neurophysiological, and neuroimaging investigations?
- Which are the presumptive mechanisms underlying PTS?
- What interventions might work?
- What do we know about the evolution of PTS after SARS-CoV-2 infection?

In order to identify the extent of the current research on PTS after SARS-CoV-2 infection, we searched LitCOVID, the World Health Organization database on COVID-19 (to 17 January 2023), using the following search strings "Parsonage AND Turner", and "brachial". As these databases are curated for SARS-CoV-2 infection articles, we did not need to use search terms like "coronavirus", "COVID-19", or "SARS-CoV-2". We screened for additional studies using the reference lists of relevant research papers. As we aimed to generate an extensive list of research suitable for answering our questions, we did not apply any search filters and language restrictions.

Two authors reviewed the title, abstract, and full text (when needed) of all retrieved articles, assessing whether the study met the inclusion criteria. A third reviewer's opinion was considered if disagreements were not solved through discussion.

The PCC mnemonics for this systematic review were children and adults (over 18 years old) (P), with studies investigating patients with PTS (C) in the context of previous or concurrent SARS-CoV-2 infection (C). We included case reports, case series, and prospective or retrospective observational and interventional studies. Conference abstracts were also included if the authors did not publish a full paper on the study.

We excluded commentaries, opinions, and narrative reviews but examined their reference lists for possible inclusions. Also, we excluded patients with COVID-19 reported to present neuropathy after prone positioning.

We extracted data to a pro forma template piloted on five randomly selected articles and adjusted the template as necessary. One reviewer extracted all relevant information, and a second reviewer checked the data.

Our primary scope was to provide an overview of the evidence reported on PTS triggered by SARS-CoV-2 infection, regardless of the risk of bias in the included studies [20]. Therefore, we did not perform a formal evaluation of the methodological quality of the included studies.

The protocol was not registered to any database.

3. Results

The literature search resulted in 470 records. After deduplication, 288 articles were included. Finally, we identified 57 papers on PTS in patients with COVID-19 to assess in full text; 21 papers were ultimately included [25–45]. The screening and selection of papers were conducted by one reviewer and cross-checked by a second author. Disagreements were managed by discussing between the two screeners or having a third author arbitrate. The PRISMA diagram with the selection process is illustrated in Figure 1.

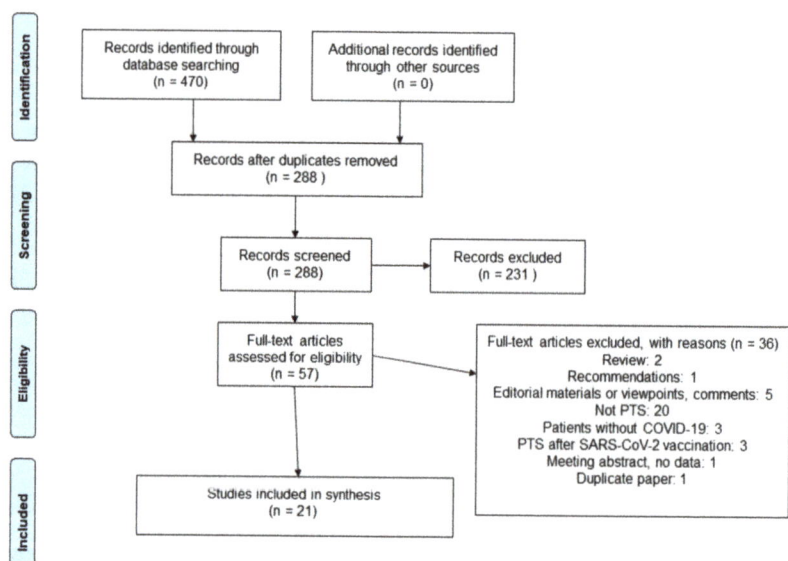

Figure 1. Flow chart showing the process for inclusion of studies. Legend: PTS: Parsonage-Turner syndrome. SARS-CoV-2: severe acute respiratory syndrome coronavirus 2.

This systematic review included 21 articles reporting on 26 cases of patients from the USA (8 cases) [25,27,32,38,40,44], France (6 patients) [34,36,41,43], Italy (3 cases) [29,31,45], Spain (1 case) [26], Germany (1 case) [42], Hong Kong (1 case) [33], Singapore [39], Kuwait (1 case) [37], Iran (1 case) [28], Chile [35], and Mexico (2 cases) [30].

The patients were aged between 17 and 76 years, most of them being males (21/26, 80.8%). The publication dates ranged from 2020 to 2022. The detailed study characteristics are presented in Supplemental Materials S2.

3.1. Medical History

Regarding the immunological status of the patients, one report notes that the patient was vaccinated a few months prior to PTS [41], but the authors provide no further information on the vaccine; another patient was vaccinated with Moderna mRNA 1273 four months prior to PTS [39], and two patients had no recent vaccination [31,35]. One case received kidney transplantation due to polycystic kidney disease and was under treatment with prednisolone, tacrolimus, and mycophenolate mofetil [28]. Two patients, a sister and a brother, had a history of steroid allergy [30]. Two patients were investigated for autoimmune diseases, but the vaccination status is not reported [34]. For the remaining 17/26 (65.4%) PTS cases, the authors did not provide information on vaccination status or other immunosuppressing states.

Nine (34.6%) patients presented significant comorbidities: clavicle fracture [25], familial history of PTS [30], history of work-related shoulder pain [32], shoulder arthroplasty [32], psoriatic arthropathy in remission [33], an episode of anterior dislocation of the shoulder [41], or prior rotator cuff repair performed 2.5 years previously [44].

3.2. Clinical Picture

The PTS had an acute onset in all cases (26/26, 100%). In two patients (2/26, 7.7%), the onset time of PTS was unclear [26,29]. The neurological complaints were reported to occur simultaneously with COVID-19 in 5/24 (20.8%) patients [30,32,41,45], and within one week of infection in 3/24 (12.5%) cases [25,37,39]. Nine individuals (9/24, 37.5%) developed PTS after more than seven days but within one month of infection [28,31–33,35,36,42,43]. In 7/24 (29.2%) patients, PTS symptom onset occurred after more than a month from COVID-19 infection [27,32,34,38,40,44]. In two patients, the time of onset of PTS was unclear.

Pain was present in most cases (25/26, 96.2%). Only one patient (1/26, 3.8%), hospitalized in the intensive care unit (ICU) with Acute Respiratory Distress Syndrome (ARDS), had neuralgic amyotrophy affecting C5–C6 nerve roots, the lateral pectoral and phrenic nerves; he presented hypoesthesia, motor deficit, muscle wasting, and diaphragmatic palsy [43]. The characteristics of pain in each case are presented in Table 1.

Table 1. Pain characteristics in PTS patients.

Study	Pain Severity	Onset Timing (Day/Night)	Location of Pain	Sleep	Mechanical Sensitivity	Time between Pain and Other PT Symptoms	Duration
Ahorukomeye 2022 [25]	Severe	N/R	Contralateral (right) shoulder	N/R	N/R	2 days	Resolved (at 12 weeks follow up)
Alvarado 2021 [26]	Severe	N/R	Both shoulders	Disrupted sleep	N/R	N/R	N/R
Alvarez 2021 [27]	Unclear	N/R	Left shoulder	N/R	N/R	N/R	Resolved (at 3 months follow-up)
Ansari 2022 [28]	Severe	N/R	Cervical spine, left scapular region	N/R	N/R	N/R	Resolved (at 2 months follow-up)
Cabona 2021 [29]	Unclear	N/R	Left shoulder	N/R	N/R	N/R	Resolved (at 1-month follow-up)
Cabrera 2022 case 1 [30]	Severe	N/R	Left shoulder	N/R	N/R	N/R	Resolved within 26 days
Cabrera 2022 case 2 [30]	Severe	N/R	Left shoulder	N/R	N/R	N/R	Resolved within 21 days

Table 1. Cont.

Study	Pain Severity	Onset Timing (Day/Night)	Location of Pain	Sleep	Mechanical Sensitivity	Time between Pain and Other PT Symptoms	Duration
Cacciavillani 2021 [31]	Severe	N/R	Left wrist and upper limb in the distribution of the lateral antebrachial cutaneous nerve	N/R	N/R	N/R	Resolved after 2 weeks
Castaneda 2022 case 1 [32]	Severe	N/R	Left shoulder	Sleep disruption	Exacerbated by movement	N/R	Occasional aching pain (at 4 months follow-up)
Castaneda 2022 case 2 [32]	Unclear	N/R	Left shoulder, radiating below elbow	Sleep disruption, worse at night	N/R	N/R	Improvement (at 9 months follow-up)
Castaneda 2022 case 3 [32]	Unclear	N/R	Left shoulder, radiating to the neck	N/R	N/R	A few weeks following onset of pain	N/R
Cheung 2022 [33]	Severe	N/R	Extended from the neck and right interscapular region to the shoulder and the ulnar side of the right arm and forearm	Sleep disruption	Aggravated by movement	N/R	Little or no pain (at 3 months follow-up)
Coll case 1 [34]	Unclear	N/R	Right shoulder	N/R	N/R	N/R	N/R
Coll case 2 [34]	Unclear	N/R	Left shoulder	N/R	N/R	N/R	N/R
Diaz 2021 [35]	Unclear	N/R	Right shoulder	N/R	N/R	7 weeks after pain onset	N/R
Fortanier 2022 case 1 [36]	Unclear	N/R	Right shoulder	N/R	N/R	Low interval	Resolution (at 3 months follow-up)
Fortanier 2022 case 2 [36]	Severe	N/R	Right shoulder	N/R	N/R	N/R	Pain persisted (4-month follow-up)
Ismail 2021 [37]	Severe	N/R	Left shoulder, followed by right shoulder one week later. Afterward, the pain intensified and progressed to both forearms and hands	N/R	Aggravated by touch and movement	2 weeks	Partial relief (8 weeks follow-up)
Mitry 2021 [38]	Severe	N/R	Multifocal joint pain, most prominent in the left shoulder and left hand. Followed by abdominal pain	N/R	Aggravated by movement	Shortly after onset	N/R
Ng 2022 [39]	Unclear	N/R	Left shoulder	N/R	N/R	N/R	Resolved (day 13)
Queler 2021 [40]	Severe	N/R	Left upper limb	N/R	N/R	N/R	N/R
Saade 2022 [41]	Unclear	N/R	Cervical spine and right upper limb	N/R	N/R	N/R	Resolved (6 months follow-up)
Siepmann 2020 [42]	Severe	N/R	Right shoulder, with a subsequent gradual shift to forearm and hand	N/R	Aggravated by arm extension	2 weeks	Partial relief (at 1.5 months after onset)
Viatgé 2021 [43]	Absent	N/A	N/A	N/A	N/A	N/A	N/A
Voss 2022 [44]	Severe	N/R	Left shoulder	Sleep disruption	Not alleviated or aggravated by shoulder movement	1 week	Important relief at 1 week
Zazzara 2022 [45]	Severe	N/R	Chest pain radiating to the proximal left arm, the shoulder and the upper region of the homolateral hemithorax	N/R	N/R	N/R	Persistence of painful dysesthesia (at 2 months from symptom onset). Improvement (at 4 months)

Notes: PTS: Parsonage-Turner syndrome; N/R: not reported; N/A not applicable.

A motor deficit was present in 21/26 (80.8%) patients [26–29,32–36,38–44,46]. Muscle strength was normal in 3/26 (11.5%) patients; two presented a pure sensory PTS [31,45], and one case is unclear: the authors report a normal motor function, but eight weeks later, he had scapula winging [25]. In addition, in two familial cases (2/26), the authors do not mention any motor deficit, but the patients presented deltoid, supraspinatus, and scapular muscle wasting [30].

Muscle wasting was reported in 14/26 (53.8%) patients [25–27,29,30,32,34,35,37,41].

Paresthesia was noted in 12/26 (46.2%) PTS individuals [25–27,30,32,33,37,39,40,42]. However, a sensory loss was reported in 9/26 (34.6%) patients [26,28,31,33,37,42–45].

The clinical picture of individual cases is presented in Table 2. The extended data can be found in Supplemental Materials S1.

Table 2. Clinical characteristics of PTS patients.

Study	Pain	Motor Deficit	Muscle Wasting	Paresthesia	Sensory Loss	Notes
Ahorukomeye 2022 [25]	Present	Absent	Present	Present	Absent	
Alvarado 2021 [26]	Present	Present	Present	Present	Present	Bilateral PTS
Alvarez 2021 [27]	Present	Present	Present	Present	Absent	Extended PTS
Ansari 2022 [28]	Present	Present	Absent	Absent	Present	
Cabona 2021 [29]	Present	Present	Present	Absent	Absent	Musculocutaneous nerve
Cabrera 2022 case 1 [30]	Present	Absent	Present	Present	Absent	Family case
Cabrera 2022 case 2 [30]	Present	Absent	Present	Present	Absent	Family case
Cacciavillani 2021 [31]	Present	Absent	Absent	Absent	Present	Pure sensory
Castaneda 2022 case 1 [32]	Present	Present	Present	Absent	Absent	
Castaneda 2022 case 2 [32]	Present	Present	Present	Present	Absent	
Castaneda 2022 case 3 [32]	Present	Present	Present	Present	Absent	
Cheung 2022 [33]	Present	Present	Absent	Present	Present	
Coll case 1 [34]	Present	Present	Present	Absent	Absent	Accessory nerve
Coll case 2 [34]	Present	Present	Present	Absent	Absent	Accessory nerve
Diaz 2021 [35]	Present	Present	Present	Absent	Absent	
Fortanier 2022 case 1 [36]	Present	Present	Absent	Absent	Absent	
Fortanier 2022 case 2 [36]	Present	Present	Absent	Absent	Absent	
Ismail 2021 [37]	Present	Present	Present	Present	Present	Bilateral PTS
Mitry 2021 [38]	Present	Present	Absent	Absent	Absent	Diaphragm
Ng 2022 [39]	Present	Present	Absent	Present	Absent	
Queler 2021 [40]	Present	Present	Absent	Present	Absent	
Saade 2022 [41]	Present	Present	Present	Absent	Absent	
Siepmann 2020 [42]	Present	Present	Absent	Present	Present	
Viatgé 2021 [43]	Absent	Present	Absent	Absent	Present	
Voss 2022 [44]	Present	Present	Absent	Absent	Present	
Zazzara 2022 [45]	Present	Absent	Absent	Absent	Present	Pure sensory

3.3. Ancillary Investigations

Among 26 patients, NCS was performed in 11 cases (11/26, 42.3%) [27,31,33–37,42,45], and EMG in 18 cases (18/26, 69.2%) [25,28,31–37,41–45]. The NCS findings varied depending on the nerve fibers affected and the timing of the investigation. The authors reported acute motor axon loss signs [26], normal latencies with an important reduction of compound action potentials (CMAP) amplitude [34], signs of subacute plexopathy [35], and normal findings three months after PTS onset [33]. In addition, a few patients also presented an absence of sensory responses [26] or reduced sensory nerve activation potential amplitude [31]. Some authors noted that they performed electrophysiological studies for four patients [26,29,30]. Likewise, the EMG results were also heterogeneous: signs of denervation [25,29,32,34,36], patchy plexopathy [40], positive sharp waves and fibrillation [35], chronic trunk plexopathy with reinnervation [27], and normal findings five weeks after PTS symptoms onset [31].

A neuromuscular ultrasound investigation was employed in 5/26 (19.2%) cases [25,29,31,42,43]. The findings included enlargement of the affected nerves [25,29,42], multifocal damage of the nerves [29], and amyotrophy [43]. Also, normal findings were reported in a patient with pure sensory PTS [31].

Diaphragmatic ultrasound was useful for assessing diaphragmatic dysfunction [43].

MRI was performed in 17/26 (65.4%) cases. The most common finding was muscle edema (10/17, 58.8% cases) [26,27,29,37,38,41–44], followed by hyperintensity of the affected fascicles (8/17, 47.1% cases) [29,33,36,39,40,43,45], and muscle atrophy (5/17, 29.4% patients) [34,41,43,44]. Contrast enhancement of the affected nerve was reported in one patient [42]. Also, on MRI diffusion neurography of the brachial plexus, the measurements of anisotropic fractions and apparent diffusion coefficient (ADC), compared with the normal side, identified a tendency to isotropy, with nervous elements structural disorganization, consistent with PTS. With contrast medium, no reinforcement foci were noted. The authors suggest this signal asymmetry was probably due to inflammation [35]. Other authors note a short inversion time inversion recovery (STIR) hypersignal on the path of the affected nerve bundles, without caliber abnormality or lesion detectable by MRI [43] or segmental diffusion-weighted imaging (DWI) restriction and corresponding apparent diffusion coefficient (ADC) low signal of the nerve trunk [45]. Also, hourglass constrictions were detected in one case [29].

A nerve biopsy from a medial brachial cutaneous nerve was performed in one case, demonstrating marked axonal loss [40].

3.4. Treatment

Non-steroidal anti-inflammatory drugs (NSAIDs) were prescribed initially for 8/26 (30.8%) cases, with minimal or no effect [25–27,30,33,44]. Two patients (2/26, 7.7%) also received muscle relaxers [25,44]. Other authors report an initial administration of acetaminophen (2/26, 7% of patients) with minimal relief [31,37].

As the patients presented with severe pain, 5/26 (19.2%) received gabapentin or gabapentin-type neuromodulators [25,30,33,45]. Pregabalin was tried for 3/26 (11.5%) cases [33,35,37], and duloxetine was given to one patient [45]. Five patients (5/26, 19.2%) were treated with opioids [26,30,37,44].

In addition, one patient also received local injections with steroids and lidocaine, leading to a slight improvement [37]. Two patients received pain medication, but the authors did not specify precisely the type of drugs (2/26, 7.7%) [34].

Corticosteroids were administered in 12/26 (46.2%) PTS cases [26,28,29,32,34,36–38,41,42,45]. One patient received intravenous methylprednisolone (1000 mg daily for 5 days), but it was stopped due to dermatological side effects. A course of intravenous immunoglobulins (IVIG) (25 g/day for 5 days) was also employed, with partial relief of pain and no improvement in muscle power [37]. The rest of the patients received oral steroids. Among the patients that received steroid therapy, the authors reported the outcome in eight cases. One patient with isolated musculocutaneous involvement fully recovered at one month [29]. Another PTS patient that received oral prednisolone (25 mg) for three weeks, followed by tapering, presented partial improvement of muscle strength at 21 days after the initiation of the treatment. At the 2-month follow-up, the patient's shoulder examination was normal, without pain or functional limitations [28]. Four patients demonstrated partial improvement on follow-up visits at different time intervals (ranging from two months to six months) [32,36,41,45]. In one individual, the neurological examination remained the same at eight weeks [37]. Another case reported pain relief at 7- and 14-days, but the motor and sensory examinations remained the same [42].

In two patients, a brother and sister with a history of steroid allergy, the authors administered extended-release pirfenidone, starting on day 22, considering its potential anti-inflammatory action [30]. On day 26 post-infection, the symptoms of neuralgia subsided [30].

Rehabilitation was recommended for 11/26 (42.3%) PTS patients [26,32–35,41,43,44].

One patient with pure motor PTS received no treatment (1/26, 3.8%). Nonetheless, the evolution was favorable, with the complete disappearance of the symptoms after three months [36]. The authors provided no information on the treatment [39,40].

3.5. Evolution

In 7/26 (26.9%) patients, the authors did not report on the evolution of PTS [26,32,34,38,40,43]. Among the 19 patients with reported outcomes, 5/19 (26.3%) had a complete remission of symptoms at 1 month [29], 2 months [28], 3 months [27,36], and 6 months follow-up visits [35], respectively.

The clinical examination was found to be improved in 11/19 (57.9%) patients. Nonetheless, the timing of the follow-up visits was heterogeneous: 13 days [39], approximately 3 weeks [30], 6 weeks [31], 2 months [25,45], 3 months [33], 4 months [32,36], 6 months [41], 8 months [44], and 9 months [32].

3.6. SARS-CoV-2 Infection

The COVID-19 diagnosis was based on a positive real-time reverse-transcription polymerase chain reaction (RT-PCR) test in 15/26 (73.1%) patients [25,27,28,30,31,34,36,37,41–43,45]. However, the cycle threshold (Ct) of the positive RT-PCR test was not specified in any cases. In 9/26 (34.6%) patients, the authors did not specify how the COVID-19 diagnosis was obtained [26,29,32,33,39,40,44]. Two patients (2/26, 7.7%) were not tested by RT-PCR and the diagnosis of SARS-CoV-2 infection was made retrospectively. One patient presented anti-SARS-CoV-2 antibodies suggesting prior infection/exposure (elevated IgG, normal IgM) [35]. Another case had a negative RT-PCR but positive IgG antibodies a few weeks after the respiratory illness [38].

Regarding the COVID-19 severity, 4/26 (15.4%) patients had mild disease [33,42,44,45], one patient presented moderate to severe infection (1/26, 3.8%), and 9/26 (34.6%) had severe illness [25–27,29,32,34,40,43]. The severity of the SARS-CoV-2 infection was not reported for 12/26 (46.2%) of cases [30–32,35–39,41]. Among the patients with severe COVID-19, eight (8/26, 30.8%) required ICU treatment [26,27,29,32,34,40,43]. Four patients (4/8, 50%) developed PTS symptoms several days or weeks after ICU discharge or extubation [26,27,32,34], including one with extended PTS [27]. The data on ICU stay and PTS symptoms is presented in Table 3.

Table 3. Characteristics of patients with PTS that necessitated ICU treatment.

Study	ICU Stay	Prone Positioning	PTS Symptoms
Alvarado 2021 [26]	Several days	On 2 occasions	During a visit to the rehabilitation department
Alvarez 2021 [27]	23 days	Intermittently	8 days after extubation
Cabona 2021 [29]	13 days	N/R	At ICU discharge
Castaneda 2022, case 2 [32]	Several weeks	N/R	Following extubation
Coll 2021, case 1 [34]	6 weeks	Present	1 month after ICU discharge
Coll 2021, case 2 [34]	5 weeks	Present	1 week after ICU discharge
Queler 2021 [40]	7 weeks	None	Following extubation
Viatgé 2021 [43]	24 days	Present	Following extubation

Notes: ICU—intensive care unit; PTS—Parsonage-Turner syndrome; N/R—not reported.

4. Discussion

The present systematic review identified 26 cases of PTS following SARS-CoV-2 infection. The study population included 80.8% males, a more significant proportion than commonly reported in the literature in PTS. For example, the cohort evaluated by van Alfen et al. consisted of 67.5% males [4]. However, as PTS is considered to present an autoimmune origin, one would expect to present a female predominance. Therefore, an unknown sex-specific factor in this pathology may make male patients more prone to attacks [4]. In addition, a family history was present in two cases [30], but no genetic testing was performed. This proportion (7.7%) is lower than reported in the general population (19%), but several authors in our review did not report on the family history of their patients.

In our series, 15/26 (57.7%) patients experienced severe pain. However, the pain intensity was not clearly presented in 10/26 (38.5%) cases. One patient did not present pain [43]. Therefore, among 16 patients with information on pain intensity, 93.8% had severe pain. This data is similar to other reports in the literature [4,6]. Usually, the pain in PTS emerges within a few hours and, in most cases, the attacks begin at night [4,15]. However, most articles in our review did not provide detailed patient pain data. Among 25 patients with pain, 22 (88%) had unilateral symptoms and three (12%) presented bilateral symptoms in an asymmetric pattern [26,37,38]. Our percentage of patients with unilateral pain is higher than the data found by other authors in patients with PTS. For example, van Alfen reported that, in 71.5% of patients, the pain was unilateral, and in 28.5%, it was bilateral [4]. In 5/25 (20%) patients with pain, the symptom caused sleep disturbances [26,32,33,44]. In our systematic review, the percentage is much lower than reported in the literature (93.5%) [4], possibly because the authors do not mention anything about sleep quality in 20/25 (80%) cases. An increased mechanical sensitivity (pain elicited by movement, pressure, or touch of the affected limb) was reported in 5/25 (20%) of patients (4 males and 1 female) [32,33,37,38,42]. In one case (1/25, 4%), the pain was not alleviated or aggravated by shoulder movement [44]. Nonetheless, these aspects are not presented in most cases (19/25, 76%).

In PTS, many patients describe three pain phases during the attack. The constant initial pain may be followed by intense neuropathic stabbing or shooting pains, often elicited by motion, lying on, or prolonged limb posturing. About two-thirds of PTS cases reported further subsequent persisting musculoskeletal pain. This later pain type is usually localized to the origin or insertion of the paretic or compensating muscles, primarily in the periscapular, cervical, and occipital regions [4]. However, such a detailed description of the patient's symptoms was unavailable in the studies included in this review.

The timing of other symptoms and signs that follow the pain was reported in 8/25 (32%) patients [25,32,35–38,42,44]. Among them, 6/8 (75%) presented additional symptoms within 2 weeks; in 2/8 (25%) patients, the motor deficit was reported after a longer time interval (seven weeks [35] or a few weeks [32]). Our findings are similar to other reports, where authors found that 27.2% of all cases of paresis did not manifest themselves until >2 weeks after the onset of pain [4]. A recent study with an in-depth analysis of PTS patients found that, in about one-third of patients, there is an increment of the motor deficit over days (8.6%), weeks (16%), or months (5.6%) [4]. However, we did not find reports on the aggravation of the motor deficit.

Among the 24 patients with a motor deficit or muscle wasting, in ten patients, the motor deficit was assessed using the Medical Research Council (MRC) grading system (see Supplemental Materials S2). The intensity varied from 1/5 to 4/5, with 7/10 (70%) of individuals presenting a maximum deficit of 3/5 or 4/5 [27,29,32,36,39,41] and 3/10 (30%) cases presenting severe paralysis with an MRC of 1/5 or 2/5 [32,35,37]. This contrasts with the literature, where about two-thirds of patients presented severe motor deficits [4]. In our review, among individuals with reported outcomes, 26.3% had a complete recovery.

In addition, the clinical assessment revealed that 53.8% of patients presented muscle atrophy, while data from the literature indicate more significant proportions, ranging from 75.4 to 88.5% [4]. This discrepancy could be due to the timing of examination, as the median time for atrophy to first appear was reported to be 5 weeks [4], or to the fact that in our series, the motor deficit was not severe in most cases. Furthermore, muscle weakness and wasting might go unnoticed. First, weakness is only sometimes appreciable in the early PTS stage if pain limits the patient's movements. Also, synergistic muscles may mask the motor deficit, or an overlying muscle may mask the muscle wasting (e.g., the trapezius muscle masks supraspinatus muscle atrophy, the biceps muscle may mask brachialis muscle atrophy) [6].

The pattern of sensory symptoms in our series also differs from the results of other studies investigating PTS. Paresthesia was noted in 12/26 (46.2%) PTS individuals [25–27,30,32,33,37,39,40,42]. However, a sensory loss was reported in 9/26 (34.6%) patients [26,28,31,33,37,42–45]. The sensory symptoms and signs were present alone or in combination with motor findings in different patterns. Although previous research demonstrated that in more than half of PTS patients, there is no recovery on follow-up [4], the evolution of sensory symptoms was poorly reported in PTS patients following SARS-CoV-2 infection, with the authors focusing on motor recovery.

In addition, in our review, no patient presented autonomic nervous system involvement (e.g., vegetative and trophic skin changes, edema, temperature dysregulation), although they have been reported in 15.4% of PTS patients [4]. Involvement of nerves outside the brachial plexus was reported in several patients, including the lumbosacral plexus [27], phrenic nerve [43], and spinal accessory nerve [34].

The lumbosacral nerves may be rarely affected in hereditary PTS forms [6], but authors investigating large series of sporadic series of PTS did not report any lower extremity muscle involvement [5]. Furthermore, when the lower extremity muscle involvement is not concomitant with the episodes of forequarter region weakness, it is uncertain that they represent the same disorder [6]. For example, lumbosacral radiculoplexus neuropathy and PTS share the same clinical features: severe pain, muscle weakness, and atrophy. For the patient with extended PTS included in the present review, although he did not present genetic testing, the authors note he had no family history of neurological diseases [27].

Phrenic nerve involvement is difficult to diagnose. For example, in a study of phrenic neuropathies due to PTS, 10 of the 17 cases were isolated, with no evidence of involvement of other concomitant nerves [47]. The patients may present with unilateral or bilateral diaphragmatic palsy. When unilateral, it may be undiagnosed. In addition, when isolated, phrenic neuropathies are likely to go unrecognized if asymptomatic or if they cause only mild and transient dyspnea. They are more likely to be diagnosed when accompanied by an antecedent event or severe shoulder pain [6]. In the present review, one patient presented phrenic nerve involvement [43], but the possibility of diaphragmatic palsy might have been overlooked.

The incidence of cranial nerve involvement varies from 0% [48] to 10% [49], being more frequent in patients with hereditary forms of PTS [4]. In a study on sporadic PTS, the spinal accessory nerve was the most commonly involved cranial nerve, accounting for approximately 2% of the total lesions [5]. Two patients in our review presented spinal accessory nerve involvement [34], but they had no genetic testing, and the family history is not mentioned.

Pulmonary imaging, including chest X-ray or computed tomography results, were reported in 9/26 (34.6%) patients. These imaging methods help investigate the differential diagnosis for PTS (e.g., Pancoast tumor) and the possibility of diaphragmatic paralysis. However, in our cases, it was performed primarily for COVID-19, with rare exceptions [34,43]. Also, an MRI of the cervical spine was performed in 8/26 (30.8%) patients in order to exclude a spinal pathology [25,27,28,33,36,39,42,44]. An MRI of the shoulder was performed in 7/26 (26.9%) cases [32,34,35,38]. Although many patients presented changes on the cervical spine MRI (see Supplemental Materials S2), the results did not explain the patients' clinical picture and course.

The most used diagnostic test was EMG (69.2% of cases), followed by MRI of the upper limb and brachial plexus (65.4% of individuals), NCS (42.3% of patients), and neuromuscular ultrasound (19.2% of cases). Only on one occasion did the authors perform a nerve biopsy (3.8% of cases). Interestingly, the MRI scan was abnormal in 16/17 (94.1%) patients. Only one case with MRI without gadolinium presented normal findings [28].

The diagnosis of PTS is primarily clinical, based on the typical history and neurologic examination findings. Nonetheless, electrodiagnostic studies are helpful. They can localize and characterize individual peripheral nervous system lesions and identify typical patterns (e.g., mononeuropathies and multiple mononeuropathies involving pure or predominantly motor nerves, severe involvement of one muscle, and spare or relative spare of others). However, a normal NCS does not exclude, with certainty, a PTS diagnosis. In addition, MRI and ultrasound studies provide information on individual lesions, potentially providing additional confirmation when required [50–53]. Although ultrasound is less valuable than MRI for brachial plexus imaging, it is much more helpful for extraplexal imaging due to its ability to follow the nerves and fascicle courses [6]. As most lesions in PTS are extraplexal, this gives ultrasonography a benefit over MRI. Other advantages of ultrasonography include better spatial resolution, lower costs, ease of side-to-side comparisons, and real-time examination [54]. Some authors prefer ultrasound imaging, considering that most PTS lesions are extraplexal [5,52] and because the MRI field of view at a given resolution restricts the detailed examination of the peripheral nervous system, with false-negative results [6].

Although there are no diagnostic blood, urine, or CSF tests for PTS, routine blood work is required to exclude emergent and treatable conditions. For example, metabolic studies may reveal increased liver enzymes, and a further hepatitis profile is warranted. Also, serology for common infections and laboratory testing for vasculitis might be required. When the patients present risk factors for specific disorders (e.g., human immunodeficiency virus infection), ancillary investigations related to these conditions are also helpful. Recent reports note that antiganglioside antibodies are present in 26% of the PTS patients tested [4]. Nonetheless, in the present review, the authors investigated the antiganglioside antibodies only in one patient [36].

During the acute phase of PTS, pain control is a priority. In general, NSAIDs and acetaminophen do not provide relief [6], and neuropathic pain medication is recommended (an antiepileptic drug, such as gabapentin or pregabalin, or a tricyclic agent, such as amitriptyline or nortriptyline) [6]. Patients with PTS following SARS-CoV-2 infection received various pain medications. Corticosteroids in different doses and regimens were administered in 46.2% of PTS cases with mixed results, from full recovery at one month to partial improvement of symptoms or no improvement. Nonetheless, randomized placebo-controlled trials are needed to evaluate the effects of corticosteroids and other medications in PTS patients.

One patient with PTS following SARS-CoV-2 infection received a course of IVIG, with partial relief of pain and no improvement in muscle power [37]. Small case series of IVIG treatment report that early treatment may shorten the disease course, being more efficient than delayed treatment [54]. Nonetheless, further research is required in this direction.

Physical therapy was recommended in 42.3% of the cases in the present review. In the acute phase, the pain is severe and may be exacerbated by limb motion. Therefore, physical therapy should be started once the pain permits movement, including range-of-motion exercises, stretching exercises, agonist muscle strengthening, and orthotic devices [6]. Surgical intervention is reserved for patients with refractory or severe disease who have failed conservative treatment. However, at least three months should be given to await any spontaneous recovery [55–57], but in cases where no constrictions are found on ancillary investigations, conservative treatment should be continued [58].

The data on the prognosis of PTS are variable. For example, some authors found that 36% of patients recover within one year, 75% within two years, and 89% within three years [48]. Other studies report that only 11 of 83 PTS patients had complete recovery over a 17-year follow-up [59]. Nonetheless, the likelihood of recovery for each unique lesion should be determined using the basic rules of reinnervation [6]. In patients with previous SARS-CoV-2 infection, the PTS symptoms, 26.3% had a complete remission by six months.

The limitations of the present review are primarily related to the quality of the included studies. The data extraction was challenging due to missing, incomplete, or unclear descriptions of the information. This could be due to the lack of standardized methodology and clear reporting criteria contributing to substantial methodological variation in SARS-CoV-2 studies. Furthermore, some included studies generated interesting scientific debates [60–63].

In addition, an increased possibility of bias associated with case reports and the limited inferences they provide may raise concerns. Our findings are confined by the quality and the extent of information in included reports, which were inconsistent among the 26 included patients. This concerns both the PTS and the SARS-CoV-2 infection. For example, information on previous COVID-19 is scarce in most patients. In addition, other PTS triggers, such as coinfections, intravenous procedures (e.g., intravenous therapy, contrast administration, or blood withdrawal), and certain medications, are not thoroughly assessed.

However, case reports are an appropriate study design, essential in advancing research, particularly for rare conditions. Despite the methodological constraints, observing individual patients provides important insights into a disease's etiology, pathogenesis, natural evolution, and treatments [24]. They play a critical role in shedding light upon new events and provide first-line evidence to further test hypotheses with statistical approaches. The present systematic review highlights the necessity of having a high index of suspicion of PTS in patients with previous SARS-CoV-2 infection, as the clinical manifestations can be variable. Our findings emphasize the need for a standardized approach to investigation and reporting on PTS. Future studies should aim for a comprehensive assessment of patients. Factors such as the baseline characteristics of the patients, evolution, and treatments should be consistently assessed across studies. Also, a thorough differential diagnosis should be employed.

5. Conclusions

To the best of our knowledge, this is the first systematic review of PTS following SARS-CoV-2 infection. We found that, to date, only 26 cases have been reported, with various clinical and paraclinical findings. The clinical and paraclinical spectrum was heterogeneous, ranging from classical PTS to pure sensory neuropathy, extended neuropathy, spinal accessory nerve involvement, and diaphragmatic palsy. Also, two familial cases were reported. The present systematic review highlights the necessity of having a high index of suspicion of PTS in patients with previous SARS-CoV-2 infection, as the clinical manifestations can be variable.

Nonetheless, a standardized approach is needed in order to investigate and report on PTS. Future studies should aim for a comprehensive assessment of patients. Factors such as the characteristics of the patients, evolution, and treatments should be consistently assessed across studies. Also, a thorough differential diagnosis should be employed.

Supplementary Materials: The following supporting information can be downloaded at: https://www.mdpi.com/article/10.3390/biomedicines11030837/s1, Supplemental Materials S1: PRISMA checklist [64]; Supplemental Materials S2: Characteristics of the included studies.

Author Contributions: Conceptualization, A.C., I.L., M.S. and E.C.R.; methodology, A.C., I.L., M.S. and E.C.R.; software, A.C. and E.C.R.; validation, A.C., I.L. and E.C.R.; formal analysis, A.C. and E.C.R.; investigation, A.C., I.L., M.S. and E.C.R.; resources, A.C., I.L., M.S. and E.C.R.; writing—original draft preparation, A.C.; writing—review and editing, A.C., I.L., M.S. and E.C.R.; visualization, A.C., I.L., M.S. and E.C.R.; supervision, M.S. and E.C.R.; project administration, E.C.R. All authors have read and agreed to the published version of the manuscript.

Funding: This research received no external funding.

Institutional Review Board Statement: Not applicable.

Informed Consent Statement: Not applicable.

Data Availability Statement: All data for the systematic review are available within the article.

Conflicts of Interest: The authors declare no conflict of interest.

References

1. Parsonage, M.J.; Turner, J.W. Neuralgic amyotrophy; the shoulder-girdle syndrome. *Lancet* **1948**, *1*, 973–978. [CrossRef]
2. Beghi, E.; Kurland, L.T.; Mulder, D.W.; Nicolosi, A. Brachial plexus neuropathy in the population of Rochester, Minnesota, 1970–1981. *Ann. Neurol.* **1985**, *18*, 320–323. [CrossRef] [PubMed]
3. Van Alfen, N.; van Eijk, J.J.; Ennik, T.; Flynn, S.O.; Nobacht, I.E.; Groothuis, J.T.; Pillen, S.; van de Laar, F.A. Incidence of neuralgic amyotrophy (Parsonage Turner syndrome) in a primary care setting–a prospective cohort study. *PLoS ONE* **2015**, *10*, e0128361. [CrossRef]
4. Van Alfen, N.; van Engelen, B.G. The clinical spectrum of neuralgic amyotrophy in 246 cases. *Brain* **2006**, *129*, 438–450. [CrossRef] [PubMed]
5. Ferrante, M.A.; Wilbourn, A.J. Lesion distribution among 281 patients with sporadic neuralgic amyotrophy. *Muscle Nerve* **2017**, *55*, 858–861. [CrossRef] [PubMed]
6. Seror, P. Neuralgic amyotrophy. An update. *Jt. Bone Spine* **2017**, *84*, 153–158. [CrossRef]
7. Porambo, M.E.; Sedarsky, K.E.; Elliott, E.J.; Theeler, B.J.; Smith, J.K. Nivolumab-induced neuralgic amyotrophy with hourglass-like constriction of the anterior interosseous nerve. *Muscle Nerve* **2019**, *59*, E40–E42. [CrossRef]
8. Cani, I.; Latorre, A.; Cordivari, C.; Balint, B.; Bhatia, K.P. Brachial Neuritis After Botulinum Toxin Injections for Cervical Dystonia: A Need for a Reappraisal? *Mov. Disord. Clin. Pract.* **2019**, *6*, 160–165. [CrossRef]
9. Ferrante, M.A. Neuralgic Amyotrophy. Available online: https://www.medlink.com/articles/neuralgic-amyotrophy (accessed on 1 February 2023).
10. Van Eijk, J.J.; Groothuis, J.T.; Van Alfen, N. Neuralgic amyotrophy: An update on diagnosis, pathophysiology, and treatment. *Muscle Nerve* **2016**, *53*, 337–350. [CrossRef]
11. Pierre, P.A.; Laterre, C.E.; Van den Bergh, P.Y. Neuralgic amyotrophy with involvement of cranial nerves IX, X, XI and XII. *Muscle Nerve* **1990**, *13*, 704–707. [CrossRef]
12. Sierra, A.; Prat, J.; Bas, J.; Romeu, A.; Montero, J.; Matos, J.A.; Bella, R.; Ferrer, I.; Buendia, E. Blood lymphocytes are sensitized to branchial plexus nerves in patients with neuralgic amyotrophy. *Acta Neurol. Scand.* **1991**, *83*, 183–186. [CrossRef] [PubMed]
13. Vriesendorp, F.J.; Dmytrenko, G.S.; Dietrich, T.; Koski, C.L. Anti-peripheral nerve myelin antibodies and terminal activation products of complement in serum of patients with acute brachial plexus neuropathy. *Arch. Neurol.* **1993**, *50*, 1301–1303. [CrossRef] [PubMed]
14. Suarez, G.A.; Giannini, C.; Bosch, E.P.; Barohn, R.J.; Wodak, J.; Ebeling, P.; Anderson, R.; McKeever, P.E.; Bromberg, M.B.; Dyck, P.J. Immune brachial plexus neuropathy: Suggestive evidence for an inflammatory-immune pathogenesis. *Neurology* **1996**, *46*, 559–561. [CrossRef]
15. Van Alfen, N. The neuralgic amyotrophy consultation. *J. Neurol.* **2007**, *254*, 695–704. [CrossRef]
16. Watts, G.D.; O'Briant, K.C.; Chance, P.F. Evidence of a founder effect and refinement of the hereditary neuralgic amyotrophy (HNA) locus on 17q25 in American families. *Hum. Genet.* **2002**, *110*, 166–172. [CrossRef]
17. Kuhlenbäumer, G.; Hannibal, M.C.; Nelis, E.; Schirmacher, A.; Verpoorten, N.; Meuleman, J.; Watts, G.D.; De Vriendt, E.; Young, P.; Stögbauer, F.; et al. Mutations in SEPT9 cause hereditary neuralgic amyotrophy. *Nat. Genet.* **2005**, *37*, 1044–1046. [CrossRef]
18. Feinberg, J. EMG: Myths and facts. *HSSJ* **2006**, *2*, 19–21. [CrossRef]
19. Van Alfen, N.; Huisman, W.J.; Overeem, S.; van Engelen, B.G.; Zwarts, M.J. Sensory nerve conduction studies in neuralgic amyotrophy. *Am. J. Phys. Med. Rehabil.* **2009**, *88*, 941–946. [CrossRef]
20. Peters, M.; Godfrey, C.; McInerney, P.; Munn, Z.; Tricco, A.; Khalil, H. Chapter 11: Scoping Reviews (2020 Version). Available online: https://jbi-global-wiki.refined.site/space/MANUAL/3283910770/Chapter+11%3A+Scoping+reviews (accessed on 22 December 2021).
21. Peters, M.D.J.; Godfrey, C.; McInerney, P.; Khalil, H.; Larsen, P.; Marnie, C.; Pollock, D.; Tricco, A.C.; Munn, Z. Best practice guidance and reporting items for the development of scoping review protocols. *JBI Evid. Synth.* **2022**, *20*, 953–968. [CrossRef]
22. Tricco, A.C.; Lillie, E.; Zarin, W.; O'Brien, K.K.; Colquhoun, H.; Levac, D.; Moher, D.; Peters, M.D.J.; Horsley, T.; Weeks, L.; et al. PRISMA Extension for Scoping Reviews (PRISMA-ScR): Checklist and Explanation. *Ann. Intern. Med.* **2018**, *169*, 467–473. [CrossRef]
23. Peters, M.D.J.; Marnie, C.; Tricco, A.C.; Pollock, D.; Munn, Z.; Alexander, L.; McInerney, P.; Godfrey, C.M.; Khalil, H. Updated methodological guidance for the conduct of scoping reviews. *JBI Evid. Synth.* **2020**, *18*, 2119–2126. [CrossRef] [PubMed]
24. Murad, M.H.; Sultan, S.; Haffar, S.; Bazerbachi, F. Methodological quality and synthesis of case series and case reports. *BMJ Evid. -Based Med.* **2018**, *23*, 60–63. [CrossRef] [PubMed]
25. Ahorukomeye, P.; Pennacchio, C.A.; Preston, D.C.; Cheng, C.W. Parsonage Turner syndrome after cervical trauma and COVID-19 infection: A case report and review of the literature. *AME Case Rep.* **2022**, *6*, 37. [CrossRef] [PubMed]
26. Alvarado, M.; Lin-Miao, Y.; Carrillo-Arolas, M. Parsonage-Turner syndrome post-infection by SARS-CoV-2: A case report. *Neurol. Engl. Ed.* **2021**, *36*, 568–571. [CrossRef] [PubMed]
27. Alvarez, A.; Amirianfar, E.; Mason, M.C.; Huang, L.; Jose, J.; Tiu, T. Extended Neuralgic Amyotrophy Syndrome in a Confirmed COVID-19 Patient After Intensive Care Unit and Inpatient Rehabilitation Stay. *Am. J. Phys. Med. Rehabil.* **2021**, *100*, 733–736. [CrossRef]

28. Ansari, B.; Eishi Oskouei, A.; Moeinzadeh, F. Parsonage-Turner Syndrome following COVID-19 Infection: A Rare and Unique Case. *Adv. Biomed. Res.* **2022**, *11*, 7. [CrossRef]
29. Cabona, C.; Zaottini, F.; Pistoia, F.; Grisanti, S.; Schenone, C.; Villani, F.; Schenone, A.; Aloé, T.; Reni, L.; Benedetti, L. Isolated musculocutaneous nerve involvement in COVID-19 related Neuralgic amyotrophy. Comment on: "Neuralgic amyotrophy and COVID-19 infection: 2 cases of spinal accessory nerve palsy" by Coll et al. Joint Bone Spine 2021;88:105196. *Jt. Bone Spine* **2021**, *88*, 105238. [CrossRef]
30. Cabrera Pivaral, C.E.; Rincon Sanchez, A.R.; Davalos Rodriguez, N.O.; Ramirez Garcia, S.A. Parsonage Turner syndrome associated with COVID-19: About 2 family cases. *Neurologia* **2022**, *38*, 59–60. [CrossRef]
31. Cacciavillani, M.; Salvalaggio, A.; Briani, C. Pure sensory neuralgic amyotrophy in COVID-19 infection. *Muscle Nerve* **2021**, *63*, E7–E8. [CrossRef]
32. Castaneda, D.M.; Chambers, M.M.; Johnsen, P.H.; Fedorka, C.J. Parsonage-Turner Syndrome following COVID-19 infection: A Report of Three Cases. *JSES Rev. Rep. Tech.* **2022**, *online ahead of print*. [CrossRef]
33. Cheung, V.Y.T.; Tsui, F.P.Y.; Cheng, J.M.K. Pain management for painful brachial neuritis after COVID-19: A case report. *Hong Kong Med. J.* **2022**, *28*, 178–180. [CrossRef] [PubMed]
34. Coll, C.; Tessier, M.; Vandendries, C.; Seror, P. Neuralgic amyotrophy and COVID-19 infection: 2 cases of spinal accessory nerve palsy. *Jt. Bone Spine* **2021**, *88*, 105196. [CrossRef]
35. Diaz, C.; Contreras, J.J.; Munoz, M.; Osorio, M.; Quiroz, M.; Pizarro, R. Parsonage-Turner syndrome association with SARS-CoV-2 infection. *JSES Rev. Rep. Tech.* **2021**, *1*, 252. [CrossRef] [PubMed]
36. Fortanier, E.; Le Corroller, T.; Hocquart, M.; Delmont, E.; Attarian, S. Shoulder palsy following SARS-CoV-2 infection: Two cases of typical Parsonage-Turner syndrome. *Eur. J. Neurol.* **2022**, *29*, 2548–2550. [CrossRef] [PubMed]
37. Ismail, I.I.; Abdelnabi, E.A.; Al-Hashel, J.Y.; Alroughani, R.; Ahmed, S.F. Neuralgic amyotrophy associated with COVID-19 infection: A case report and review of the literature. *Neurol. Sci.* **2021**, *42*, 2161–2165. [CrossRef]
38. Mitry, M.A.; Collins, L.K.; Kazam, J.J.; Kaicker, S.; Kovanlikaya, A. Parsonage-turner syndrome associated with SARS-CoV2 (COVID-19) infection. *Clin. Imaging* **2020**, *72*, 8–10. [CrossRef]
39. Ng, G.J.; Chiew, Y.R.; Kong, Y.; Koh, J.S. Neuralgic amyotrophy in COVID-19 infection and after vaccination. *Ann. Acad. Med. Singap.* **2022**, *51*, 376–377. [CrossRef]
40. Queler, S.; Sneag, D.; Geannette, C.; Shin, S.; Winfree, C.; Simpson, D. Long-Segment peripheral neuropathies after COVID-19: Magnetic resonance neurography findings. *Neurology* **2021**, *96*, 4645.
41. Saade, F.; Bouteille, C.; Quemener-Tanguy, A.; Obert, L.; Rochet, S. Parsonage-Turner syndrome and SARS-CoV-2 infection: A case report. *Hand. Surg. Rehabil.* **2022**, *42*, 90–92. [CrossRef]
42. Siepmann, T.; Kitzler, H.H.; Lueck, C.; Platzek, I.; Reichmann, H.; Barlinn, K. Neuralgic amyotrophy following infection with SARS-CoV-2. *Muscle Nerve* **2020**, *62*, E68–E70. [CrossRef]
43. Viatge, T.; Noel-Savina, E.; Prevot, G.; Faviez, G.; Plat, G.; De Boissezon, X.; Cintas, P.; Didier, A. Parsonage-Turner syndrome following severe SARS-CoV-2 infection. *Rev. Mal. Respir.* **2021**, *38*, 853–858. [CrossRef] [PubMed]
44. Voss, T.G.; Stewart, C.M. Parsonage-Turner syndrome after COVID-19 infection. *JSES Rev Rep Tech* **2022**, *2*, 182–185. [CrossRef] [PubMed]
45. Zazzara, M.B.; Modoni, A.; Bizzarro, A.; Lauria, A.; Ciciarello, F.; Pais, C.; Galluzzo, V.; Landi, F.; Tostato, M. COVID-19 atypical Parsonage-Turner syndrome: A case report. *BMC Neurol.* **2022**, *22*, 96. [CrossRef] [PubMed]
46. Ismail, Z.; Rajji, T.K.; Shulman, K.I. Brief cognitive screening instruments: An update. *Int. J. Geriatr. Psychiatry* **2010**, *25*, 111–120. [CrossRef]
47. Tsao, B.E.; Ostrovskiy, D.A.; Wilbourn, A.J.; Shields, R.W., Jr. Phrenic neuropathy due to neuralgic amyotrophy. *Neurology* **2006**, *66*, 1582–1584. [CrossRef]
48. Tsairis, P.; Dyck, P.J.; Mulder, D.W. Natural history of brachial plexus neuropathy. Report on 99 patients. *Arch. Neurol.* **1972**, *27*, 109–117. [CrossRef]
49. Cruz-Martínez, A.; Barrio, M.; Arpa, J. Neuralgic amyotrophy: Variable expression in 40 patients. *J. Peripher. Nerv. Syst.* **2002**, *7*, 198–204. [CrossRef]
50. Arányi, Z., Csillik, A., Dévay, K., Rosero, M., Barsi, P., Böhm, J.; Schelle, T. Ultrasonographic identification of nerve pathology in neuralgic amyotrophy: Enlargement, constriction, fascicular entwinement, and torsion. *Muscle Nerve* **2015**, *52*, 503–511. [CrossRef]
51. ArÁnyi, Z.; Csillik, A.; DéVay, K.; Rosero, M.; Barsi, P.; BÖhm, J.; Schelle, T. Ultrasonography in neuralgic amyotrophy: Sensitivity, spectrum of findings, and clinical correlations. *Muscle Nerve* **2017**, *56*, 1054–1062. [CrossRef]
52. Sneag, D.B.; Rancy, S.K.; Wolfe, S.W.; Lee, S.C.; Kalia, V.; Lee, S.K.; Feinberg, J.H. Brachial plexitis or neuritis? MRI features of lesion distribution in Parsonage-Turner syndrome. *Muscle Nerve* **2018**, *58*, 359–366. [CrossRef]
53. Van Rosmalen, M.; Lieba-Samal, D.; Pillen, S.; van Alfen, N. Ultrasound of peripheral nerves in neuralgic amyotrophy. *Muscle Nerve* **2019**, *59*, 55–59. [CrossRef] [PubMed]
54. Shanina, E.; Liao, B.; Smith, R.G. Brachial Plexopathies: Update on Treatment. *Curr. Treat. Options Neurol.* **2019**, *21*, 24. [CrossRef]
55. Nagano, A.; Shibata, K.; Tokimura, H.; Yamamoto, S.; Tajiri, Y. Spontaneous anterior interosseous nerve palsy with hourglass-like fascicular constriction within the main trunk of the median nerve. *J. Hand. Surg. Am.* **1996**, *21*, 266–270. [CrossRef] [PubMed]

56. Wu, P.; Yang, J.Y.; Chen, L.; Yu, C. Surgical and conservative treatments of complete spontaneous posterior interosseous nerve palsy with hourglass-like fascicular constrictions: A retrospective study of 41 cases. *Neurosurgery* **2014**, *75*, 250–257; discussion 257. [CrossRef] [PubMed]
57. Ochi, K.; Horiuchi, Y.; Tazaki, K.; Takayama, S.; Nakamura, T.; Ikegami, H.; Matsumura, T.; Toyama, Y. Surgical treatment of spontaneous posterior interosseous nerve palsy: A retrospective study of 50 cases. *J. Bone Jt. Surg. Br.* **2011**, *93*, 217–222. [CrossRef]
58. Gstoettner, C.; Mayer, J.A.; Rassam, S.; Hruby, L.A.; Salminger, S.; Sturma, A.; Aman, M.; Harhaus, L.; Platzgummer, H.; Aszmann, O.C. Neuralgic amyotrophy: A paradigm shift in diagnosis and treatment. *J. Neurol. Neurosurg. Psychiatry* **2020**, *91*, 879–888. [CrossRef]
59. Huffmann, G. Neuralgic shoulder amyotrophy: Clinical analysis and development (author's transl). *Z. Neurol.* **1973**, *206*, 79–83.
60. Coll, C.; Tessier, M.; Vandendries, C.; Seror, P. Answer to Cabona et al « Isolated musculocutaneous nerve involvement in COVID-19 related Neuralgic amyotrophy » Joint Bone Spine 2021;88:105238 and to Finsterer and Scorza « SARS-CoV-2 or SARS-CoV-2 vaccination associated Parsonage-Turner syndrome ». Joint Bone Spine 2021;88:105239. *Jt. Bone Spine* **2021**, *88*, 105240. [CrossRef]
61. Finsterer, J.; Scorza, F.A. SARS-CoV-2 or SARS-CoV-2 vaccination associated Parsonage-Turner syndrome. Comment on: "Neuralgic amyotrophy and COVID-19 infection: 2 cases of spinal accessory nerve palsy" by Coll et al. Joint Bone Spine 2021;88:105196. *Jt. Bone Spine* **2021**, *88*, 105239. [CrossRef]
62. Finsterer, J. Anatomy and physiology argue against SARS-CoV-2-associated Parsonage-Turner syndrome if the accessory nerve is affected. *Hand. Surg. Rehabil.* **2023**, *in press*. [CrossRef]
63. Siepmann, T.; Kitzler, H.H.; Reichmann, H.; Barlinn, K. Variability of symptoms in neuralgic amyotrophy following infection with SARS-CoV-2. *Muscle Nerve* **2021**, *63*, E8–E9. [CrossRef] [PubMed]
64. Page, M.J.; McKenzie, J.E.; Bossuyt, P.M.; Boutron, I.; Hoffmann, T.C.; Mulrow, C.D.; Shamseer, L.; Tetzlaff, J.M.; Akl, E.A.; Brennan, S.E.; et al. The PRISMA 2020 statement: An updated guideline for reporting systematic reviews. *BMJ* **2021**, *372*, n71. [CrossRef]

Disclaimer/Publisher's Note: The statements, opinions and data contained in all publications are solely those of the individual author(s) and contributor(s) and not of MDPI and/or the editor(s). MDPI and/or the editor(s) disclaim responsibility for any injury to people or property resulting from any ideas, methods, instructions or products referred to in the content.

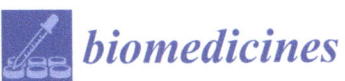

Article

SARS-CoV-2 Affects Thyroid and Adrenal Glands: An ^{18}F-FDG PET/CT Study

Chiara Lauri [1,*], Giuseppe Campagna [1], Andor W. J. M. Glaudemans [2], Riemer H. J. A. Slart [2], Bram van Leer [2,3], Janesh Pillay [3], Marzia Colandrea [4], Chiara Maria Grana [4], Antonio Stigliano [5] and Alberto Signore [1]

1. Nuclear Medicine Unit, Department of Medical-Surgical Sciences and of Translational Medicine, Sant'Andrea University Hospital, "Sapienza" University of Rome, 00161 Rome, Italy; giuseppe.campagna@uniroma1.it (G.C.); alberto.signore@uniroma1.it (A.S.)
2. Department of Nuclear Medicine and Molecular Imaging, University Medical Center Groningen, 9713 GZ Groningen, The Netherlands; a.w.j.m.glaudemans@umcg.nl (A.W.J.M.G.); r.h.j.a.slart@umcg.nl (R.H.J.A.S.); b.van.leer@umcg.nl (B.v.L.)
3. Department of Critical Care, University Medical Center Groningen, University of Groningen, 9713 GZ Groningen, The Netherlands; j.pillay@umcg.nl
4. Nuclear Medicine Division, European Institute of Oncology—IRCCS, 20141 Milan, Italy; marzia.colandrea@ieo.it (M.C.); chiara.grana@ieo.it (C.M.G.)
5. Endocrinology, Department of Clinical and Molecular Medicine, Sant'Andrea University Hospital, "Sapienza" University of Rome, 00161 Rome, Italy; antonio.stigliano@uniroma1.it
* Correspondence: chiara.lauri@uniroma1.it

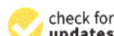

Citation: Lauri, C.; Campagna, G.; Glaudemans, A.W.J.M.; Slart, R.H.J.A.; van Leer, B.; Pillay, J.; Colandrea, M.; Grana, C.M.; Stigliano, A.; Signore, A. SARS-CoV-2 Affects Thyroid and Adrenal Glands: An ^{18}F-FDG PET/CT Study. *Biomedicines* 2023, 11, 2899. https://doi.org/10.3390/biomedicines11112899

Academic Editors: Elena Cecilia Rosca and Amalia Cornea

Received: 26 September 2023
Revised: 12 October 2023
Accepted: 23 October 2023
Published: 26 October 2023

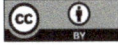

Copyright: © 2023 by the authors. Licensee MDPI, Basel, Switzerland. This article is an open access article distributed under the terms and conditions of the Creative Commons Attribution (CC BY) license (https:// creativecommons.org/licenses/by/ 4.0/).

Abstract: Background: Since most endocrine glands express ACE-2 receptors and can be infected by SARS-CoV-2 virus, this retrospective multicentre observational study aims to assess the metabolic activity of thyroid and adrenal glands of COVID-19 patients by ^{18}F-FDG PET/CT. Methods: We retrospectively evaluated the ^{18}F-FDG PET/CT scans of COVID-19 patients admitted by three different centres, either in a low-intensity department or in the intensive care unit (ICU). A visual assessment and a semi-quantitative evaluation of areas of interest in thyroid and adrenal glands were performed by recording SUVmax and SUVmean. The ^{18}F-FDG PET/CT uptake in COVID-19 patients was compared with those observed in normal age-matched controls. Results: Between March 2020 and March 2022, 33 patients from three different centres (twenty-eight patients in a low-intensity department and five patients in ICU), were studied by ^{18}F-FDG PET/CT during active illness. Seven of them were also studied after clinical remission (3–6 months after disease onset). Thirty-six normal subjects were used as age-matched controls. In the thyroid gland, no statistically significant differences were observed between control subjects and COVID-19 patients at diagnosis. However, at the follow-up PET/CT study, we found a statistically higher SUVmax and SUVmean ($p = 0.009$ and $p = 0.004$, respectively) in the thyroid of COVID-19 patients. In adrenal glands, we observed lower SUVmax and SUVmean in COVID-19 patients at baseline compared to control subjects ($p < 0.0001$) and this finding did not normalize after clinical recovery ($p = 0.0018$ for SUVmax and $p = 0.002$ for SUV mean). Conclusions: In our series, we observed persistent low ^{18}F-FDG uptake in adrenal glands of patients at diagnosis of COVID-19 and after recovery, suggesting a chronic hypofunction. By contrast, thyroid uptake was comparable to normal subjects at disease onset, but after recovery, a subgroup of patients showed an increased metabolism, thus possibly suggesting the onset of an inflammatory thyroiditis. Our results should alert clinicians to investigate the pituitary–adrenal axis and thyroid functionality at the time of infection and to monitor them after recovery.

Keywords: COVID-19 patients; SARS-CoV-2; thyroid gland; adrenal glands; ^{18}F-FDG PET/CT; ICU

1. Introduction

Since the outbreak of coronavirus disease 2019 (COVID-19) pandemic, increasing evidence in the literature highlights that severe acute respiratory syndrome coronavirus 2 (SARS-CoV-2) does not show a selective tropism on the respiratory system. It is, indeed, now well known that SARS-CoV-2 variants have widespread effects on many tissues and organs, including central nervous, cardiovascular and digestive systems, thus shifting COVID-19 from a respiratory syndrome to a systemic disease [1,2]. A large body of literature also describes endocrine gland impairment deriving from several factors: a direct gland damage induced by the virus, an indirect effect on hypothalamus–pituitary gland axis, a massive production of inflammatory cytokines and chemokines and virus-triggered inflammation [3,4].

SARS-CoV-2 mainly uses angiotensin-converting enzyme 2 (ACE-2) receptors to gain cellular access, causing tissue damage [3]. ACE-2 receptors are variably expressed in pituitary, thyroid, adrenal, pancreatic and gonadal glands; therefore, the endocrine system offers several potential targets for viral-induced damage [5–7]. It is now clear that endocrine disorders contribute to the complex and varied symptoms experienced by infected patients and that some of them may take a long time to normalize endocrine functionality [5–7].

It has been reported that 13 to 64% of COVID-19 patients are affected by thyroid dysfunctions [4], with a higher prevalence compared to non-COVID-19 subjects [8–10]. Transient thyrotoxicosis has been mainly described in patients admitted to the intensive care unit (ICU) [11] and it has been associated with high interleukin 6 (IL-6) levels [12]. This would increase cardiovascular risks, such as arrhythmias, that have been frequently reported in COVID-19 patients. Sub-acute thyroiditis and Graves' thyrotoxicosis have also been described [13,14] as well as hypothyroidism, with the majority of patients reverting to normal thyroid function after several months post infection [8].

Similar findings have been described after SARS-CoV-2 vaccination, thus suggesting a direct role of spike protein interaction with ACE-2 receptors, cross reactivity with thyroid proteins and immune-mediated phenomena triggered by the vaccine itself [15–17].

Adrenal impairment has also been frequently reported. Its aetiology is multifactorial. Several case reports described adrenal insufficiency due to adrenal infarction or haemorrhage [18–22]. Moreover, it has been postulated that SARS-CoV-2 is able to impair the stress-induced cortisol production by expressing several amino acid sequences that mimic human adrenocorticotropic hormone (ACTH). Therefore, the host's antibodies produced against the virus will also cross-react and inactivate endogenous circulating ACTH [23,24]. This "immune-invasive strategy" may result in the development of corticosteroid insufficiency and could predispose to more critical clinical presentation of respiratory tract infection and persisting symptoms [23,24]. In addition to this, a direct injury on the adrenal cortex, due to the expression of ACE2 receptors in the *zona fasciculata* and *reticularis*, impairs the glucocorticoid synthesis [25]. The indiscriminate use of high doses of exogenous corticosteroids, which have been largely used for therapy, determines a suppression of hypothalamus–pituitary–adrenal (HPA) axis, thus contributing to hypocortisolism [23,26–29].

As the acute and devasting phase of SARS-CoV-2 pandemic is passed, "long COVID" is becoming the new challenge facing clinicians. This condition, due to a multi-systemic involvement, is characterized by persistent malaise, fatigue, dizziness, myalgia and joint pain, headache and possible cognitive disturbances affecting the patient for a long time after COVID-19 diagnosis [30–32]. It has been postulated that adrenal insufficiency concurs in the development and maintenance of fatigue, myalgia and arthralgia, which have been reported in 65%, 50.6%, and 54.7%, respectively, of long COVID patients [33,34]. Nevertheless, data on cortisol levels in COVID-19 patients are rarely reported and provide discordant findings [34,35] and, in general, the long-term impact of endocrine dysfunction still needs to be further elucidated.

Fluorine-18 fluorodeoxyglucose positron emission tomography/computed tomography (^{18}F-FDG PET/CT) is not recommended for diagnosis or for follow-up of COVID-19 patients despite the literature having extensively described incidental cases of SARS-CoV-2 infection diagnosed in patients undergoing ^{18}F-FDG PET/CT for other reasons [36–40].

Moreover, with the increasing awareness that SARS-CoV-2 infection is not only confined to the respiratory tract, but rather showing a multi-systemic tropism, several papers have described the ^{18}F-FDG uptake in extra-thoracic tissues and organs during SARS-CoV-2 infection or vaccination [41–49]. During the early months of the COVID-19 pandemic, after observing the first two patients affected by SARS-CoV-2 infection [42], we performed a qualitative and semi-quantitative analysis of ^{18}F-FDG uptake in several organs/tissues, in addition to lungs, and correlated these measurements with patients' haematological parameters [43]. Given the increasing evidence of endocrine gland involvement, our attention now focuses on the analysis of ^{18}F-FDG uptake in the thyroid and adrenal glands. Therefore, the aim of this retrospective multicentre observational study is to describe ^{18}F-FDG uptake in thyroid and adrenal glands in COVID-19 patients at baseline, during follow-up, and in comparison to normal age-matched subjects.

2. Materials and Methods

2.1. Patients

Inclusion criteria for patients in this retrospective study were:
- Positivity to nasopharyngeal swab with real time polymerase chain reaction (RT-PCR) test for SARS-CoV-2 between 2020 and 2022;
- Patients admitted in low intensity departments or intensive care unit (ICU);
- Availability of at least one ^{18}F-FDG PET/CT scan during the active SARS-CoV-2 infection performed in order to assess the extent of the disease.

Exclusion criteria were:
- Patients with pre-existing structural and/or functional alterations of thyroid and adrenal glands;
- Patients who previously received chemotherapy or biologic therapies for oncologic reasons;
- Pregnancy or nursing women;
- Age < 18 years.

For the control group, we retrospectively evaluated ^{18}F-FDG PET/CT studies performed for several oncologic and non-oncologic clinical indications between 2020 and 2022. Patients without a history of thyroid and adrenal dysfunctions, based on the electronic patient file, and showing a normal ^{18}F-FDG biodistribution without any pathological uptake were enrolled. Patients receiving chemotherapy or immune check-point inhibitors at the time of the study were excluded from the analysis.

2.2. The ^{18}F-FDG PET/CT Studies

The ^{18}F-FDG PET/CT scans at diagnosis, and at recovery when available, were acquired at Sant'Andrea University Hospital of Rome (Rome, Italy), International European Oncology hospital in Milan (Milan, Italy), and University Medical Centre Groningen (Groningen, The Netherlands) by using a hybrid PET/CT system (Siemens, Germany).

The ^{18}F-FDG (3–5 MBq/Kg) was administered 1 h before imaging from pelvis to head as per standardized EARL procedures [50,51]. After image acquisition, attenuation corrected PET images were automatically fused with CT images and displayed in maximum intensity projection (MIP) in axial, coronal and sagittal plane.

To minimize mismatches between CT and PET scans, CT images were obtained with a slice thickness of 3.75 mm. Moreover, immediately after CT acquisition, PET scan started from the pelvic region (therefore, less than 2 min delay from CT to pelvic PET).

Patient data were retrospectively collected via electronic patient files. Given the retrospective nature of this study, the local Ethical Committee waived the need for approval, but written informed consent was obtained from all non-ICU patients. For ICU patients, written informed consent was obtained from their closest relatives.

2.3. Analysis of ^{18}F-FDG PET/CT Studies

A visual analysis of ^{18}F-FDG metabolic activity on lungs and mediastinal lymph-nodes was performed to assess the severity of the infection [43,52–55] and to meet the clinical need of each patient. The ^{18}F-FDG biodistribution in both thyroid and adrenal glands was retrospectively visually evaluated.

A semi-quantitative analysis on axial sections of EARL reconstructed images was also performed by drawing circular regions of interest (ROIs) in right and left thyroid lobe and on both adrenal glands and by calculating the maximum and mean standardized uptake value (SUVmax and SUVmean). The whole glands' activity was calculated as the mean of right and left lobe of thyroid gland and as the mean of left and right adrenal gland. In patients with the right adrenal gland too close to the liver, the measurement was not performed due to overlap of liver metabolic activity.

2.4. Statistical Analysis

Continuous variables are presented as mean ± standard deviation (SD) and 95% confidence interval (95% CI).

Comparisons between control subjects, COVID-19 at diagnosis and COVID-19 ICU of SUVmax and SUVmean of thyroid and adrenal glands were evaluated by generalized linear mixed model (GLIMMIX) with Gaussian distribution.

Normality residuals were tested by Shapiro–Wilk test and checking the Q-Q plot. Homoscedasticity was evaluated by checking the studentized residuals vs. fitted values plot.

Post-hoc analysis was performed using the Tukey method.

The differences between thyroid and adrenal glands in control subjects versus COVID-19 subjects after recovery were estimated by the Student's t-test (normality verified) or Brunner–Munzel test (normality failed).

COVID-19 at diagnosis versus COVID-19 after recovery of thyroid and adrenal glands was tested by paired Student's t-test.

The cut-offs of thyroid and adrenal gland uptake were obtained using Youden index, as described elsewhere [56,57].

Statistical analysis was performed using the SAS v.9.4 TS level 1M8 (SAS Institute Inc., Cary, NC, USA). A p-value < 0.05 was considered statistically detectable.

3. Results

3.1. Patients

Between March 2020 and March 2022, we enrolled 33 patients (twenty-four males and nine females, mean age 57.67 ± 14 years) with SARS-CoV-2 infection admitted to three centres and studied with ^{18}F-FDG PET/CT (fourteen patients were studied at Sant'Andrea hospital in Rome; four patients were recruited by IEO in Milan; and fifteen patients were studied at UMC Groningen). Five out of these fifteen patients were mechanically ventilated and admitted to ICU for their critical illness at the time of ^{18}F-FDG PET/CT.

Seven patients were studied twice, at diagnosis and after complete clinical recovery, which occurred between 3 and 6 months after diagnosis, and a double negative RT-PCR test for SARS-CoV-2.

Respiratory symptoms (mainly dyspnoea), anosmia and persistent fever were the main causes for hospitalization of these patients. These clinical manifestations appeared on average 5 to 7 days before ^{18}F-FDG PET/CT. Therapies varied amongst the different centres and according to the severity of patients' clinical manifestations, and mainly included personalized doses of corticosteroids, remdesivir, tocilizumab, paracetamol and hydroxychloroquine.

One critically ill patient admitted in ICU died due to progressive respiratory failure and extra-pulmonary organ failure. Another five patients died for unrelated complications.

For the control group, we identified 36 age-matched patients (17 males and 19 females, mean age 59.40 ± 15.73 years) without known thyroid and adrenal dysfunctions that underwent ^{18}F-FDG PET/CT for oncological and non-oncological reasons and who showed no pathologic metabolic lesions at scan analysis.

3.2. Thyroid and Adrenal Gland Analysis

Semi-quantitative results of thyroid and adrenal gland ^{18}F-FDG uptake in control group (group A), non-critical COVID-19 patients (group B) and ICU group (group C) are reported in Table 1.

Table 1. Differences between control group, non-critical COVID-19 patients and the ICU group, in terms of SUVmax and SUVmean of thyroid and adrenal glands.

Variable	A Control Subjects (n = 36) Mean ± SD (95% CI)	B COVID-19 at Diagnosis (n = 28) Mean ± SD (95% CI)	C COVID-19 ICU (n = 5) Mean ± SD (95% CI)	p	p (A vs. B)	p (A vs. C)	p (B vs. C)
Thyroid (SUVmax)	1.36 ± 0.18 (1.30 to 1.42)	1.55 ± 0.47 (1.37 to 1.73)	1.31 ± 0.24 (1.02 to 1.61)	0.06	--	--	--
Thyroid (SUVmean)	1.24 ± 0.16 (1.19 to 1.30)	1.35 ± 0.38 (1.21 to 1.50)	1.18 ± 0.22 (0.90 to 1.45)	0.19	--	--	--
Adrenal (SUVmax)	2.16 ± 0.32 (2.05 to 2.27)	1.65 ± 0.26 (1.55 to 1.75)	1.73 ± 0.26 (1.40 to 2.06)	<0.0001	<0.0001	0.003	0.58
Adrenal (SUVmean)	1.94 ± 0.30 (1.84 to 2.04)	1.51 ± 0.27 (1.40 to 1.61)	1.64 ± 0.23 (1.35 to 1.93)	<0.0001	<0.0001	0.03	0.34

When examining thyroid ^{18}F-FDG uptake (Figure 1), no differences were observed among the three groups of patients in terms of pattern distribution. Non-critical patients showed slightly higher SUVmax and SUVmean compared to normal subjects.

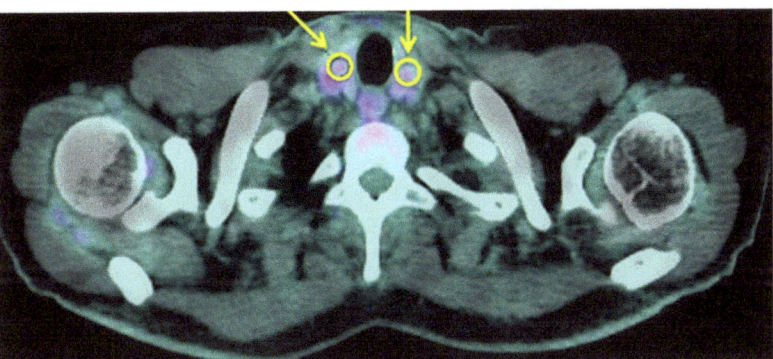

Figure 1. Example of calculation of quantitative parameters on thyroid gland of one COVID-19 patient. Yellow circles and arrows show the regions of interest drawn on thyroid tissue. In this patient, the right lobe had an SUVmax of 2.18 and an SUVmean of 2.05; the left lobe had an SUVmax of 2.10 and an SUVmean of 1.94.

No statistically significant differences were observed comparing basal and follow-up study in the seven patients who repeated PET/CT scan, but interestingly, they showed higher SUVmax (p = 0.009) and SUVmean (p = 0.004) at follow-up study compared to control subjects (Table 2). Despite mean values that were significantly higher at follow-up scan, only three patients showed an increased thyroid uptake, thus suggesting that thyroid inflammation or thyroid hyperfunction may appear evident several months after COVID-19 diagnosis, but not in all patients.

Table 2. Differences between control group and COVID-19 patients after recovery in terms of SUVmax and SUVmean of thyroid gland.

Thyroid Uptake	Control Group (n = 36) Mean ± SD (95% CI)	COVID-19 after Recovery (n = 7) Mean ± SD (95% CI)	p
SUVmax	1.36 ± 0.18 (1.30 to 1.42)	1.65 ± 0.30 (1.37 to 1.93)	0.009
SUVmean	1.24 ± 0.16 (1.19 to 1.30)	1.46 ± 0.22 (1.25 to 1.66)	0.004

For thyroid gland in control subjects, a cut-off of 1.56 for SUVmax showed a sensitivity of 42.4% and a specificity of 94.4%; for SUVmean, a cut-off of 1.41 provided 39.4% of sensitivity and 91.7% of specificity. SUVmax was higher than the cut-off in 14/33 COVID-19 patients at diagnosis (42.4%) and in 2/36 controls (5.56%) ($p = 0.0003$). SUVmean was higher than the cut-off in 13/33 COVID-19 patients at diagnosis (39.4%) and in 3/36 controls (8.3%) ($p = 0.002$) (Figures 2 and 3).

Only two patients were excluded from the analysis of right gland because it was too close to the liver.

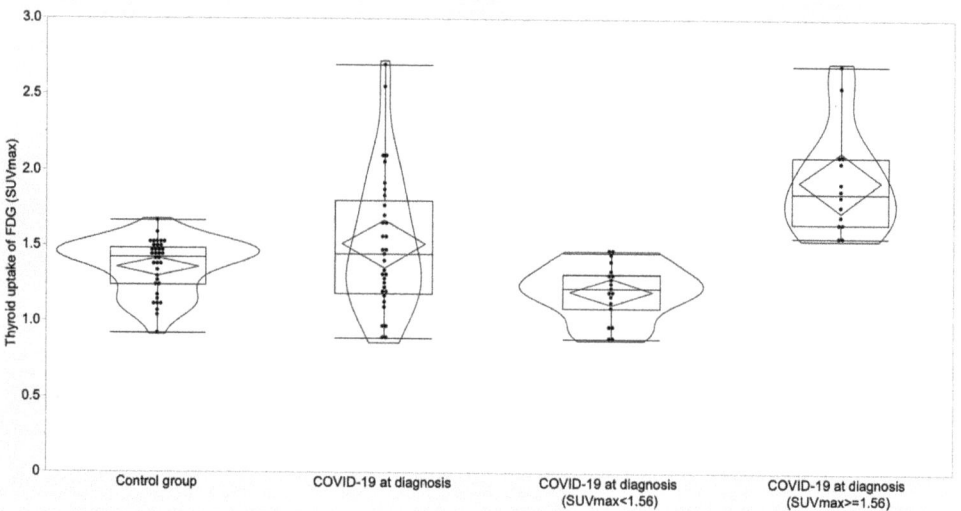

Figure 2. Boxplots and violin plots of SUVmax in thyroid glands of control group vs. COVID-19 patients at the diagnosis and distribution of SUVmax of COVID-19 patients according to the cut-off.

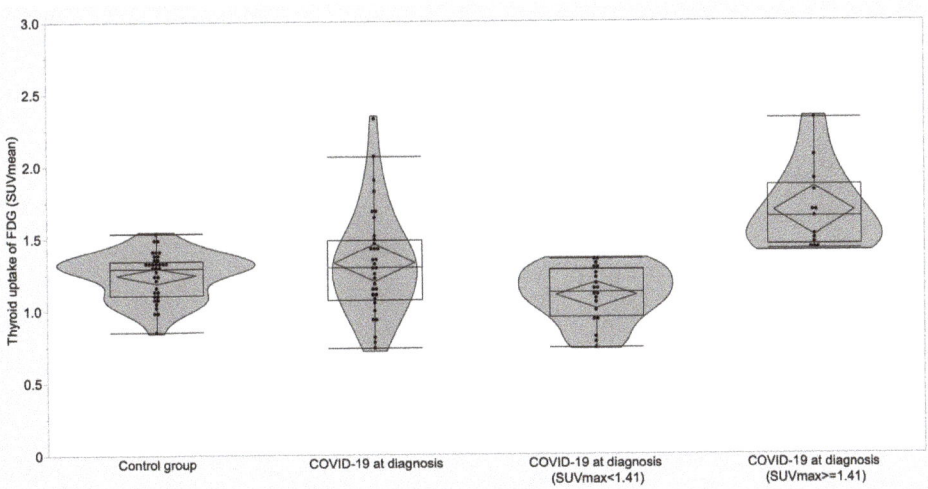

Figure 3. Boxplots and violin plots of SUVmean in thyroid glands of control group vs. COVID-19 patients at the diagnosis and distribution of SUVmean of COVID-19 patients according to the cut-off.

Similar to the thyroid gland, no correlation was detected between the uptake distribution pattern of adrenal glands and disease severity (Figure 4). As reported in Table 1, the adrenal glands of COVID-19 patients, either admitted in low-intensity unit or in ICU, showed statistically lower SUVmax and SUVmean than control subjects.

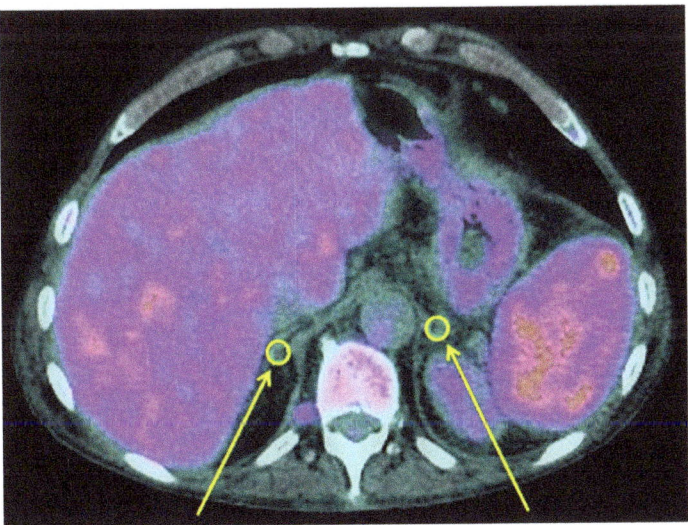

Figure 4. Example of calculation of quantitative parameters on adrenal glands of one COVID-19 patient. Yellow circles and arrows show the regions of interest. In this patient, the right adrenal gland had an SUVmax of 1.33 and an SUVmean of 1.21; the left adrenal gland had an SUVmax of 1.26 and an SUVmean of 1.20.

The post-hoc analysis showed lower SUVmax and SUVmean in patients with moderate infection (group B; $p < 0.0001$ for both SUVmax and SUVmean) and in ICU patients (group C; $p = 0.003$ for SUVmax and $p = 0.03$ for SUVmean) compared to the control group.

No statistically significant differences were observed when comparing the basal study and the follow-up study in the seven patients who repeated PET/CT scan, but after recovery, they showed persistently lower ^{18}F-FDG uptake in adrenal glands compared to healthy control subjects, in terms of SUVmax and SUVmean (Table 3).

Table 3. Differences between control group and COVID-19 patients after recovery in terms of SUVmax, SUVmean of adrenal glands.

Adrenal Glands' Uptake	Control Group (n = 36) Mean ± SD (95% CI)	COVID-19 after Recovery (n = 7) Mean ± SD (95% CI)	p
SUVmax	2.16 ± 0.32 (2.05 to 2.27)	1.66 ± 0.26 (1.57 to 1.75)	<0.0001
SUVmean	1.94 ± 0.30 (1.84 to 2.04)	1.53 ± 0.26 (1.43 to 1.62)	<0.0001

For adrenal glands, a cut-off of 1.99 for SUVmax showed a sensitivity of 93.9% and specificity of 66.7%; for SUVmean, a cut-off of 1.88 provided 97% of sensitivity and 52.8% of specificity (Figures 3 and 4). SUVmax was lower than the cut-off in 31/33 COVID-19 patients at diagnosis (93.9%) and in 12/36 controls (33.3%) ($p < 0.0001$).

SUVmean was lower than the cut-off in all but one of the COVID-19 patients at diagnosis (97%) and in 17/36 controls (47.2%) ($p < 0.0001$) (Figures 5 and 6).

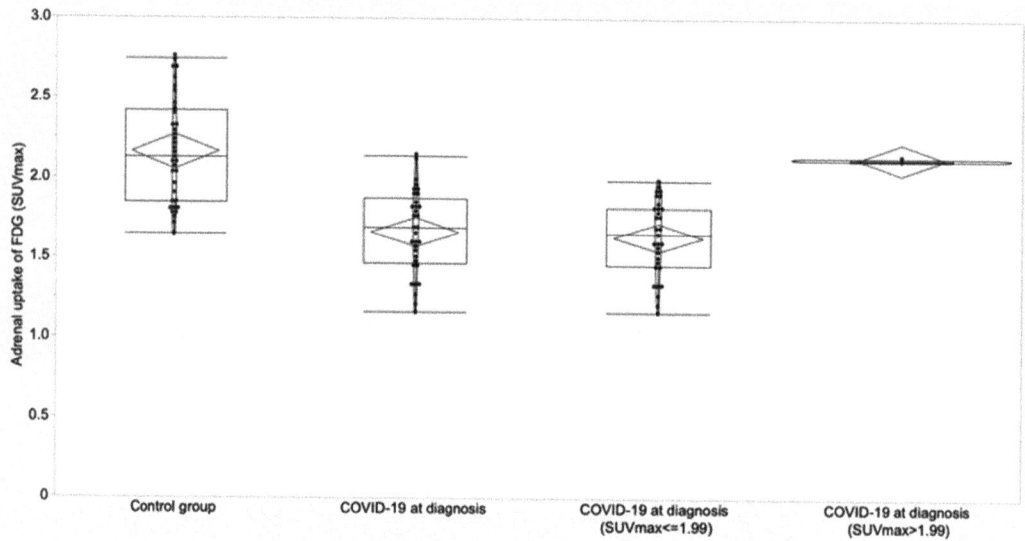

Figure 5. Boxplots and violin plots of SUVmax in adrenal glands of control group vs. COVID-19 patients at the diagnosis and distribution of SUVmax of COVID-19 patients according to the cut-off.

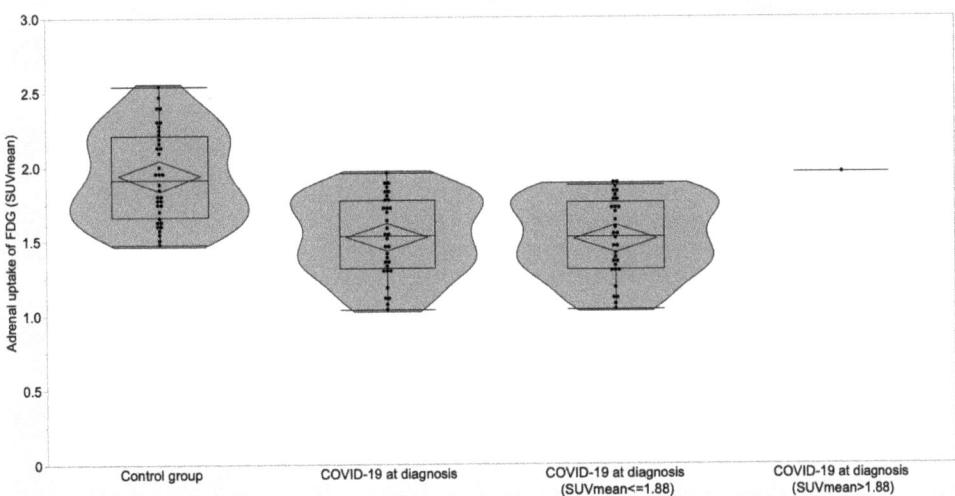

Figure 6. Boxplots and violin plots of SUVmean in adrenal glands of control group vs. COVID-19 patients at the diagnosis and distribution of SUVmean of COVID-19 patients according to the cut-off.

4. Discussion

Endocrine glands represent a potential target of SARS-CoV-2 infection, and thyroid dysfunctions and adrenal insufficiency have been largely described in the literature [4–27,58–61]. Their impairment takes part of the complex and variegated symptomatology experienced by the patients and might influence the clinical course of the disease [62].

It is well known that this virus is able to trigger long-term immune activation thus being responsible for latent or overt inflammatory and autoimmune phenomena or hypofunctionality [63,64]. Drugs may also indirectly impair endocrine glands by exerting a suppressive effect, and this especially, holds true for HPA axis due to the large use of steroids, which may turn in the development of hypocortisolism [23,27–29]. It is, indeed well known that a prolonged treatment with high corticosteroid doses leads to high risk of adrenal insufficiency that may take up to 6 months to revert [29]. In COVID-19 patients, both the virus itself and steroid treatment could contribute to the development of cortisol deficiency and to understand which of these aspects has a major role, deserves further speculations.

As opposed to thyroid dysfunctions, which usually revert after a variable time from the infection, adrenal insufficiency might persist for several months after the recovery, thus having a potential role in long-COVIDsyndrome. In particular, HPA axis impairment and hypothyroidism are, in part, implied in persistent fatigue reported by the majority of patient with long-COVID [58–62].

Although ^{18}F-FDG PET/CT plays only a marginal role in the diagnosis and monitoring of COVID-19 patients, the increasing evidence of incidental findings detected by this imaging modality further supports the awareness that SARS-CoV-2 infection is not only confined to the respiratory tract, but rather it may involve several other organs and apparatuses [36–43,65,66].

Therefore, this retrospective multicentre study aimed at comparing the ^{18}F-FDG uptake in thyroid and adrenal glands in patients affected by SARS-CoV-2 infection and in normal control subjects. Moreover, we compared the ^{18}F-FDG uptake in seven patients who performed an ^{18}F-FDG PET/CT study at both basal time and after recovery.

For thyroid gland we did not observe any difference in ^{18}F-FDG uptake between control subjects and newly diagnosed COVID-19 patients (either admitted in low-intensity departments or in ICU). Neither was a difference observed from basal PET/CT scan and follow-up study in the subgroup of patients who performed a double scan. However, we found statistically higher metabolic activity in the follow-up PET/CT as compared to control group, thus potentially suggesting an inflammatory status or hyperfunction of thyroid gland. Unfortunately, given the retrospective nature of this study, data on thyroid function were not collected; therefore, we are not able to correlate ^{18}F-FDG uptake with the hormonal status of these patients. It would have been very interesting to investigate whether these patients experienced a thyroiditis or changes in thyroid hormone function during and after SARS-CoV-2 infection.

As far as adrenal glands are concerned, we found interesting results. COVID-19 patients (either admitted in low-intensity departments or in ICU) showed statistically lower SUVmax and SUVmean than control subjects. No differences were observed from basal PET/CT scan and follow-up study, the metabolic activity did not normalize at recovery but was persistently lower than activity observed in healthy controls. This would potentially suggest a suppressive state of adrenal glands, which may persist for a long time after recovery, thus negatively influencing patients' quality of life [67]. As previously mentioned, given the observational retrospective nature of this study, we are not able to correlate PET/CT findings with pituitary and adrenal function, but this aspect deserves further speculation, especially considering the role of adrenal insufficiency in the development of long-COVID syndrome. Furthermore, we are not able to determine the contribution of direct gland damage due to the virus or the possible role of steroid therapies in adrenal glands of COVID-19 patients. We can only speculate that in our population, a combination of both aspects would have contributed to low ^{18}F-FDG uptake in adrenal glands, but this requires further investigations.

Similar to our findings, Sollini et al. recently analysed ^{18}F-FDG uptake in several organs in patients suffering from long-COVID, reporting lower adrenal uptake in COVID-19 patients than in control subjects and speculating that hypocortisolism might play a role in long-COVID syndrome [68].

Conversely, Bülbül and colleagues recently assessed ^{18}F-FDG uptake in several endocrine glands including pituitary, thyroid, adrenal glands, testis and pancreas. Although they found a statistically higher SUVmean in the pancreas of COVID-19 patients compared to non-COVID-19 patients, they did not observe statistical differences in thyroid, adrenal, pituitary glands and testis [69].

Despite the multicentre nature, our study has several limitations. First of all, as previously mentioned, it has a retrospective design. All ^{18}F-FDG PET/CT scans were performed during the pandemic wave and, in that period, the restrictions due to spreading of SARS-CoV-2 infection in the many departments had a negative impact on the working quality also in Nuclear Medicine Units and did not allow the clinician to deeply assess the whole status of the patients [70–73].

Moreover, the number of examined patients is limited; however, ^{18}F-FDG PET/CT is not included as a crucial imaging modality for the assessment of COVID-19 severity, rather it retains a supportive role over conventional radiological scans, and it is justified only in selected patients. Indeed, despite the large number of COVID-19 patients admitted in our three centres during the pandemic waves, only a small percentage of them required a PET/CT study to assess the severity of the infection, to detect possible involvement of other organs or when clinical symptoms did not match CT findings. Another limitation is the lack of pituitary, thyroid and adrenal function assessment in COVID-19 patients. We, therefore, herein only describe the ^{18}F-FDG uptake in thyroid and adrenal gland, opening new questions about the different behaviour of different endocrine glands. Some may show an inflammatory or autoimmune status and hyper-functionality; some others may be downregulated and lead to hypofunctionality. The availability of laboratory tests would have allowed a correlation between hormonal status of these patients and ^{18}F-FDG uptake and would have laid the basis for further speculations. Moreover, we cannot exclude that the use of high-dose glucocorticoids, which has been largely adopted during the SARS outbreak, might be responsible of the reduced metabolism observed in adrenal glands.

Despite these limitations, our observation should alert clinicians about excluding a cortisol deficiency or a thyroid impairment in these kinds of patients in order to promptly start supportive therapies [23,74].

The correlation between hormonal status of COVID-19 patients, in particular on the HPA axis and ^{18}F-FDG uptake deserves further speculations and might be relevant in preventing long-COVID syndrome and improving patients' quality of life.

5. Conclusions

Despite the observation that thyroid uptake was comparable to normal subjects at disease onset, after recovery, a subgroup of patients showed an increased metabolic activity, thus possibly suggesting the onset of an inflammatory thyroiditis. Moreover, we observed lower ^{18}F-FDG uptake in adrenal glands of COVID-19 patients compared to normal subjects and this finding did not normalize after recovery. This would potentially suggest a persistent hypofunctionality and would alert clinicians to investigate the endocrine status at both basal time and after the recovery. In the long-COVID era, this aspect should be one of the priority areas for future research.

Author Contributions: Conceptualization, A.S. (Alberto Signore) and C.L.; methodology, A.S. (Alberto Signore), C.L., G.C., R.H.J.A.S., A.W.J.M.G., B.v.L., J.P., C.M.G., M.C. and A.S. (Antonio Stigliano); software, A.W.J.M.G.; validation, A.S. (Alberto Signore) and C.L.; formal analysis, A.W.J.M.G.; investigation, C.L., R.H.J.A.S., A.W.J.M.G., B.v.L., J.P., C.M.G. and M.C.; resources, C.L., R.H.J.A.S., A.W.J.M.G., B.v.L., J.P., C.M.G. and M.C.; data curation, C.L.; writing—original draft preparation, C.L.; writing—review and editing, A.S. (Alberto Signore); supervision, A.S. (Alberto Signore). All authors have read and agreed to the published version of the manuscript.

Funding: This research received no external funding.

Institutional Review Board Statement: Ethical review and approval were waived for this study due to the retrospective nature of this paper.

Informed Consent Statement: Informed consent was obtained from all subjects involved in the study.

Data Availability Statement: Data are available upon request.

Conflicts of Interest: The authors declare no conflict of interest.

References

1. Huang, C.; Wang, Y.; Li, X.; Ren, L.; Zhao, J.; Hu, Y.; Zhang, L.; Fan, G.; Xu, J.; Gu, X.; et al. Clinical features of patients infected with 2019 novel coronavirus in Wuhan, China. *Lancet* **2020**, *395*, 497–506. [CrossRef] [PubMed]
2. Chen, N.; Zhou, M.; Dong, X.; Qu, J.; Gong, F.; Han, Y.; Qiu, Y.; Wang, J.; Liu, Y.; Wei, Y.; et al. Epidemiological and clinical characteristics of 99 cases of 2019 novel coronavirus pneumonia in Wuhan, China: A descriptive study. *Lancet* **2020**, *395*, 507–513. [PubMed]
3. Hossain, M.F.; Hasana, S.; Mamun, A.A.; Uddin, M.S.; Wahed, M.I.I.; Sarker, S.; Behl, T.; Ullah, I.; Begum, Y.; Bulbul, I.J.; et al. COVID-19 outbreak: Pathogenesis, current therapies, and potentials for future management. *Front. Pharmacol.* **2020**, *11*, 563478.
4. Giovanella, L.; Ruggeri, R.M.; Ovčariček, P.P.; Campenni, A.; Treglia, G.; Deandreis, D. Prevalence of thyroid dysfunction in patients with COVID-19: A systematic review. *Clin. Transl. Imaging* **2021**, *9*, 233–240. [PubMed]
5. Marazuela, M.; Giustina, A.; Puig-Domingo, M. Endocrine and metabolic aspects of the COVID-19 pandemic. *Rev. Endocr. Metab. Disord.* **2020**, *21*, 495–507.
6. Parolin, M.; Parisotto, M.; Zanchetta, F.; Sartorato, P.; De Menis, E. Coronaviruses and endocrine system: A systematic review on evidence and shadows. *Endocr. Metab. Immune Disord. Drug Targets* **2021**, *21*, 1242–1251.
7. Clarke, S.A.; Abbara, A.; Dhillo, W.S. Impact of COVID-19 on the Endocrine System: A Mini-review. *Endocrinology* **2021**, *163*, bqab203.
8. Chen, M.; Zhou, W.; Xu, W. Thyroid function analysis in 50 patients with COVID-19: A retrospective study. *Thyroid* **2021**, *31*, 8–11. [CrossRef]
9. Khoo, B.; Tan, T.; Clarke, S.A.; Mills, E.G.; Patel, B.; Modi, M.; Phylactou, M.; Eng, P.C.; Thurston, L.; Alexander, E.C.; et al. Thyroid function before, during, and after COVID-19. *J. Clin. Endocrinol. Metab.* **2021**, *106*, e803–e811.

10. Lui, D.T.W.; Lee, C.H.; Chow, W.S.; Lee, A.C.H.; Tam, A.R.; Fong, C.H.Y.; Law, C.Y.; Leung, E.K.H.; To, K.K.W.; Tan, K.C.B.; et al. Thyroid dysfunction in relation to immune profile, disease status, and outcome in 191 patients with COVID-19. *J. Clin. Endocrinol. Metab.* **2021**, *106*, e926–e935.
11. Muller, I.; Cannavaro, D.; Dazzi, D.; Covelli, D.; Mantovani, G.; Muscatello, A.; Ferrante, E.; Orsi, E.; Resi, V.; Longari, V.; et al. SARS-CoV-2-related atypical thyroiditis. *Lancet Diabetes Endocrinol.* **2020**, *8*, 739–741. [CrossRef] [PubMed]
12. Lania, A.; Sandri, M.T.; Cellini, M.; Mirani, M.; Lavezzi, E.; Mazziotti, G. Thyrotoxicosis in patients with COVID-19: The THYRCOV study. *Eur. J. Endocrinol.* **2020**, *183*, 381–387. [CrossRef] [PubMed]
13. Mateu-Salat, M.; Urgell, E.; Chico, A. SARS-COV-2 as a trigger for autoimmune disease: Report of two cases of Graves' disease after COVID-19. *J. Endocrinol. Investig.* **2020**, *43*, 1527–1528. [CrossRef] [PubMed]
14. Jiménez-Blanco, S.; Pla-Peris, B.; Marazuela, M. COVID-19: A cause of recurrent Graves' hyperthyroidism? *J. Endocrinol. Investig.* **2021**, *44*, 387–388. [CrossRef]
15. Morita, S.; Takagi, T.; Inaba, H.; Furukawa, Y.; Kishimoto, S.; Uraki, S.; Shimo, N.; Takeshima, K.; Uraki, S.; Doi, K.; et al. Effect of SARS-CoV-2 BNT162b2 mRNA vaccine on thyroid autoimmunity: A twelve-month follow-up study. *Front. Endocrinol.* **2023**, *14*, 1058007. [CrossRef]
16. Muller, I.; Consonni, D.; Crivicich, E.; Di Marco, F.; Currò, N.; Salvi, M. Increased risk of Thyroid Eye Disease following Covid-19 Vaccination. *J. Clin. Endocrinol. Metab.* **2023**, *25*, dgad501.
17. Mainieri, F.; Chiarelli, F.; Betterle, C.; Bernasconi, S. Graves' disease after COVID mRNA vaccination for the first time diagnosed in adolescence-case report. Cause and effect relationship or simple coincidence? *J. Pediatr. Endocrinol. Metab.* **2023**, *36*, 993–997. [CrossRef]
18. Kumar, R.; Guruparan, T.; Siddiqi, S.; Sheth, R.; Jacyna, M.; Naghibi, M.; Vrentzou, E. A case of adrenal infarction in a patient with COVID 19 infection. *BJR Case Rep.* **2020**, *6*, 20200075. [CrossRef]
19. Elkhouly, M.M.N.; Elazzab, A.A.; Moghul, S.S. Bilateral adrenal hemorrhage in a man with severe COVID-19 pneumonia. *Radiol. Case Rep.* **2021**, *16*, 1438–1442.
20. Sharrack, N.; Baxter, C.T.; Paddock, M.; Uchegbu, E. Adrenal haemorrhage as a complication of COVID-19 infection. *BMJ Case Rep.* **2020**, *13*, 5–8. [CrossRef]
21. Álvarez-Troncoso, J.; Zapatero Larrauri, M.; Montero Vega, M.D.; Vallano, R.G.; Pelaez, E.P.; Rojas-Marcos, P.M.; Martin-Luengo, F.; Del Campo, P.L.; Gil, C.R.H.; Esteban, E.T.; et al. Case report: COVID-19 with bilateral adrenal hemorrhage. *Am. J. Trop. Med. Hyg.* **2020**, *103*, 1156–1157. [CrossRef] [PubMed]
22. Hashim, M.; Athar, S.; Gaba, W.H. New onset adrenal insufficiency in a patient with COVID-19. *BMJ Case Rep.* **2021**, *14*, e237690. [CrossRef] [PubMed]
23. Pal, R.; Banerjee, M. COVID-19 and the endocrine system: Exploring the unexplored. *J. Endocrinol. Investig.* **2020**, *43*, 1027–1031. [CrossRef] [PubMed]
24. Wheatland, R. Molecular mimicry of ACTH in SARS-implications for corticosteroid treatment and prophylaxis. *Med. Hypotheses* **2004**, *63*, 855–862. [CrossRef] [PubMed]
25. Mao, Y.; Xu, B.; Guan, W.; Xu, D.; Li, F.; Ren, R.; Zhu, X.; Gao, Y.; Jiang, L. The Adrenal Cortex, an Underestimated Site of SARS-CoV-2 Infection. *Front. Endocrinol.* **2021**, *11*, 593179. [CrossRef]
26. Piticchio, T.; Le Moli, R.; Tumino, D.; Frasca, F. Relationship between betacoronaviruses and the endocrine system: A new key to understand the COVID-19 pandemic—A comprehensive review. *J. Endocrinol. Investig.* **2021**, *44*, 1553–1570. [CrossRef]
27. Lisco, G.; De Tullio, A.; Stragapede, A.; Solimando, A.G.; Albanese, F.; Capobianco, M.; Giagulli, V.A.; Guastamacchia, E.; de Pergola, G.; Vacca, A. COVID-19 and the Endocrine System: A Comprehensive Review on the Theme. *J. Clin. Med.* **2021**, *10*, 2920. [CrossRef]
28. Brender, E.; Lynm, C.; Glass, R.M. JAMA patient page. Adrenal insufficiency. *JAMA* **2005**, *294*, 2528. [CrossRef]
29. Broersen, L.H.; Pereira, A.M.; Jørgensen, J.O.; Dekkers, O.M. Adrenal Insufficiency in Corticosteroids Use: Systematic Review and Meta-Analysis. *J. Clin. Endocrinol. Metab.* **2015**, *100*, 2171–2180. [CrossRef]
30. Davis, H.E.; Assaf, G.S.; McCorkell, L.; Wei, H.; Low, R.J.; Re'em, Y.; Redfield, S.; Austin, J.P.; Akrami, A. Characterizing long COVID in an international cohort: 7 months of symptoms and their impact. *EClinicalMedicine* **2021**, *38*, 101019. [CrossRef]
31. Ladds, E.; Rushforth, A.; Wieringa, S.; Taylor, S.; Rayner, C.; Husain, L.; Greenhalgh, T. Persistent symptoms after Covid-19: Qualitative study of 114 "long Covid" patients and draft quality principles for services. *BMC Health Serv. Res.* **2020**, *20*, 1144. [CrossRef] [PubMed]
32. Mendelson, M.; Nel, J.; Blumberg, L.; Madhi, S.A.; Dryden, M.; Stevens, W. Long-COVID: An evolving problem with an extensive impact. *S. Afr. Med. J.* **2020**, *111*, 10–12. [CrossRef]
33. Lopez-Leon, S.; Wegman-Ostrosky, T.; Perelma, C.; Sepulveda, R.; Rebolledo, P.A.; Cuapio, A.; Villapol, S. More than 50 long-term effects of COVID-19: A systematic review and meta-analysis. *Sci. Rep.* **2021**, *11*, 16144. [CrossRef]
34. Clarke, S.A.; Phylactou, M.; Patel, B.; Mills, E.G.; Muzi, B.; Izzi-Engbeaya, C.; Choudhury, S.; Khoo, B.; Meeran, K.; Comninos, A.N.; et al. Normal adrenal and thyroid function in patients who survive COVID-19 infection. *J. Clin. Endocrinol. Metab.* **2021**, *106*, 2208–2220. [CrossRef] [PubMed]
35. Salzano, C.; Saracino, G.; Cardillo, G. Possible adrenal involvement in long COVID syndrome. *Medicina* **2021**, *57*, 1087. [CrossRef] [PubMed]

36. Olivari, L.; Riccardi, N.; Rodari, P.; Buonfrate, D.; Diodato, S.; Formenti, F.; Angheben, A.; Salgarello, M. Accidental diagnosis of COVID-19 pneumonia after 18F FDG PET/CT: A case series. *Clin. Transl. Imaging* 2020, *8*, 393–400. [CrossRef] [PubMed]
37. Albano, D.; Bertagna, F.; Bertoli, M.; Bosio, G.; Lucchini, S.; Motta, F.; Panarotto, M.B.; Peli, A.; Camoni, L.; Bengel, F.M.; et al. Incidental findings suggestive of COVID-19 in asymptomatic patients undergoing nuclear medicine procedures in a high-prevalence region. *J. Nucl. Med.* 2020, *61*, 632–636. [CrossRef]
38. Setti, L.; Kirienko, M.; Dalto, S.C.; Bonacina, M.; Bombardieri, E. FDG-PET/CT findings highly suspicious for COVID-19 in an Italian case series of asymptomatic patients. *Eur. J. Nucl. Med. Mol. Imaging* 2020, *47*, 1649–1656. [CrossRef]
39. Qin, C.; Liu, F.; Yen, T.C.; Lan, X. 18F-FDG PET/CT findings of COVID-19: A series of four highly suspected cases. *Eur. J. Nucl. Med. Mol. Imaging* 2020, *47*, 1281–1286. [CrossRef]
40. Colandrea, M.; Gilardi, L.; Travaini, L.L.; Fracassi, S.L.V.; Funicelli, L.; Grana, C.M. 18F-FDG PET/CT in asymptomatic patients with COVID-19: The submerged iceberg surfaces. *Jpn. J. Radiol.* 2020, *38*, 1007–1011. [CrossRef]
41. Bai, Y.; Xu, J.; Chen, L.; Fu, C.; Kang, Y.; Zhang, W.; Fakhri, G.E.; Gu, J.; Shao, F.; Wang, M. Inflammatory response in lungs and extrapulmonary sites detected by [18F] fluorodeoxyglucose PET/CT in convalescing COVID-19 patients tested negative for coronavirus. *Eur. J. Nucl. Med. Mol. Imaging* 2021, *9*, 1–12. [CrossRef] [PubMed]
42. Signore, A.; Lauri, C.; Bianchi, M.P.; Pelliccia, S.; Lenza, A.; Tetti, S.; Martini, M.L.; Franchi, G.; Trapasso, F.; De Biase, L.; et al. [18F]FDG PET/CT in Patients Affected by SARS-CoV-2 and Lymphoproliferative Disorders and Treated with Tocilizumab. *J. Pers. Med.* 2022, *12*, 1839. [CrossRef] [PubMed]
43. Signore, A.; Lauri, C.; Colandrea, M.; Di Girolamo, M.; Chiodo, E.; Grana, C.M.; Campagna, G.; Aceti, A. Lymphopenia in patients affected by SARS-CoV-2 infection is caused by margination of lymphocytes in large bowel: An [18F]FDG PET/CT study. *Eur. J. Nucl. Med. Mol. Imaging* 2022, *29*, 1–11. [CrossRef] [PubMed]
44. Nawwar, A.A.; Searle, J.; Hagan, I.; Lyburn, I.D. COVID-19 vaccination induced axillary nodal uptake on [18F] FDG PET/CT. *Eur. J. Nucl. Med. Mol. Imaging* 2021, *48*, 2655–2656. [CrossRef] [PubMed]
45. Nawwar, A.A.; Searle, J.; Hopkins, R.; Lyburn, I.D. False-positive axillary lymph nodes on FDG PET/CT resulting from COVID-19 immunization. *Clin. Nucl. Med.* 2021, *46*, 1004–1005. [CrossRef]
46. Doss, M.; Nakhoda, S.K.; Li, Y.; Jian, Q.Y. COVID-19 vaccine–related local FDG uptake. *Clin. Nucl. Med.* 2021, *46*, 439–441.7. [CrossRef]
47. Eifer, M.; Eshet, Y. Imaging of COVID-19 vaccination at FDG PET/CT. *Radiology* 2021, *299*, E248. [CrossRef]
48. McIntosh, L.J.; Bankier, A.A.; Vijayaraghavan, G.R.; Licho, R.; Rosen, M.P. COVID-19 vaccination-related uptake on FDG PET/CT: An emerging dilemma and suggestions for management. *Am. J. Roentgenol.* 2021, *217*, 975–983. [CrossRef]
49. Moghimi, S.; Wilson, D.; Martineau, P. FDG PET Findings Post–COVID Vaccinations: Signs of the Times? *Clin. Nucl. Med.* 2021, *46*, 437–438. [CrossRef]
50. Jamar, F.; Buscombe, J.; Chiti, A.; Delbeke, D.; Donohoe, K.J.; Signore, A. EANM/SNMMI guideline for 18F-FDG use in inflammation and infection. *J. Nucl. Med.* 2013, *54*, 647–658. [CrossRef]
51. Boellaard, R.; Delgado-Bolton, R.; Oyen, W.J.; Giammarile, F.; Tatsch, K.; Eschner, W.; Verzijlbergen, F.J.; Barrington, S.F.; Pike, L.C.; Weber, W.A.; et al. FDG PET/CT: EANM procedure guidelines for tumour imaging: Version 2.0. *Eur. J. Nucl. Med. Mol. Imaging* 2015, *42*, 328–354. [CrossRef] [PubMed]
52. Inoue, K.; Goto, R.; Okada, K.; Kinomura, S.; Fukuda, H. A bone marrow F-18 FDG uptake exceeding the liver uptake may indicate bone marrow hyperactivity. *Ann. Nucl. Med.* 2009, *23*, 643–649. [CrossRef] [PubMed]
53. Ahn, S.S.; Hwang, S.H.; Jung, S.M.; Lee, S.-W.; Park, Y.-B.; Yun, M.; Song, J.J. Evaluation of spleen glucose metabolism using 18F-FDG PET/CT in patients with febrile autoimmune disease. *J. Nucl. Med.* 2017, *58*, 507–513. [CrossRef] [PubMed]
54. Ahn, S.S.; Hwang, S.H.; Jung, S.M.; Lee, S.-W.; Park, Y.-B.; Yun, M.; Song, J.J. The clinical utility of splenic fluorodeoxyglucose uptake for diagnosis and prognosis in patients with macrophage activation syndrome. *Medicine* 2017, *96*, e7901. [CrossRef] [PubMed]
55. Boursier, C.; Duval, X.; Mahida, B.; Hoen, B.; Goehringer, F.; Selton-Suty, C.; Chevalier, E.; Roch, V.; Lamiral, Z.; Bourdon, A.; et al. Hypermetabolism of the spleen or bone marrow is an additional albeit indirect sign of infective endocarditis at FDG-PET. *J. Nucl. Cardiol.* 2021, *28*, 2533–2542. [CrossRef] [PubMed]
56. Youden, W.J. Index for rating diagnostic tests. *Cancer* 1950, *3*, 32–35. [CrossRef] [PubMed]
57. Perkins, N.J.; Schisterman, E.F. The Youden Index and the optimal cut-point corrected for measurement error. *Biom. J.* 2005, *47*, 428–441. [CrossRef]
58. Alzahrani, A.S.; Mukhtar, N.; Aljomaiah, A.; Aljamei, H.; Bakhsh, A.; Alsudani, N.; Elsayed, T.; Alrashidi, N.; Fadel, R.; Alqahtani, E.; et al. The Impact of COVID-19 Viral Infection on the Hypothalamic-Pituitary-Adrenal Axis. *Endocr. Pract.* 2021, *27*, 83–89. [CrossRef]
59. Siejka, A.; Barabutis, N. Adrenal insufficiency in the COVID-19 era. *Am. J. Physiol. Endocrinol. Metab.* 2021, *320*, E784–E785. [CrossRef]
60. Akbas, E.M.; Akbas, N. COVID-19, adrenal gland, glucocorticoids, and adrenal insufficiency. *Biomed. Pap. Med. Fac. Univ. Palacky. Olomouc Czech Repub.* 2021, *165*, 1–7. [CrossRef]
61. Kanczkowski, W.; Evert, K.; Stadtmüller, M.; Haberecker, M.; Laks, L.; Chen, L.S.; Frontzek, K.; Pablik, J.; Hantel, C.; Beuschlein, F.; et al. COVID-19 targets human adrenal glands. *Lancet Diabetes Endocrinol.* 2022, *10*, 13–16. [CrossRef] [PubMed]

62. Daraei, M.; Hasibi, M.; Abdollahi, H.; Mirabdolhagh Hazaveh, M.; Zebaradst, J.; Hajinoori, M.; Asadollahi-Amin, A. Possible role of hypothyroidism in the prognosis of COVID-19. *Intern. Med. J.* **2020**, *50*, 1410–1412. [CrossRef] [PubMed]
63. Acosta-Ampudia, Y.; Monsalve, D.M.; Rojas, M.; Rodríguez, Y.; Zapata, E.; Ramírez-Santana, C.; Anaya, J.M. Persistent autoimmune activation and proinflammatory state in post-coronavirus disease 2019 syndrome. *J. Infect. Dis.* **2022**, *225*, 2155–2162. [CrossRef] [PubMed]
64. Mongioì, L.M.; Barbagallo, F.; Condorelli, R.A.; Cannarella, R.; Aversa, A.; La Vignera, S.; Calogero, A.E. Possible long-term endocrine-metabolic complications in COVID-19: Lesson from the SARS model. *Endocrine* **2020**, *68*, 467–470. [CrossRef]
65. Albano, D.; Treglia, G.; Giovanella, L.; Giubbini, R.; Bertagna, F. Detection of thyroiditis on PET/CT imaging: A systematic review. *Hormones* **2020**, *19*, 341–349. [CrossRef]
66. Van Leer, B.; van Snick, J.H.; Londema, M.; Nijsten, M.W.N.; Kasalak, O.; Slart, R.H.J.A.; Glaudemans, A.W.J.M.; Pillay, J. [18F]FDG-PET/CT in mechanically ventilated critically ill patients with COVID-19 ARDS and persistent inflammation. *Clin. Transl. Imaging* **2023**, *11*, 297–306. [CrossRef]
67. Frara, S.; Allora, A.; Castellino, L.; di Filippo, L.; Loli, P.; Giustina, A. COVID-19 and the pituitary. *Pituitary* **2021**, *24*, 465–481. [CrossRef]
68. Sollini, M.; Morbelli, S.; Ciccarelli, M.; Cecconi, M.; Aghemo, A.; Morelli, P.; Chiola, S.; Gelardi, F.; Chiti, A. Long COVID hallmarks on [18F] FDG-PET/CT: A case-control study. *Eur. J. Nucl. Med. Mol. Imaging* **2021**, *48*, 3187–3197. [CrossRef]
69. Bülbül, O.; Göksel, S.; Demet, N.A.K. Effect of Coronavirus Disease 2019 on Fluorine-18 fluorodeoxyglucose Uptake of Endocrine Organs. *Cumhur. Med. J.* **2023**, *45*, 81–86. [CrossRef]
70. Annunziata, S.; Bauckneht, M.; Albano, D.; Argiroffi, G.; Calabro, D.; Abenavoli, E.; Linguanti, F.; Laudicella, R.; Young Committee of the Italian Association of Nuclear Medicine (AIMN). Impact of the COVID-19 pandemic in nuclear medicine departments: Preliminary report of the first international survey. *Eur. J. Nucl. Med. Mol. Imaging* **2020**, *47*, 2090–2099. [CrossRef]
71. Freudenberg, L.S.; Paez, D.; Giammarile, F.; Cerci, J.; Modiselle, M.; Pascual, T.N.B.; El-Haj, N.; Orellana, P.; Pynda, Y.; Carrio, I.; et al. Global impact of COVID-19 on nuclear medicine departments: An international survey in April 2020. *J. Nucl. Med.* **2020**, *61*, 1278–1283. [CrossRef] [PubMed]
72. Freudenberg, L.S.; Dittmer, U.; Herrmann, K. Impact of COVID-19 on nuclear medicine in Germany, Austria and Switzerland: An international survey in April 2020. *Nuklearmedizin* **2020**, *59*, 294–299. [CrossRef] [PubMed]
73. Annunziata, S.; Albano, D.; Laudicella, R.; Bauckneht, M.; Young Committee of the Italian Association of Nuclear Medicine (AIMN). Surveys on COVID-19 in nuclear medicine: What happened and what we learned. *Clin. Transl. Imaging* **2020**, *8*, 303–305. [CrossRef] [PubMed]
74. Pal, R. COVID-19, hypothalamo-pituitary-adrenal axis and clinical implications. *Endocrine* **2020**, *68*, 251–252. [CrossRef]

Disclaimer/Publisher's Note: The statements, opinions and data contained in all publications are solely those of the individual author(s) and contributor(s) and not of MDPI and/or the editor(s). MDPI and/or the editor(s) disclaim responsibility for any injury to people or property resulting from any ideas, methods, instructions or products referred to in the content.

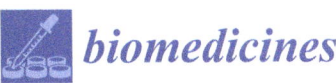

Article

Viral Coinfection of Children Hospitalized with Severe Acute Respiratory Infections during COVID-19 Pandemic

Célia Regina Malveste Ito [1,*], André Luís Elias Moreira [1], Paulo Alex Neves da Silva [1], Mônica de Oliveira Santos [1], Adailton Pereira dos Santos [1], Geovana Sôffa Rézio [2], Pollyanna Neta de Brito [2], Alana Parreira Costa Rezende [2], Jakeline Godinho Fonseca [2], Fernanda Aparecida de Oliveira Peixoto [3], Isabela Jubé Wastowski [4], Viviane Monteiro Goes [5], Mariely Cordeiro Estrela [5], Priscila Zanette de Souza [5], Lilian Carla Carneiro [1] and Melissa Ameloti Gomes Avelino [6]

1. Microorganism Biotechnology Laboratory, Institute of Tropical Pathology and Public Health, Federal University of Goiás, 235 St. Leste Universitário, Goiânia 74605-050, GO, Brazil
2. State Emergency Hospital of the Northwest Region of Goiânia Governador Otávio Lage de Siqueira (HUGOL), Anhanguera Avenue, 14.527–Santos Dumont, Goiânia 74463-350, GO, Brazil
3. Neonatal ICU of Clinical Hospital of Federal University of Goiás/EBSERH, 1st Avenue Leste Universitário, Goiânia 74605-020, GO, Brazil
4. Molecular Immunology Laboratory, Goiás State University, Laranjeiras Unity Prof. Alfredo de Castro St., 9175, Parque das Laranjeiras, Goiânia 74855-130, GO, Brazil
5. Institute of Molecular Biology of Paraná (IBMP), Professor Algacyr Munhoz Mader St, 3775–Industrial City of Curitiba, Curitiba 81350-010, PR, Brazil
6. Departament of Pediatrics, Federal University of Goiás, Universitaria Avenue, Leste Universitário, Goiânia 74605-050, GO, Brazil
* Correspondence: crmalveste@gmail.com

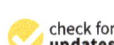

Citation: Malveste Ito, C.R.; Moreira, A.L.E.; Silva, P.A.N.d.; Santos, M.d.O.; Santos, A.P.d.; Rézio, G.S.; Brito, P.N.d.; Rezende, A.P.C.; Fonseca, J.G.; Peixoto, F.A.d.O.; et al. Viral Coinfection of Children Hospitalized with Severe Acute Respiratory Infections during COVID-19 Pandemic. *Biomedicines* 2023, 11, 1402. https://doi.org/10.3390/biomedicines11051402

Academic Editors: Elena Cecilia Rosca and Amalia Cornea

Received: 2 January 2023
Revised: 24 April 2023
Accepted: 26 April 2023
Published: 9 May 2023

Copyright: © 2023 by the authors. Licensee MDPI, Basel, Switzerland. This article is an open access article distributed under the terms and conditions of the Creative Commons Attribution (CC BY) license (https://creativecommons.org/licenses/by/4.0/).

Abstract: The main pathogens of severe respiratory infection in children are respiratory viruses, and the current molecular technology allows for a rapid and simultaneous detection of a wide spectrum of these viral pathogens, facilitating the diagnosis and evaluation of viral coinfection. Methods: This study was conducted between March 2020 and December 2021. All children admitted to the ICU with a diagnosis of SARI and who were tested by polymerase chain reaction on nasopharyngeal swabs for SARS-CoV-2 and other common respiratory viral pathogens were included in the study. Results: The result of the viral panel identified 446 children, with one infected with a single virus and 160 co-infected with two or more viruses. This study employed descriptive analyses, where a total of twenty-two coinfections among SARI-causing viruses were identified. Thus, the five most frequent coinfections that were selected for the study are: hRV/SARS-CoV-2 (17.91%), hRV/RSV (14.18%), RSV/SARS-CoV-2 (12.69%), hRV/BoV (10.45%), and hRV/AdV (8.21%). The most significant age group was 38.1%, representing patients aged between 24 and 59 months (61 individuals). Patients older than 59 months represented a total of 27.5%, comprising forty-four patients. The use of oxygen therapy was statistically significant in coinfections with Bocavirus, other CoVs, Metapneumovirus, and RSV. Coinfections with SARS-CoV-2 and the other different coinfections presented a similar time of use of oxygen therapy with a value of ($p > 0.05$). In the year 2020, hRV/BoV was more frequent in relation to other types of coinfections, representing a total of 35.1%. The year 2021 presented a divergent profile, with hRV/SARS-CoV-2 coinfection being the most frequent (30.8%), followed by hRV/RSV (28.2%). Additionally, 25.6% and 15.4% represented coinfections between RSV/SARS-CoV-2 and hRV/AdV, respectively. We saw that two of the patients coinfected with hRV/SARS-CoV-2 died, representing 9.52% of all deaths in the study. In addition, both hRV/hBoV and hRV/RSV had death records for each case, representing 8.33% and 6.67% of all deaths, respectively. Conclusion: Coinfections with respiratory viruses, such as RSV and hBoV, can increase the severity of the disease in children with SARI who are admitted to the ICU, and children infected with SARS-CoV-2 have their clinical condition worsened when they have comorbidities.

Keywords: viruses; SARI; comorbidities; epidemiology; sickness

1. Introduction

The main pathogens of severe respiratory infection in children are respiratory viruses, and the use of real-time polymerase chain reaction (PCR) technology allows a rapid and simultaneous detection of a wide spectrum of these viral pathogens, facilitating the diagnosis and evaluation of viral coinfection in severe respiratory syndromes [1].

Viral coinfections are present in severe acute respiratory infections (SARI) in a substantial proportion of children, with a rate of 14% to 44% [2,3]. During the pandemic period, the coinfections had a potential role in increased morbidity and mortality rates in the world [4].

Many respiratory viruses can cause coinfection, such as Human Metapneumovirus (hMPV), Respiratory Syncytial Virus (RSV), and Human Rhinovirus (hRV), and data on these viruses in the COVID-19 pandemic help in the diagnosis of patients, as well as determining which follow-up for the propaedeutic clinical signs presented may be of paramount importance in choosing the optimal antiviral therapy [4,5].

In the beginning of the COVID-19 pandemic, in March 2020, when the first cases of SARS-CoV-2 appeared in Brazil, the number of SARI registered was 68,100, and in 2021, there were 62,772 cases registered in children and adolescents [6].

In the city of Goiânia, capital of Goiás State, located in the center of western Brazil, 11,509 cases of SARI were recorded in 2020, 7911 by SARS-CoV-19, 22 by Influenza, 112 by other viruses, and 3419 by unspecified SARI, in the age groups <02 to ≤60. In 2021, 17,576 cases of SARS were reported, by SARS-CoV-2 (14,775), Influenza (57), other respiratory viruses (187), and unspecified (2530), in the age groups from <02 to ≤60. In the age group <2 to 19 years of age, the cases of SARI reported in the State of Goiás in the years 2020 and 2021 were 5078 cases in total, 1042 by SARS-CoV-2, 63 cases by influenza, 1002 by other respiratory viruses, and 2903 by unspecified SARI [7].

Blocking and closing borders between countries are strict health measures that help contain the spread of SARS-CoV-2 and decrease other respiratory infections caused by other viruses in children [8]. During the COVID-19 pandemic period, in the United Kingdom, a rate of 2% of viral coinfections associated with a wide variety of respiratory viruses was found [9].

This work was carried out with children and adolescents hospitalized in an intensive care unit with severe respiratory infection or with suspected COVID-19, with the objective of describing the viral coinfections detected, comparing the clinical epidemiology of children due to viral coinfection, and to determine whether viral coinfections contributed to disease severity.

2. Methods

2.1. Ethical Aspects and Hospitals Participating in the Study

All procedures and protocols for sample collection and processing were submitted and approved, under registration number 33540320.7.0000.5078 by the Research Ethics Committee of Hospital das Clínicas–GO of Federal University of Goiás, located in Goiânia-Goiás, Brazil. All parents of sick patients and voluntary donors signed the informed consent form.

The hospital unit responsible for the collection of samples and the availability of medical records for the study was the State Emergency Hospital of the Northwest Region of Goiânia Governador Otávio Lage de Siqueira (HUGOL).

2.2. Target Population

This study included 606 pediatrics patients with SARI patients due to viral contamination. The samples were collected in one hospital in a capital in the Center-West region of Brazil in the period from March 2020 to December 2021. We considered the following eligibility criteria: children (≤14 years old) admitted to emergency pediatric intensive care units (ICU). The coinfections and clinical aspects related to them were also analyzed such as: sex, age, comorbidities, fever, dyspnea, respiratory distress, wheezing, cough, chest X-ray, chest computed tomography, use of corticosteroids, use of antibiotics, salbutamol, antivirals, oxygen therapy, non-invasive ventilation (NIV), invasive mechanical ventilation (IMV), and the outcomes, for the five main coinfections mentioned. In addition, all subjects were tested by RT-qPCR (TaqMan—Thermo Fisher®, Boston, MA, USA, EUA).

2.3. Collection and Processing of Samples

For viral identification, 606 samples were collected using Rayon swabs of nasal secretion of the 606 hospitalized children. The swabs were stored in 15 mL Falcon tubes containing 3 mL of viral transport medium (VTM) and sent to the laboratory. The samples were transferred to tubes to transport samples of 5 mL containing 750 µL of TRIzol-LS reagent (Invitrogen®, New York, NY, USA, EUA) and 250 µL of the sample collected. Then, the tubes with the samples were stored in a freezer at −80 °C until the moment of ribonucleic acid extraction.

The amplification of the genetic material was performed with the kits of the Thermo Fisher Scientific (Applied Biosystems TrueMarkTM Respiratory I Combo Kit [A56284C] and Applied Biosystems TrueMarkTM Respiratory II Combo Kit [A56286C]). Both kits contained primer/probe sets specific to genomic regions of adenovirus, enterovirus, influenza A (Pan), influenza B, respiratory syncytial virus A/B, rhinovirus, human metapneumovirus, SARS-CoV-2 and primer/probe specific to conjoint coronavirus 229E, HKU1 coronavirus, NL63 coronavirus, OC43 coronavirus, parainfluenza virus 1, parainfluenza virus 2, parainfluenza virus 3, parainfluenza virus 4, and RNase P genomic regions.

The steps of experiments followed the manufacturer's instructions. A cycle threshold between 8 and 35 was considered a detected virus (positive); for greater than 40, undetected viruses (negative); and between 35 and 40 required confirmations.

2.4. Statistical Analysis

All analyzed data were deposited in Excel, version 2016 (Microsoft Windows™, Washington, DC, USA) and the data analyses were performed in the R software (R Core Team, Vienna, Austria), version 4.2.1 with the dplyr library. While the statistical analyses were performed with the aid of the R software, descriptive analyses of absolute and relative frequencies were performed with the standard functions of R Studio. To verify the association of variables, Pearson's chi-square test was used, and the Student's test was used to compare the means. Statistical modeling with binomial logistic regression, odds ratio calculations, and confidence intervals (95%) were performed using the "mfx" libraries. All graphical analyses were built using the ggplot2 and plotly libraries.

3. Results

A total of 606 children admitted to pediatric intensive care units with severe acute respiratory infection (SARI) were screened for the viral panel. The result of the viral panel identified 446 children with one infected with a single virus and 160 co-infected with two or more viruses. Among the viruses detected, Human Rhinovirus (hRV) was the most prevalent (30%), followed by Respiratory Syncytial Virus RSV (17%), SARS-CoV-2 (13%), and coinfections 24% (Figure 1).

Viral coinfections accounted for 24% of all samples studied, and among these, 79.4% of the patients analyzed had coinfections with only two viruses, and 20.6% of the affected patients had coinfections caused by three or more viruses (multiple virus).

This study employed descriptive analyses where a total of twenty-two coinfections among SARI-causing viruses were identified. Thus, the five most frequent coinfections that were selected for the study are: hRV/SARS-CoV-2 (17.91%), hRV/RSV (14.18%), RSV/SARS-CoV-2 (12.69%), hRV/BoV (10.45%), and hRV/AdV (8.21%) (Figure 2).

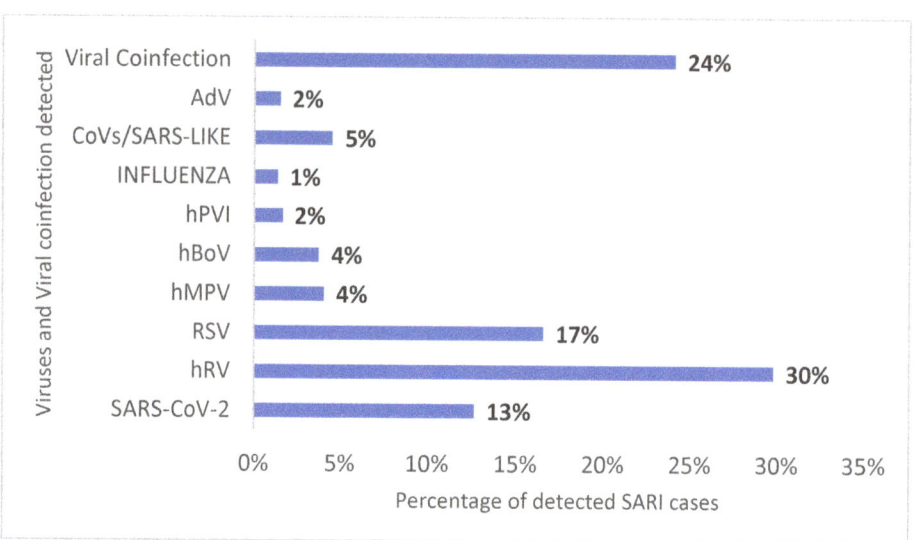

Figure 1. Profile of the virus found in the viral panel of 606 children hospitalized with SARI in the years 2020 and 2021 in a tertiary hospital. Legend: hRV (Human Rhinovirus), RSV (Respiratory Syncytial Virus), hMPV (Human Metapneumovirus), hBoV (Human Bocavirus), hPVI (Human Parainfluenza), CoVs (Coronavirus), and AdV (Adenovirus).

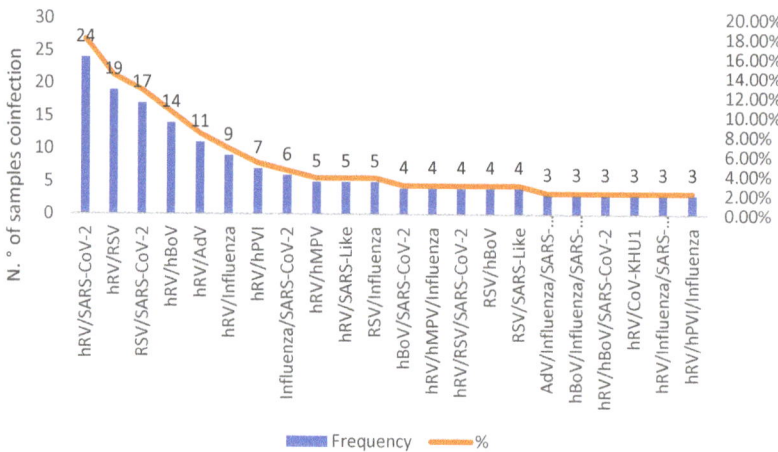

Figure 2. Comparative analysis of twenty-two respiratory coinfections caused by viruses. Legend: (hRV—Human Rhinovirus; HBoV—Human Bocavirus; AdV—Adenovirus; RSV—Respiratory Syncytial Virus; FLU—Influenza; hPVI—Human Parainfluenza Virus; CoV—Coronavirus; hMPV—Human Metapneumovirus).

It was analyzed which coinfections were more prevalent among age groups, and it was verified that the most affected of the public were children aged between 0.1 and 2 years old, with virus coinfections such as RSV/SARS-CoV-2 (7%) for 0.1 and 2 years old and hRV/RSV (9.1%) for 0.1 and 2 years old (Figure 3). It is worth mentioning that the coinfection caused by hRV/SARS-CoV-2 also stands out, where it was possible to verify its involvement in the age groups of 0–2 years (5.6%), 2–5 years (6.6 %), and 5–14 years old (3%) (Figure 3).

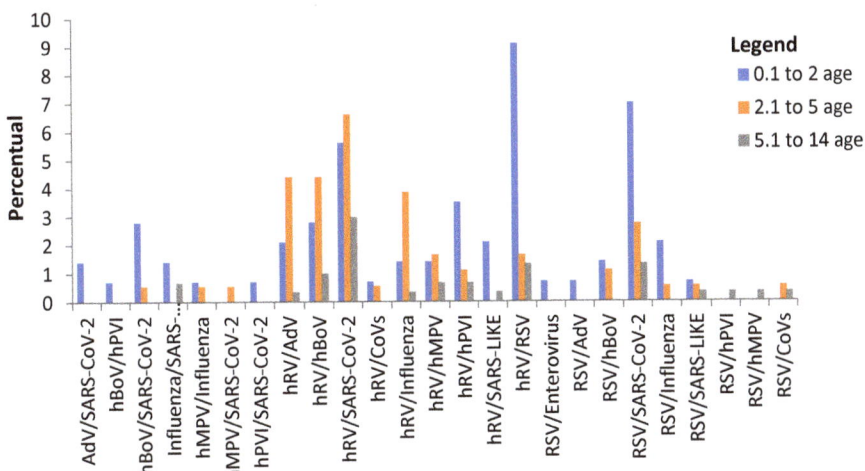

Figure 3. Analysis of involvement of coinfections according to age group. Legend: 0,1–2 years (blue), 2,1–5 years (orange), and 5,1–14 years (gray). Rhinovirus (hRV), Bocavirus (hBoV), SARS-CoV-2, Respiratory Syncytial Virus (RSV), Adenovirus (AdV), Coronavirus (CoVs), Human Metapneumovirus (hMPV), Parainfluenza (hPVI).

It was also evaluated whether there were differences in the length of stay of patients in intensive care units (ICU), in patients who were hospitalized with two viral types, and patients who were co-infected with several types of viruses. Patients co-infected with two viral types were hospitalized for a period of 161 h (6.7 days) and children co-infected with several viral types remained hospitalized for a period of 147 h (6.1 days), but despite verifying a reduction in the length of hospital stay of patients affected by multiple types of viruses, there were no statistically significant differences when compared with the group co-infected with only two types of viruses ($p > 0.005$) (Figure 4).

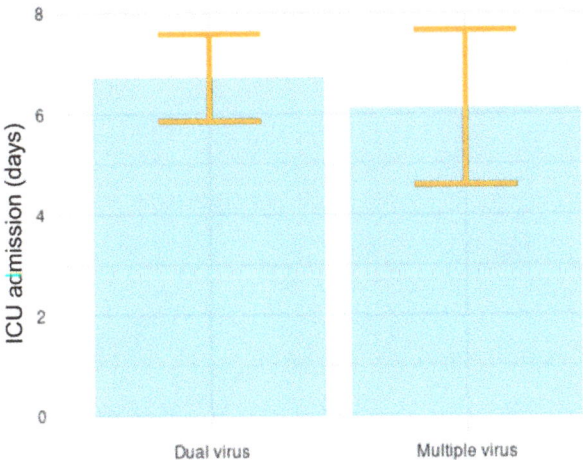

Figure 4. Analysis of length of stay in intensive care units (ICU) caused by viral coinfections.

The age range of coinfected patients has been analyzed based on data obtained previously. Thus, the most significant age group was 38.1%, representing patients aged between 24 and 59 months (61 individuals). Patients older than 59 months represented a total of

27.5%, comprising forty-four patients (Figure 5A). Then, evaluations of the age groups affected by the five most frequent coinfections were carried out. For the group representing co-infections caused by hRV/SARS-CoV-2, the age group with the highest frequency (33.3%) was patients aged over 59 months (Figure 5B).

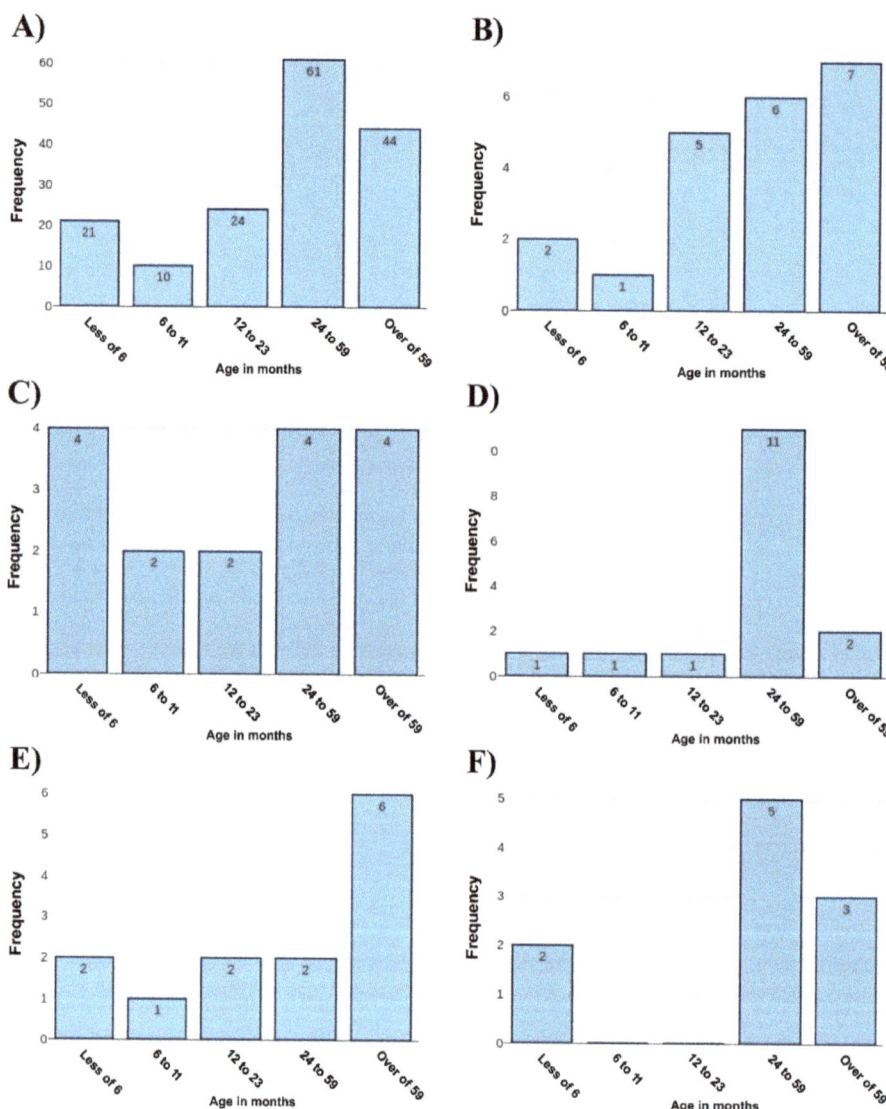

Figure 5. Analysis of the age group of co-infected patients. Legend: (A) representation of the age group of patients in relation to all coinfections analyzed during the study. (B) The age range of patients co-infected with hRV and SARS-CoV-2. (C) The age group of individuals co-infected with RSV and SARS-CoV-2. (D) The age group of patients co-infected with Rhinovirus and RSV. (E) Individuals affected by hRV and hBoV. In (F), individuals affected by coinfections caused by hRV and AdV had their age profile highlighted.

For the group of patients co-infected with RSV/SARS-CoV-2, three groups showed the same rates of frequency of involvement. Thus, patients younger than 6 months, between 24 to 59 months, and older than 59 months represented an individual percentage of 25% for each group (Figure 5C). The most representative age group of patients affected by hRV/RSV was from 24 to 59 months, totaling 68.75%. The other age groups had low frequencies of coinfection (Figure 5D). When analyzing the coinfections caused by hRV/hBoV, the most affected age group was those aged over 59 months, representing a total of 46.2% of the cases (Figure 5E). The highest frequency of patients affected by hRV/AdV were those aged between 24 to 49 months, which totaled 50% of cases (Figure 5F).

Another variable evaluated was the percentage of patients who required Invasive Mechanical Ventilation (IMV) and Non-Invasive Mechanical Ventilation (NIV): 16.25% of co-infected patients underwent IMV and 18.13% underwent NIV (Table 1).

Table 1. Analysis of the need for IMV and NIV during ICU stay.

Variables	IMV	NIV
YES	26 (16.25%)	29 (18.13%)
NO	126 (78.75%)	123 (76.88%)
N/A	8 (5%)	8 (5%)

Invasive Mechanical Ventilation (IMV); Non-Invasive Mechanical Ventilation (NIV).

When the duration of oxygen therapy was observed for patients with different coinfections, only patients with Rhinovirus/SARS-CoV-2 coinfection had a shorter oxygen therapy time when compared to patients with Rhinovirus/Bocavirus ($p < 0.001$), Rhinovirus/CoVs ($p < 0.01$), Rhinovirus/Metapneumovirus ($p < 0.02$), and Rhinovirus/VSR ($p < 0.02$). All patients with the other different coinfections had similar oxygen therapy use time ($p > 0.05$) (Figure 6).

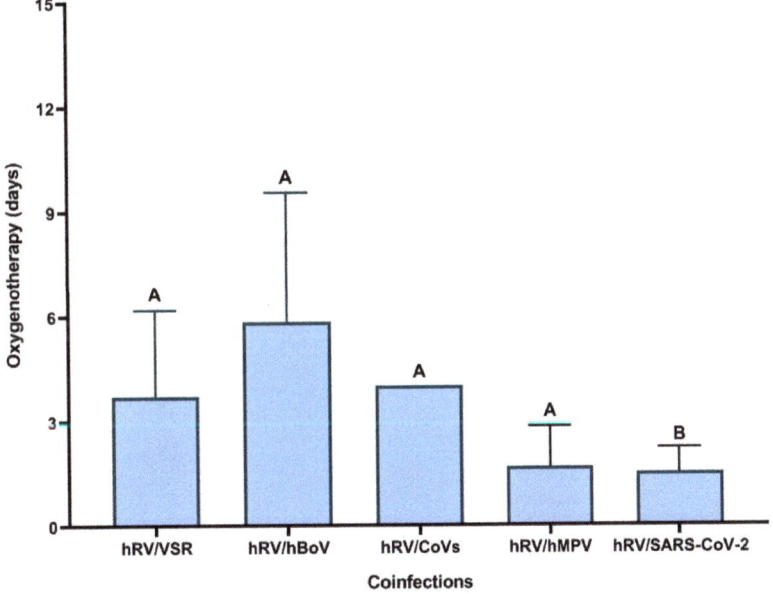

Figure 6. Time of use of oxygen therapy in children with viral coinfection with SARI. (hRV—Rhinovirus; hBoV: Bocavirus; CoVs: Coronavirus; hMPV: Metapneumovirus). Legend: letter (**A**) means all the virus types were statistically significant with relation to oxygenotherapy; letter (**B**) the virus type have no significant statistic with relation to oxygenotherapy.

Although the number of hospitalization days between those infected with RSV and non-infected with this virus did not have a statistically significant difference ($p > 0.36$), we compared the number of hospitalization days of children co-infected with RSV and other children co-infected with other viruses and demonstrated that children coinfected with RSV spent more days in the hospital (7.6 days) than uninfected children (6 days) (Table 2).

Table 2. Comparison between the length of stay of patients co-infected with RSV in the ICU and those not co-infected with RSV.

Statistic/Coinfection	Coinfection with RSV	Coinfection without RSV
Average ICU days	7.69	6.00
Standard Error	0.72	1.65
p-value	0.36	

A descriptive analysis demonstrated the clinical outcome for all cases related to the five most frequent coinfections; unfortunately, due to the severity of the infection, some children died. Thus, we saw that two of the patients co-infected with hRV/SARS-CoV-2 died, representing 9.52% of all deaths in the study. In addition, both hRV/hBoV and hRV/RSV had death records for each case, representing 8.33% and 6.67% of all deaths, respectively (Table 3).

Table 3. Descriptive analysis of the clinical outcome of co-infected patients.

Outcome	General	hRV/SARS-CoV-2	RSV/SARS-CoV-2	hRV/RSV	hRV/hBoV	hRV/AdV
Hospital discharge	152 (95.0%)	19 (90.48%)	11 (100%)	14 (93.34%)	11 (91.67%)	10 (100%)
Death	8 (5.00%)	2 (9.52%)	0 (0.0%)	1 (6.67%)	1 (8.33%)	0 (0.0%)

Legends: hRV—Human Rhinovirus; RSV—Respiratory Syncytial Virus; hBoV—Human Bocavirus; AdV—Adenovirus.

We compared age groups versus clinical course, and identified eight deaths of five children aged over 59 months (3.13%), one aged between 12 and 23 months (0.63%), and two aged between 24 and 59 months (1.25%). For the proportion of deaths versus comorbidities, we observed that 50% of the dead children had some type of comorbidity, and neurological disease was the most prevalent. The other 50% of children who died were due to the severity of SARS symptoms caused by viruses (Table 4).

Table 4. Characteristics of patients with coinfection by two or more viruses who died during the COVID-19 pandemic.

Age/Months	Comorbidities	*ICU Days	*IMV–O2 Days	Viruses
20	Neurological	22	19	SARS-CoV-2/Influenza/Rhinovirus
31	Neurological	15	15	SARS-CoV-2/Rhinovirus
36	No comorbidity	9	9	RSV/Rhinovirus
63	Neurological	20	18	Bocavirus/Rhinovirus
84	No comorbidity	9	9	RSV/Metapneumovirus
108	No comorbidity	26	25	Rhinovirus/Metapneumovirus
132	No comorbidity	1	1	SARS-CoV-2/RSV
144	Endocrine	7	7	SARS-CoV-2/Influenza/Rhinovirus

Legend: IMV—Invasive Mechanical Ventilation; O2: oxygen; ICU—Intensive Care Unit.

The analysis was conducted between the years 2020 and 2021. In the year 2020, hRV/BoV was more frequent in relation to other types of coinfections, representing a total of 35.1%. Then, hRV/SARS-CoV-2 represented a total of 24.3% in relation to the other coinfections analyzed during this period. RSV/SARS-CoV-2, hRV/RSV, and hRV/AdV had a total of 16.2%, 13.5%, and 10.8% of coinfections, respectively (Figure 7A).

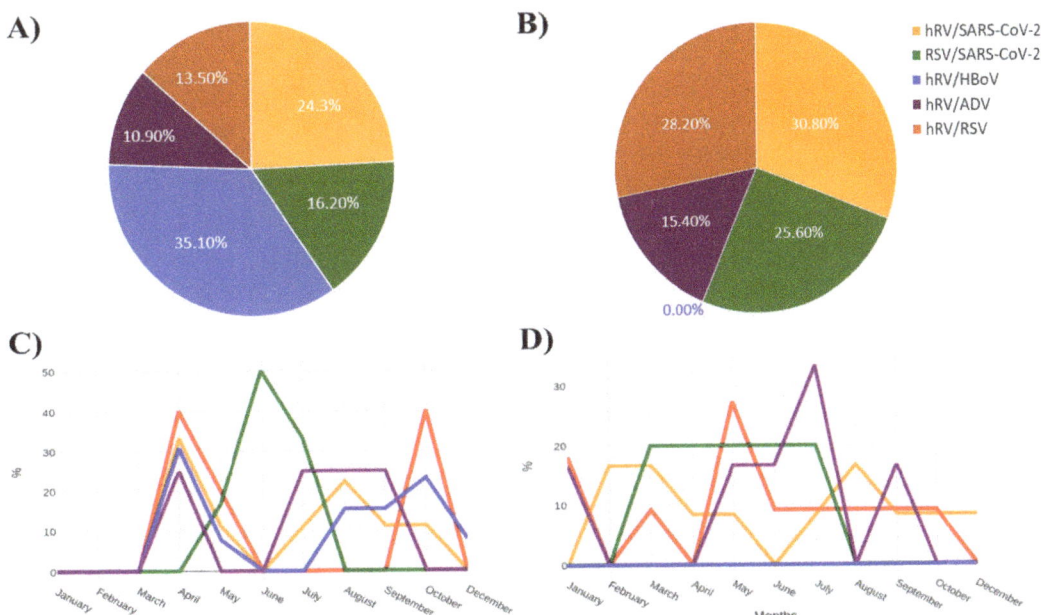

Figure 7. Analysis of the seasonality profile of the most frequent viral coinfections in the years 2020 and 2021. Legend: (**A**) the percentage of the five most frequent coinfections in 2020 is observed. (**B**) Refers to the percentages of the five most frequent coinfections in 2021. (**C**) Analysis of the frequency of coinfections in relation to the months of the year in 2020. (**D**) Characterization of the most frequent coinfections in relation to the months of 2021.

Moreover, the year 2021 presented a divergent profile, with hRV/SARS-CoV-2 coinfection being the most frequent (30.8%), followed by hRV/RSV (28.2%). Additionally, 25.6% and 15.4% represented coinfections between RSV/SARS-CoV-2 and hRV/AdV, respectively. Interestingly, hRV/BoV presented the highest rates of coinfection during the year 2020. However, this type of coinfection was not recorded in the year 2021 (Figure 7B).

Coinfection frequency levels have also been evaluated in relation to the months of the year. For the year 2020, the coinfection that presented the highest rate of involvement in the months of April, September, and October was hRV/BoV. Rhinovirus/SARS-CoV-2 also had elevated levels of coinfection for the months of April and August 2020. In the month of April, an exponential increase in coinfection caused by RSV/SARS-CoV-2 was observed until the month of June, followed by a decline in cases until the month of August (Figure 7C).

When analyzing the coinfection rates for the months of 2021, two main types of coinfections have been highlighted. Initially, there was an increase in coinfections caused by hRV/SARS-CoV-2 between January and March, followed by a decline until June. Subsequently, increases in rates of hRV/SARS-CoV-2 coinfections were again observed in August, and an exponential increase in hRV/RSV coinfections between April and May, a decrease in cases until June, and stabilizing coinfection rates up to October 2021 (Figure 7D).

4. Discussion

Since the beginning of the COVID-19 pandemic, several measures have been taken by the government of Brazilian states to assist the population with SARI suspected of being contaminated by SARS-CoV-2. Our findings are important to demonstrate the circulation of respiratory viruses and their interactions with other viruses that caused severe acute respiratory infection in children during the period of health mitigation to contain COVID-19.

In this study, we detected 22 variations with two viruses (79.4%) or three viruses or more (20.6%), and the most prevalent viral coinfections were hRV/SARS-CoV-2, hRV/RSV, RSV/SARS-CoV-2, hRV/BoV, and hRV/AdV. Silva et al. [10] studied viral panels in children of ages between 18 days and 13 years old. The results indicated that rhinoviruses, adenoviruses, metapneumoviruses, and influenza were among the most important agents of ARI in pediatrics; equal results were found in this work. In a study prior to the COVID-19 pandemic, coinfection rates varied. Paulis et al. [11] found a rate of 31.2% of viral coinfection in children and A. Martínez-Roig et al. [12] found a rate of 61.81% (36.36% with two, 16.10% and 9.35% with more than two viruses). Already during the pandemic, some studies have demonstrated lower rates of coinfection. Elen Vink et al. [9] found a 2% coinfection rate, which claimed to be a rare event during the pandemic. Varella et al. [13] described an 8.9% rate of viral coinfection in children hospitalized in the pandemic. Nihan Şık and colleagues [14] found a rate of 86% coinfection with hRV and enterovirus being the most prevalent.

The highest proportion of coinfection in this study was between hRV and SARS-CoV-2, which we believe to be due to the high spread of the two viruses in the same period. Varela et al. [13], in a study like ours, found a rate of 7.1% of coinfection of hRV with SARS-CoV-2 and described that the viral occurrence was totally indistinct in epidemiological levels during the COVID-19 pandemic, since hRV was the most frequent virus co-circulating with SARS-CoV-2 in hospitalized children. Le Glass et al. [15] also described SARS-CoV-2 coinfection with hRV as more frequent, with patients presenting more respiratory distress and a greater chance of being admitted to ICUs.

When we analyzed only the year 2020, the most frequent coinfection was hRV and hBoV. Wang et al. [16] detected a high rate of patients co-infected with hBoV and other viruses, with hRV and RSV being the most frequent, and suggested that hBoV is often associated with coinfection, stating that the acute infection was caused by this virus inducing responses in the immune system in children with respiratory diseases. HBoV can be detected alone in respiratory samples from children with acquired pneumonia, and the high incidence of severe pneumonia found in HBoV patients demonstrates that this virus is a major contributor to severe respiratory disease [17].

Li et al. [18] suggested that seasonal respiratory viruses decreased significantly in 2020, except for hBoV, which in late autumn and winter 2020 was very prevalent, compared to the last 10 years which was 0.7% to 13.3%, and at the beginning of the third wave of COVID-19 in South Korea, where the scenario was of intense social distancing measures.

In a study by Kim et al. [19], it was described that in 2020, there was a decrease in the circulation of some enveloped viruses such as influenza, metapneumovirus, parainfluenza, and RSV, but that there was a significant increase in the circulation of hRV and hBoV, which are non-enveloped viruses; these findings agree with our study.

Coinfection of RSV/hRV viruses was more prevalent in children aged 0 to 2 years, and the length of hospital stay was longer for children affected with RSV, although there was no statistically significant difference. These two viruses are the main agents that cause respiratory tract infection in children for all years [20,21].

Hanchi et al. [22], in research conducted in Marrakech, studied double or multiple coinfections and found a percentage of 38.8% of positivity in the tested samples. The authors indicated that there was a significant difference when comparing the pandemic period and the period before the pandemic ($p < 0.001$). They found a predominance of SARI during COVID-19. It was equal to our results; the most detected virus was HRV, followed by RSV. The authors believe that the results found before and during the COVID-19 pandemic could be explained by the impact of implementing preventive measures.

In a study carried out by Calvo et al. [23], the coinfections between hRV and RSV were in children around one year of age, and the ages have different characteristics in relation to the unique infections of each virus; where RSV affected babies up to one year of age and hRV was detected in children almost two years of age; and whether in simple infection or coinfection, contamination with RSV implies a worse prognosis with increased duration of both hypoxia and hospitalization days.

Costa et al. [24] described that single hRV infections were less severe, as they had a lower proportion of hospital admissions than hRV-RSV coinfections, and hRV-only patients were older than RSV patients with simple infection and coinfections. They concluded that severe illness in hRV infections is caused by other risk factors concurrent with risk factors for RSV-induced hospitalization.

The coinfection between RSV and SARS-CoV-2 affected all age groups, with a slightly greater difference in the 2- to 5-year-old age group, and it was observed that the use of oxygen therapy devices was statistically significant. Alvares [25], analyzing the hospitalization of 32 children of 2 years of age with COVID-19, found a rate of 18.7% of coinfection with RSV and that these children remained hospitalized longer.

Children are affected with respiratory infections by both SARS-CoV-2 and RSV, and coinfection with these two viruses can generate a serious problem in the scenario of the COVID-19 pandemic, as both viruses represent significant challenges in terms of diagnosis and treatment in children. It is not clear how severe the pathogenicity of SARS-CoV-2 is for children, but coinfection of RSV with SARS-CoV-2 can be serious and affect clinical prognosis, making treatment difficult [26].

In the hospitalization of children with severe SARS-CoV-2 infection, 32% required some form of respiratory support. RSV can cause severe respiratory illness in children that require hospitalization and, in some cases, can lead to death [25,26]; therefore, coinfection with the two viruses can worsen the clinical condition of the child with SARI. Despite not having a statistically significant result, Lee et al. [27] reported that SARS-CoV-2–positive patients with coinfection had a higher prevalence of hospitalization, with a significantly longer hospital stay.

In this study, 3.75% of children died during the period of hospitalization. Of these children, 50% had some type of comorbidity, with an exceptionally long hospital stay, and neurological damage was the highest rate.

In three patients who died, there was SARS-CoV-2 coinfection with other viruses, two of whom had underlying neurological diseases and one who had an endocrine disease. Some studies have shown that there is an extremely high association between a severe course of COVID-19 in children and some risk factors including cancer, immunodeficiency, chronic lung and heart disease, genetic and neurological diseases, diabetes, and obesity [28,29]. In a literary review conducted by Tsankov et al. [30], they examined the severity of COVID-19 infection among pediatric patients with comorbidities and concluded that children with pre-existing conditions are at increased risk of severe COVID-19 and associated mortality.

Most children do not require hospitalization for COVID-19 as SARS-CoV-2 causes mild symptoms in this age range, but the need for ICU admission depends on the comorbidities and complex medical history of the children evaluated [31,32]. The influence of comorbidities and SARS-CoV-2 infection on clinical outcome may be combined, and this virus may exacerbate coexisting chronic disease or be an additional factor in the severity of a clinical outcome in a patient [31].

In Brazil, a total of 1439 children under 5 years of age died because of COVID-19 during the first two years of the pandemic. For these deaths, SARS-CoV-2 made the infection worse for cases with pre-existing risk conditions and was associated with the leading cause of death; that is, SARS-CoV-2 aggravated a pre-existing problem [33].

A child who had no comorbidity had brain death decreed after 9 days of hospitalization, due to RSV/hRV coinfection, where he developed hypoxic encephalopathy and severe ischemia. Wouk et al. [34], in a literature review study, concluded that the appearance of neurological disorders in viral infections can cause neurological symptoms or lead to immune responses that trigger these pathological signs, since irreversible damage and cell death can occur if there is chronic dysfunction of the cells. Neuronal cells, both central and peripheral, can influence the development and progression of these disorders.

Neurological disorders can be caused by pathogens that cross the intact blood barrier, causing severe encephalitis or acute infections progressing to chronic disease or leading to death; these disorders can also occur indirectly through accumulation of protein aggregates, elevated levels of oxidative stress, alterations in autophagic mechanisms, synaptopathy, and neural destruction [33,35,36].

The seasonality of coinfections was evaluated, demonstrating that there was a difference between the years 2020 and 2021. In 2020, hRV/hBoV were detected in April, September, and October, and hRV/SARS-CoV-2 and RSV/SARS-CoV-2 detected in the months of April and August. In 2021, hRV/SARS-CoV-2 coinfection had peaks from January to March and August, and hRV/RSV peaked between April and May.

The epidemiological bulletin for COVID-19, in December 2020 in the state of Goiás/Brazil, showed the distribution of confirmed cases with severe acute respiratory infection (SARI) by date of hospitalization and moving average, where cases started in March and there were high peaks in June, July, and August [37]. In 2021, with the new wave of SARS-CoV-2, it did not differ from the previous year; the hospitalization rate increased in January, growing significantly in March [38].

Our study shows that more children in 2021 were infected with SARS-CoV-2, but it was also a period when mitigation measures were more lenient, and children were also returning to school.

We emphasize that according to research, in Brazil, there have been changes in the frequency of SARS-CoV-2 strains. At the beginning of the pandemic, strains B.1.1.28 and B.1.1.33 were more prevalent until October 2020, and then there was a predominance of two Brazilian variants, P.1 and P.2, originating from the lineage B.1.1.28. In just four months, these two Brazilian variants represented 75% of sequencing in Brazil. In terms of public health in Brazil, during the study period, four variants classified as variants of concern (VOC) and two (Zeta and Lambda) of the seven variants classified as variants of interest (VOI) by the WHO [39–42] were registered.

This study had limitations. The first limitation could indicate a bias in the results, the fact that we did not have viral panel data of the children evaluated in the outpatient clinic or ward. However, we believe that our data represent important data and do not agree with bias, since all were hospitalized with SARI and a viral panel was performed in all children. Because it was a pandemic season, it was recommended that children with mild flu symptoms stay at home. Another limitation would be to prove whether a co-infected child had a worse prognosis than children with single virus infection. Data such as blood tests and X-rays were not described in a cohesive manner in all medical records analyzed.

5. Conclusions

Coinfections with respiratory viruses, such as RSV and hBoV, can increase the severity of the disease in children with SARI who are admitted to the ICU, and children infected with SARS-CoV-2 have their clinical condition worsened when they have comorbidities.

Author Contributions: C.R.M.I., M.A.G.A. and L.C.C. conceived and designed the study. F.A.d.O.P., G.S.R., P.N.d.B., A.P.C.R. and J.G.F. collected the samples. M.d.O.S., A.P.d.S., P.A.N.d.S., A.L.E.M., V.M.G., M.C.E., P.Z.d.S. and C.R.M.I. performed the experiments, analyzed the data, and drafted the manuscript. I.J.W., L.C.C., C.R.M.I. and M.A.G.A. revised the manuscript. All authors have read and agreed to the published version of the manuscript.

Funding: This study was supported in part by donations from CAPES Coordination for the Improvement of Higher Education Personnel [Aid n°: 0678/2020/88881.504906/2020-01], PROJECT: Differential Diagnosis and Pediatric Clinical Evolution of COVID-19 in the Context of Seasonality of Respiratory Viruses in a Capital of the Brazilian Midwest, coordinated by Doctor and Professor Melissa A. Gomes Avelino Ferri.

Institutional Review Board Statement: Ethics Committee of the Federal University of Goiás. Protocol number: 33540320.7.0000.5078.

Informed Consent Statement: Not applicable.

Data Availability Statement: Data sharing is not applicable to this article as no new data were created or analyzed in this study.

Acknowledgments: We would like to thank all healthcare professionals at the Pediatric Intensive Care Unit of Governador Otávio Lage de Siqueira Emergency Hospital (HUGOL) for their assistance in collecting demographic data and blood and airway secretion swab samples. We thank all study participants for conducting the molecular tests. We thank and sympathize with all the family members who lost their loved ones during the COVID-19 pandemic.

Conflicts of Interest: The authors declare no conflict of interest.

References

1. Bonzel, L.; Tenenbaum, T.; Schroten, H.; Schildgen, O.; Schweitzer-Krantz, S.; Adams, O. Frequent Detection of Viral Coinfection in Children Hospitalized With Acute Respiratory Tract Infection Using a Real-Time Polymerase Chain Reaction. *Pediatr. Infect. Dis. J.* **2008**, *27*, 589–594. [CrossRef] [PubMed]
2. Kouni, S.; Karakitsos, P.; Chranioti, A.; Theodoridou, M.; Chrousos, G.; Michos, A. Evaluation of viral co-infections in hospitalized and non-hospitalized children with respiratory infections using microarrays. *Clin. Microbiol. Infect.* **2013**, *19*, 772–777. [CrossRef] [PubMed]
3. Sly, P.D.; Jones, C.M. Viral co-detection in infants hospitalized with respiratory disease: Is it important to detect? *J. Pediatr.* **2011**, *87*, 277–280. [CrossRef] [PubMed]
4. Malekifar, P.; Pakzad, R.; Shahbahrami, R.; Zandi, M.; Jafarpour, A.; Rezayat, S.A.; Akbarpour, S.; Shabestari, A.N.; Pakzad, I.; Hesari, E.; et al. Viral Coinfection among COVID-19 Patient Groups: An Update Systematic Review and Meta-Analysis. *BioMed. Res. Int.* **2021**, *2021*, 5313832. [CrossRef] [PubMed]
5. Kim, D.; Quinn, J.; Pinsky, B.; Shah, N.H.; Brown, I. Rates of Co-infection Between SARS-CoV-2 and Other Respiratory Pathogens. *J. Am. Med. Assoc.* **2020**, *323*, 2085–2086. [CrossRef] [PubMed]
6. Ito, C.R.M.; Jas, S.; Gonçalves, L.C.; Pan, S.; Santos, M.O.; Ale, M. The Epidemiology of Viruses Causing Acute and Severe Respiratory Diseases in Children, before and during the COVID-19 Pandemic. *Austin J. Infect. Dis.* **2022**, *9*, 1070.
7. Bulletins and Reports. SRAG Epidemiological Bulletins. Goiás State Department of Health. Available online: https://www.saude.go.gov.br/boletins-e-informes (accessed on 11 February 2022).
8. Abo, Y.; Clifford, V.; Lee, L.; Costa, A.; Crawford, N.; Wurzel, D.; Daley, A.J. COVID-19 public health measures and respiratory viruses in children in Melbourne. *J. Paediatr. Child Health* **2021**, *57*, 1886–1892. [CrossRef]
9. Vink, E.; Davis, C.; MacLean, A.; Pascall, D.; McDonald, S.E.; Gunson, R.; Hardwick, H.E.; Oosthuyzen, W.; Openshaw, P.J.M.; Baillie, J.K.; et al. Viral Coinfections in Hospitalized Coronavirus Disease 2019 Patients Recruited to the International Severe Acute Respiratory and Emerging Infections Consortium WHO Clinical Characterisation Protocol UK Study. *Open Forum Infect. Dis.* **2022**, *9*, ofac531. [CrossRef]
10. Silva, P.A.N.; Ito, C.R.M.; Moreira, A.L.E.; Santos, M.O.; Barbosa, L.C.G.; Wastowski, I.J.; Carneiro, L.C.; Avelino, M.A.G. Influenza and other respiratory viruses in children: Prevalence and clinical features. *Eur. J. Clin. Microbiol. Infect. Dis.* **2022**, *41*, 1445–1449. [CrossRef]
11. Ferraro, A.A.; Ferronato, A.E.; Sacramento, P.R.D.; Botosso, V.F.; De Oliveira, D.B.L.; Marinheiro, J.C.; Hársi, C.M.; Durigon, E.L.; Vieira, S.E.; De Paulis, M.; et al. Severity of viral coinfection in hospitalized infants with respiratory syncytial virus infection. *J. Pediatr.* **2011**, *87*, 307–313. [CrossRef]
12. Martínez-Roig, A.; Salvadó, M.; Caballero-Rabasco, M.; Sánchez-Buenavida, A.; López-Segura, N.; Bonet-Alcaina, M. Viral Coinfection in Childhood Respiratory Tract Infections. *Viruses* **2014**, *51*, 5–9. [CrossRef]
13. Varela, F.H.; Sartor, I.T.S.; Polese-Bonatto, M.; Azevedo, T.R.; Kern, L.B.; Fazolo, T.; de David, C.N.; Zavaglia, G.O.; Fernandes, I.R.; Krauser, J.R.M.; et al. Rhinovirus as the main co-circulating virus during the COVID-19 pandemic in children. *J. Pediatr.* **2022**, *98*, 579–586. [CrossRef] [PubMed]
14. Sik, N.; Baserdem, K.A.C.; Baserdem, O.; Appak, O.; Sayiner, A.A.; Yilmaz, D.; Duman, M. Distribution of Viral Respiratory Pathogens During the COVID-19 Pandemic: A Single-Center Pediatric Study from Turkey. *Turk. Arch. Pediatr.* **2022**, *57*, 354–359. [CrossRef]
15. Le Glass, E.; Hoang, V.T.; Boschi, C.; Ninove, L.; Zandotti, C.; Boutin, A.; Bremond, V.; Dubourg, G.; Ranque, S.; Lagier, J.-C.; et al. Incidence and Outcome of Coinfections with SARS-CoV-2 and Rhinovirus. *Viruses* **2021**, *13*, 2528. [CrossRef] [PubMed]
16. Wang, K.; Wang, W.; Yan, H.; Ren, P.; Zhang, J.; Shen, J.; Deubel, V. Correlation between bocavirus infection and humoral response, and co-infection with other respiratory viruses in children with acute respiratory infection. *J. Clin. Virol.* **2010**, *47*, 148–155. [CrossRef]

17. Ji, K.; Sun, J.; Yan, Y.; Han, L.; Guo, J.; Ma, A.; Hao, X.; Li, F.; Sun, Y. Epidemiologic and clinical characteristics of human bocavirus infection in infants and young children suffering with community acquired pneumonia in Ningxia, China. *Virol. J.* **2021**, *18*, 212. [CrossRef]
18. Li, Y.; Wang, X.; Nair, H. Global Seasonality of Human Seasonal Coronaviruses: A Clue for Postpandemic Circulating Season of Severe Acute Respiratory Syndrome Coronavirus 2? *J. Infect. Dis.* **2020**, *222*, 1090–1097. [CrossRef]
19. Kim, H.M.; Lee, E.J.; Lee, N.; Woo, S.H.; Kim, J.; Rhee, J.E.; Kim, E. Impact of coronavirus disease 2019 on respiratory surveillance and explanation of high detection rate of human rhinovirus during the pandemic in the Republic of Korea. *Influ. Other Respir. Viruses* **2021**, *15*, 721–731. [CrossRef]
20. Yoshida, L.-M.; Suzuki, M.; Nguyen, H.A.; Le, M.N.; Vu, T.D.; Yoshino, H.; Schmidt, W.-P.; Nguyen, T.T.A.; Le, H.T.; Morimoto, K.; et al. Respiratory syncytial virus: Co-infection and paediatric lower respiratory tract infections. *Eur. Respir. J.* **2013**, *42*, 461–469. [CrossRef] [PubMed]
21. Costa, L.F.; Queiróz, D.A.O.; da Silveira, H.L.; Neto, M.B.; de Paula, N.T.; Oliveira, T.F.M.S.; Tolardo, A.L.; Yokosawa, J. Human Rhinovirus and Disease Severity in Children. *Pediatrics* **2014**, *133*, e312–e321. [CrossRef]
22. Hanchi, A.L.; Guennouni, M.; Ben Houmich, T.; Echchakery, M.; Draiss, G.; Rada, N.; Younous, S.; Bouskraoui, M.; Soraa, N. Changes in the Epidemiology of Respiratory Pathogens in Children during the COVID-19 Pandemic. *Pathogens* **2022**, *11*, 1542. [CrossRef]
23. Calvo, C.; García-García, M.L.; Pozo, F.; Paula, G.; Molinero, M.; Calderón, A.; González-Esguevillas, M.; Casas, I. Respiratory Syncytial Virus Coinfections With Rhinovirus and Human Bocavirus in Hospitalized Children. *Medicine* **2015**, *94*, e1788. [CrossRef]
24. Alvares, P.A. SARS-CoV-2 and Respiratory Syncytial Virus Coinfection in Hospitalized Pediatric Patients. *Pediatr. Infect. Dis. J.* **2021**, *40*, e164–e166. [CrossRef]
25. Zandi, M.; Soltani, S.; Fani, M.; Abbasi, S.; Ebrahimi, S.; Ramezani, A. Severe acute respiratory syndrome coronavirus 2 and respiratory syncytial virus coinfection in children. *Osong Public Health Res. Perspect.* **2021**, *12*, 286–292. [CrossRef] [PubMed]
26. Zachariah, P.; Johnson, C.L.; Halabi, K.C.; Ahn, D.; Sen, A.I.; Fischer, A.; Banker, S.L.; Giordano, M.; Manice, C.S.; Diamond, R.; et al. Epidemiology, Clinical Features, and Disease Severity in Patients With Coronavirus Disease 2019 (COVID-19) in a Children's Hospital in New York City, New York. *JAMA Pediatr.* **2020**, *174*, e202430, Erratum in *JAMA Pediatr.* **2021**, *175*, 871. [CrossRef]
27. Lee, B.R.; Harrison, C.J.; Myers, A.L.; Jackson, M.A.; Selvarangan, R. Differences in pediatric SARS-CoV-2 symptomology and Co-infection rates among COVID-19 Pandemic waves. *J. Clin. Virol.* **2022**, *154*, 105220. [CrossRef] [PubMed]
28. Oualha, M.; Bendavid, M.; Berteloot, L.; Corsia, A.; Lesage, F.; Vedrenne, M.; Salvador, E.; Grimaud, M.; Chareyre, J.; de Marcellus, C.; et al. Severe and fatal forms of COVID-19 in children. *Arch Pediatr.* **2020**, *27*, 235–238. [CrossRef]
29. Castagnoli, R.; Votto, M.; Licari, A.; Brambilla, I.; Bruno, R.; Perlini, S.; Rovida, F.; Baldanti, F.; Marseglia, G.L. Severe Acute Respiratory Syndrome Coronavirus 2 (SARS-CoV-2) Infection in Children and Adolescents: A Systematic Review. *JAMA Pediatr.* **2020**, *174*, 882. [CrossRef] [PubMed]
30. Kompaniyets, L.; Agathis, N.T.; Nelson, J.M.; Preston, L.E.; Ko, J.Y.; Belay, B.; Pennington, A.F.; Danielson, M.L.; DeSisto, C.L.; Chevinsky, J.R.; et al. Underlying Medical Conditions Associated With Severe COVID-19 Illness Among Children. *JAMA Netw. Open* **2021**, *4*, e2111182. [CrossRef]
31. Tsankov, B.K.; Allaire, J.M.; Irvine, M.A.; Lopez, A.A.; Sauvé, L.J.; Vallance, B.A.; Jacobson, K. Severe COVID-19 Infection and Pediatric Comorbidities: A Systematic Review and Meta-Analysis. *Int. J. Infect. Dis.* **2021**, *103*, 246–256. [CrossRef]
32. Mania, A.; Pokorska-Śpiewak, M.; Figlerowicz, M.; Pawłowska, M.; Mazur-Melewska, K.; Faltin, K.; Talarek, E.; Zawadka, K.; Dobrzeniecka, A.; Ciechanowski, P.; et al. Pneumonia, gastrointestinal symptoms, comorbidities, and coinfections as factors related to a lengthier hospital stay in children with COVID-19—Analysis of a paediatric part of Polish register SARSTer. *Infect. Dis.* **2021**, *54*, 196–204. [CrossRef] [PubMed]
33. Pathak, E.B.; Salemi, J.L.; Sobers, N.; Menard, J.; Hambleton, I.R. COVID-19 in Children in the United States: Intensive Care Admissions, Estimated Total Infected, and Projected Numbers of Severe Pediatric Cases in 2020. *J. Public Health Manag. Pract.* **2020**, *26*, 325–333. [CrossRef]
34. COVID-19 Kills Two Children under 5 Years Old Every Day in Brazil. Fiocruz. 2022. Available online: https://portal.fiocruz.br/en/news/covid-19-kills-two-children-under-5-years-old-every-day-brazil (accessed on 30 September 2022).
35. Wouk, J.; Rechenchoski, D.Z.; Rodrigues, B.C.D.; Ribelato, E.V.; Faccin-Galhardi, L.C. Viral infections and their relationship to neurological disorders. *Arch. Virol.* **2021**, *166*, 733–753. [CrossRef] [PubMed]
36. McGavern, D.B.; Kang, S.S. Illuminating viral infections in the nervous system. *Nat. Rev. Immunol.* **2011**, *11*, 318–329. [CrossRef] [PubMed]
37. Epidemiological Report—COVID-19 Edition n°. 272—Preliminary Data, Updated on 12.30.2020 at 12:00 pm Municipal Health Secretariat Health Surveillance Directory Epidemiological Surveillance Management Diseases and Diseases Management Information and Strategies Center Health Surveillance. Available online: https://saude.goiania.go.gov.br/wp-uploads/sites/3/2020/12/Informe-COVID-19-no-272-30.12.2020.pdf (accessed on 30 September 2022).
38. Epidemiological Report-COVID-19 Total Confirmed Cases of Individuals Residents in Goiânia. Available online: https://saude.goiania.go.gov.br/wp-content/uploads/sites/3/2022/01/Informe-648-31.12.2021.pdf (accessed on 30 September 2022).
39. Michelon, C.M. Main SARS-CoV-2 variants notified in Brazil. *Rev. Bras. Anal. Clin.* **2021**, *53*, 109–116. [CrossRef]

40. Candido, D.S.; Claro, I.M.; De Jesus, J.G.; Souza, W.M.; Moreira, F.R.R.; Dellicour, S.; Mellan, T.A.; Du Plessis, L.; Pereira, R.H.M.; Sales, F.C.S.; et al. Evolution and epidemic spread of SARS-CoV-2 in Brazil. *Science* **2020**, *369*, 1255–1260. [CrossRef]
41. Atualização Epidemiológica: Variantes do SARS-CoV-2 nas Américas. Brasília-DF: Organização Pan-Americana da Saúde—OPAS. 2021, pp. 1–9. Available online: https://iris.paho.org/handle/10665.2/53376 (accessed on 6 June 2022).
42. Freitas, R.R.A.; Giovanetti, M.; Alcantara, L.C.J. Variantes Emergentes do SARS-CoV-2 e Suas Implicações na Saúde Coletiva. *Interam. J. Med. Health* **2021**, *4*, 1–8. Available online: http://www.ncbi.nlm.nih.gov/pubmed/33890566 (accessed on 6 June 2022).

Disclaimer/Publisher's Note: The statements, opinions and data contained in all publications are solely those of the individual author(s) and contributor(s) and not of MDPI and/or the editor(s). MDPI and/or the editor(s) disclaim responsibility for any injury to people or property resulting from any ideas, methods, instructions or products referred to in the content.

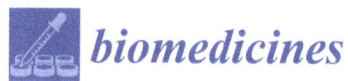

Review

SARS-CoV-2 Antibody Responses in Pediatric Patients: A Bibliometric Analysis

Ionela Maniu [1,2,*], George Constantin Maniu [1], Elisabeta Antonescu [3,4], Lavinia Duica [3,4,*], Nicolae Grigore [3,4] and Maria Totan [3,5]

1. Mathematics and Informatics Department, Research Center in Informatics and Information Technology, Faculty of Sciences, "Lucian Blaga" University, 5-7 Ion Ratiu Str., 550025 Sibiu, Romania; george.maniu@ulbsibiu.ro
2. Pediatric Research Team, Clinical Pediatric Hospital, 2-4 Pompeiu Onofreiu Str., 550166 Sibiu, Romania
3. Faculty of Medicine, Lucian Blaga University of Sibiu, 2A Lucian Blaga Str., 550169 Sibiu, Romania; elisabeta.antonescu@ulbsibiu.ro (E.A.); nicolae.grigore@ulbsibiu.ro (N.G.); maria.totan@ulbsibiu.ro (M.T.)
4. County Clinical Emergency Hospital, 2-4 Corneliu Coposu Str., 550245 Sibiu, Romania
5. Clinical Laboratory, Clinical Pediatric Hospital, 2-4 Pompeiu Onofreiu Str., 550166 Sibiu, Romania
* Correspondence: ionela.maniu@ulbsibiu.ro (I.M.); lavinia.duica@ulbsibiu.ro (L.D.)

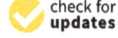

Citation: Maniu, I.; Maniu, G.C.; Antonescu, E.; Duica, L.; Grigore, N.; Totan, M. SARS-CoV-2 Antibody Responses in Pediatric Patients: A Bibliometric Analysis. *Biomedicines* **2023**, *11*, 1455. https://doi.org/10.3390/biomedicines11051455

Academic Editors: Elena Cecilia Rosca and Amalia Cornea

Received: 21 April 2023
Revised: 10 May 2023
Accepted: 12 May 2023
Published: 16 May 2023

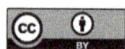

Copyright: © 2023 by the authors. Licensee MDPI, Basel, Switzerland. This article is an open access article distributed under the terms and conditions of the Creative Commons Attribution (CC BY) license (https://creativecommons.org/licenses/by/4.0/).

Abstract: The characteristics, dynamics and mechanisms/determinants of the immune response to SARS-CoV-2 infection are not fully understood. We performed a bibliometric review of studies that have assessed SARS-CoV-2 antibody responses in the pediatric population using Web of Science online databases, VOSviewer and Bibliometrix tools. The analysis was conducted on 84 publications, from 310 institutions located in 29 countries and published in 57 journals. The results showed the collaboration of scientists and organizations, international research interactions and summarized the findings on (i) the measured titers of antibodies (total antibody and/or individual antibody classes IgG, IgM, IgA) against different antigens (C-terminal region of N (N CT), full-length N protein (N FL), RBD, RBD Alpha, RBD Beta, RBD Gamma, RBD Delta, spike (S), S1, S2) in the case of different clinical forms of the disease; and (ii) the correlations between SARS-CoV-2 antibodies and cytokines, chemokines, neutrophils, C-reactive protein, ferritin, and the erythrocyte sedimentation rate. The presented study offers insights regarding research directions to be explored in the studied field and may provide a starting point for future research.

Keywords: antibodies; COVID-19; bibliometric analysis; disease severity; inflammatory markers; VOSviewer; Bibliometrix

1. Introduction

The virus that caused the pandemic at the end of 2019 is SARS-CoV-2 (Severe Acute Respiratory Syndrome coronavirus 2). SARS-CoV-2 is a single-stranded RNA virus belonging to the B lineage of the beta-coronavirus family with the ability to encode 14 open reading frames (ORFs). The ORFs have the capacity to encode 4 structural proteins (tip [S], nucleocapsid [N], envelope [E], and membrane [M] proteins), 16 nonstructural proteins, and 9 putative accessory proteins (ORF3a, 3b, 6, 7a, 7b, 8, 9b, 9c and 10) [1].

When the SARS-CoV-2 virus enters the human body, the host's immune system recognizes it, initiates and induces an immune response (develops proteins called antibodies) in order to attack/eliminate the virus [1–3].

The characteristics, dynamics and mechanisms/determinants of the immune response to SARS-CoV-2 infection are not fully understood. Understanding the antibody response to SARS-CoV-2 infection might provide important insights for planning clinical interventions/therapeutics and policy interventions (identifying individuals at risk of adverse outcomes, preventing progression to severe disease, improving treatment, cost-effectiveness/advantages of vaccination). The immune response to SARS-CoV-2 infection is generally determined by the antibodies developed against COVID-19 (specific immunoglobulin M (IgM), A (IgA) and G (IgG)) against different antigens (spike (and its subunits S1, S2), nucleocapsid, receptor-binding domain (RBD)).

There have been a number of research studies (and are continually being updated) that have included analyses of the human immune response to SARS-CoV-2 in adult patients; this is in comparison with the pediatric population, where the evidence is more scarce.

The aim of this study was to perform a bibliometric review of studies that have assessed SARS-CoV-2 antibody responses in the pediatric population in order to provide a comprehensive overview of the state of, and trends observed in, the research conducted in the analyzed field. We identify the main areas of research, the collaboration of scientists and organizations, international research interactions and the immunological features associated with the different clinical forms of SARS-CoV-2 infection and its inflammatory markers.

2. Materials and Methods

For this study, a search of the literature was performed using the Web of Science Core Collection (WoS) online databases in November 2022 in order to identify scientific contributions, including the assessment of SARS-CoV-2 antibody responses in pediatric patients. The search strategy included the keywords (antibod* or IgA or IgG OR IgM) and COVID and (pediatric OR children) and (prevalence or leve* or tite*). The search identified publications that contained the mentioned terms in their title, abstract or keywords. The retrieved studies were than evaluated by the authors to ensure that only articles related to the SARS-CoV-2 antibody responses in children were included in the analysis. Only article-type documents that measured the titres of antibodies against different tested antigens were included. For each included study, the publication title, abstract, keyword/keyword plus, authorship, publication year, journal title, language, journal category and number of total citations were extracted. The process of study selection is described using a PRISMA flow diagram in Figure 1.

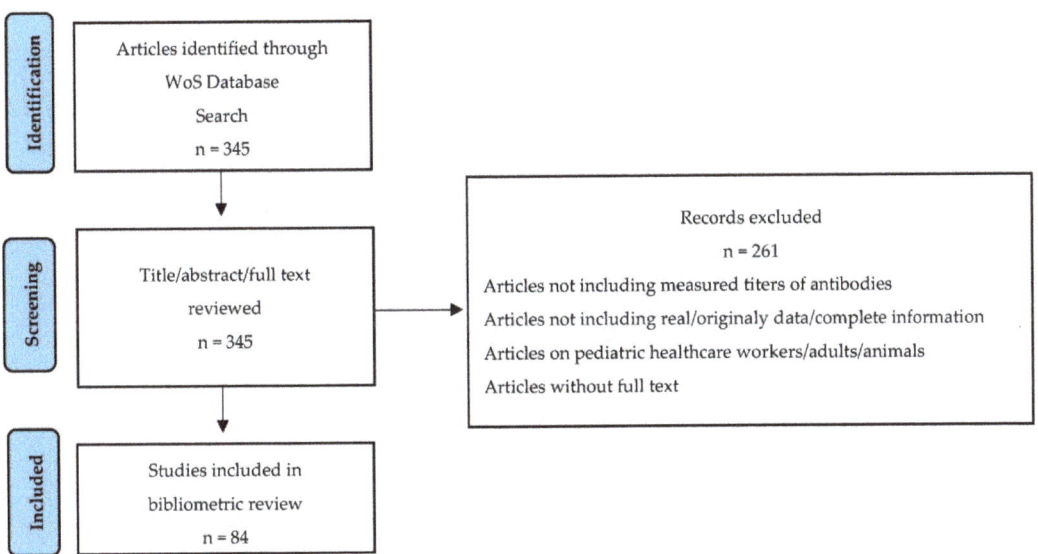

Figure 1. PRISMA flow chart of the study selection process.

The bibliometric analysis and visualizations were performed by using Visualization of Similarities viewer (VOSviewer) software (VanEck andWaltman, Center for Science and Technology Studies of Leiden University [4,5]), a tool that has been used in studies in various areas of research [6–17]. Bibliographic techniques, such as citation and co-citation analysis, bibliographic coupling and co-occurrence analysis, were used to create collaboration networks and text mining. In the case of inter-institutional or country collaboration networks, the number of publications (that have authors from different institutes or countries) was considered as a metric for collaboration. The Bibliometrix 3.1 package (Aria and Cuccurullo, University of Naples and University of Campania's Luigi Vanvitelli, Italy, [18]) and RStudio environment (CRAN, https://cran.r-project.org/ (accessed on 1 November 2022)) were used to create the historiographical citation network, the co-citations network statistics, and the top authors' production over time plots.

3. Results

Of the 345 studies retrieved from the search, 84 were included in the bibliometric analysis. A total of 29 countries had published documents in the research field. Among the most productive countries were North American countries (USA, Canada), Asian countries (China, Israel), European countries (Italy, UK, Poland, Spain, France, Germany, Netherlands, Turkey, and Russia), one Oceania country (Australia), and one South American country (Argentina). The scientific collaboration between countries is presented in Figure 2. The links between the countries represent co-authorships and the widths of the links represent the different frequencies of collaboration (thicker links reflect more collaboration between the two countries). As indicated in the graph, clusters of interconnected countries (marked with different colors—purple, red, blue, green, orange), but also isolated/unconnected countries (those that did not have any international collaboration, although some of them, such as Turkey, had four publications), can be observed.

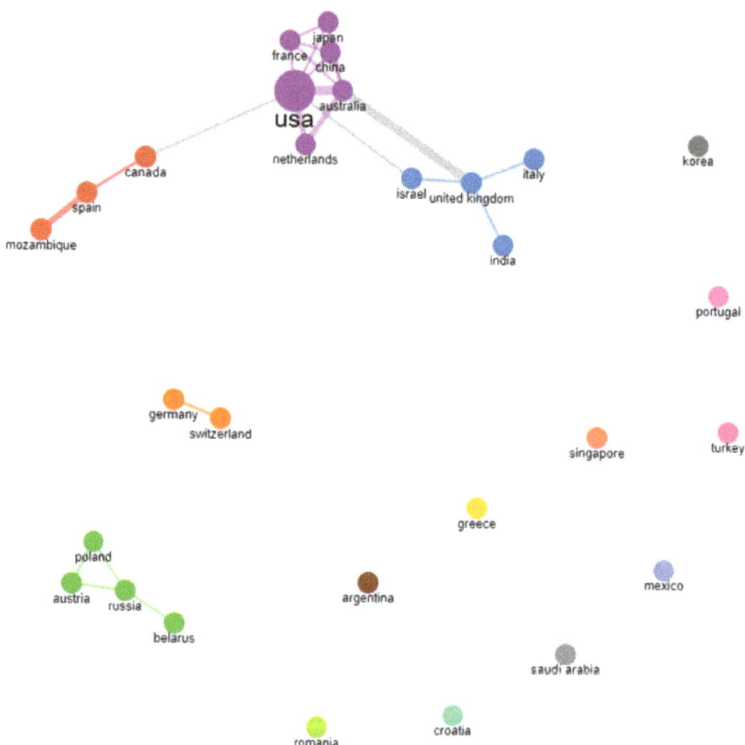

Figure 2. Bibliometrix collaboration network between countries.

A total number of 310 organizations were found to have published papers related to the topic of SARS-CoV-2 antibody responses in pediatric patients. The most productive and cited organizations are presented in Table 1 and Figure 3.

Table 1. Top productive and cited organizations.

Rank	Organizations Publications	Rank	Organizations Citations	Rank	Organizations Affiliations
1	Univ Melbourne (5)	1	Harvard Med Sch (257)	1	Emory Univ (18)
1	Emory Univ (5)	2	Brigham and Women's Hospital (252)	2	Univ Hong Kong (17)
1	Univ Hong Kong (5)	2	Massachusetts Gen Hosp (252)	3	Johns Hopkins Univ (16)
2	Chinese Univ Hong Kong (4)	3	Albert Einstein Coll Med (214)	4	Inst Pasteur (14)
2	Childrens Healthcare Atlanta (4)	3	Child. Hosp Montefiore (214)	5	Univ Bristol (11)
3	Harvard Med Sch (3)	3	Montefiore Med Ctr (214)	5	Univ Melbourne (11)
3	Univ Amsterdam (3)	3	Yale Univ (214)	5	Univ Penn (11)
3	Murdoch Child. Res Inst (3)	4	Harvard Th Chan Sch Publ Hlth (192)	6	Univ Barcelona (10)
3	Royal Child. Hosp (3)	5	Hosp Sick Child. (167)	7	Univ Med Ctr Hamburg Eppendorf (8)
3	Hosp Author Hong Kong (3)	6	Icahn Sch Med Mt Sinai (163)	8	Hosp Author Hong Kong (7)
3	London Sch Hyg and Trop med (3)	7	Univ Melbourne (128)	8	Hosp Infantil Mexico Dr Federico Gomez (7)
3	Univ Bristol (3)	8	Univ Calif Merced (119)	8	Med Univ Lublin (7)
3	Barcelona Inst Sci and Techno (3)	9	Univ Amsterdam (113)	8	Royal Child. Hosp (7)
3	Huazhong Univ Sci and Techno (3)	10	Murdoch Child. Res Inst (109)		
3	Queen Mary Hosp (3)				

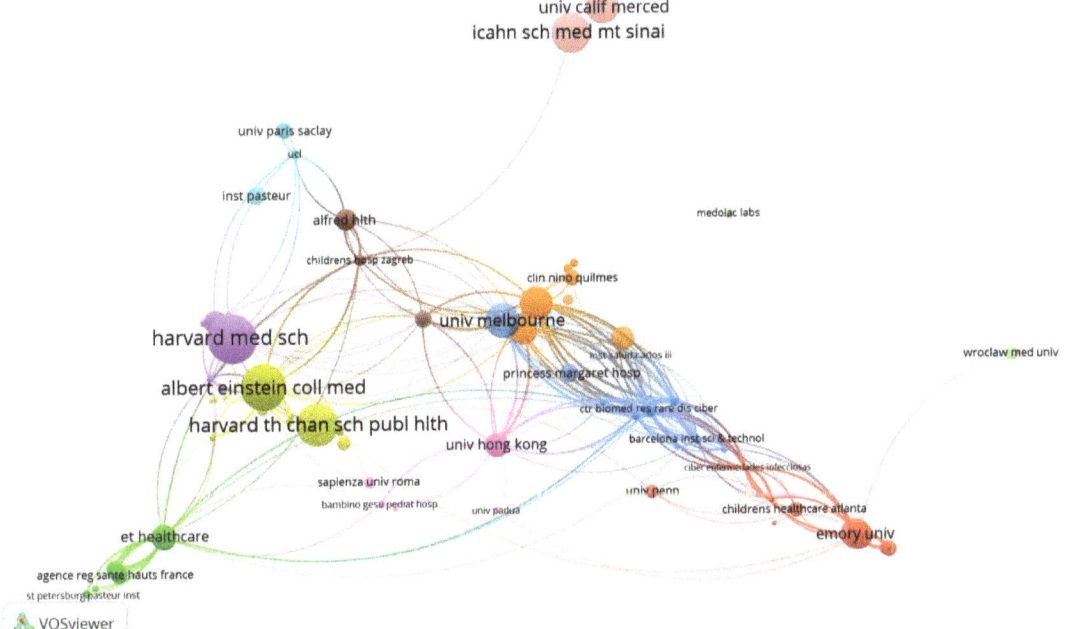

Figure 3. VOSviewer network visualization map of institutions/organizations (type of analysis: citations, weights—citations, largest set of connected items—236).

The University of Melbourne (Australia) was found to have published 5 related papers, with 128 citations. The main partners of the organization are the Royal Children's Hospital and Murdoch Childrens Res. Inst., and other organizations also from Australia, but also organizations from the USA (Univ. of Michigan, Washington Univ. School of Medicine in St. Louis, Icahn School of Medicine at Mount Sinai), UK (London Sch Hyg and Trop med), China (Univ. Hong Kong, Chinese Univ. of Hong Kong), Netherlands (University of Amsterdam), France (Univ. de Versailles Saint-Quentin, Univ. Paris Descartes), and Japan (Ishikawa Prefectural Univ.). The researches focused on a comparative analysis between the coronavirus antibody responses present in children and adults/elderly people with COVID-19 and/or healthy patients.

Emory University (Atlanta, Georgia, USA) was also found to have published 5 related papers with 93 citations. The main partner of the organization is the Children's Healthcare Atlanta hospital and other organizations also from Atlanta or from other USA states (Missouri, Arizona, Florida, Tennessee, Virginia, Georgia, Texas); the researches mainly concentrated on inflammatory markers and the SARS-CoV-2 antibody profiles of children with multisystem inflammatory syndrome (MIS-C) (and/or comparison with patients with acute/symptomatic COVID-19, healthy controls, Kawasaki disease, and also with a mouse model).

Next in the hierarchy of the top productive organizations were two universities from China: the University of Hong Kong and the Chinese University of Hong Kong, with 5/4 related publications, of which 4 are joint articles (62/61 citations). The main partners of the organization are the Hospital Authority of Hong Kong, the Queen Mary/Princess Margaret/Prince of Wales/Queen Elizabeth hospitals and other organizations also from China or from the USA and Australia. The researchers investigated humoral and cellular (T cell) responses and the long-term persistence of SARS-CoV-2-neutralizing antibody responses in recovered children and adolescents.

The collaboration between several American institutions, Harvard Medical School, Massachusetts General Hospital and Brigham and Women's Hospital, led to the publication of two of the top ten most cited articles related to the analyzed topic [19,20] and implicitly to the positioning of these institutions in the top of the most cited organizations. In addition, the next four (also American) institutions in this hierarchy were as follows: the Albert Einstein College of Medicine, the Children's Hospital at Montefiore, Montefiore Medical Center and Yale University. These institutions collaborated in the creation of another two of the top ten most cited articles [21,22].

The top 20 highly cited articles are presented in Table 2. The historiographic analysis presented in Figure 4 shows the genealogic structure mapping of the cited papers (bibliographic antecedents and descendants). The relevant authors, based on their publication number, are presented in Figure 5.

Table 2. Top 20 highly cited articles.

First Author Year [Ref.]	Document Title	Journal	Citations
Yonker 2020 [19]	Pediatric Severe Acute Respiratory Syndrome Coronavirus 2 (SARS-CoV-2): Clinical Presentation, Infectivity, and Immune Responses	JOURNAL OF PEDIATRICS	192
Pierce 2020 [21]	Immune responses to SARS-CoV-2 infection in hospitalized pediatric and adult patients	SCIENCE TRANSLATIONAL MEDICINE	167
Fox 2020 [23]	Robust and Specific Secretory IgA Against SARS-CoV-2 Detected in Human Milk	ISCIENCE	119
Rostad 2020 [24]	Quantitative SARS-CoV-2 Serology in Children With Multisystem Inflammatory Syndrome (MIS-C)	PEDIATRICS	71
Yang 2021 [25]	Association of Age With SARS-CoV-2 Antibody Response	JAMA NETWORK OPEN	68
Bartsch 2021 [20]	Humoral signatures of protective and pathological SARS-CoV-2 infection in children	NATURE MEDICINE	60
Tosif 2020 [26]	Immune responses to SARS-CoV-2 in three children of parents with symptomatic COVID-19	NATURE COMMUNICATIONS	56

Table 2. Cont.

First Author Year [Ref.]	Document Title	Journal	Citations
Pierce 2021 [22]	Natural mucosal barriers and COVID-19 in children	JCI INSIGHT	47
Selva 2021 [27]	Systems serology detects functionally distinct coronavirus antibody features in children and elderly	NATURE COMMUNICATIONS	44
Cohen 2021 [28]	SARS-CoV-2 specific T cell responses are lower in children and increase with age and time after infection	NATURE COMMUNICATIONS	37
Anderson 2021 [29]	Severe Acute Respiratory Syndrome-Coronavirus-2 (SARS-CoV-2) Antibody Responses in Children With Multisystem Inflammatory Syndrome in Children (MIS-C) and Mild and Severe Coronavirus Disease 2019 (COVID-19)	JOURNAL OF THE PEDIATRIC INFECTIOUS DISEASES SOCIETY	21
Isoldi 2021 [30]	The comprehensive clinic, laboratory, and instrumental evaluation of children with COVID-19: A 6-months prospective study	JOURNAL OF MEDICAL VIROLOGY	19
Lau 2021 [31]	Long-term persistence of SARS-CoV-2 neutralizing antibody responses after infection and estimates of the duration of protection	ECLINICALMEDICINE	19
Woudenberg 2021 [32]	Humoral immunity to SARS-CoV-2 and seasonal coronaviruses in children and adults in north-eastern France	EBIOMEDICINE	18
Shrwani 2021 [33]	Detection of Serum Cross-Reactive Antibodies and Memory Response to SARS-CoV-2 in Prepandemic and Post-COVID-19 Convalescent Samples	JOURNAL OF INFECTIOUS DISEASES	17
Sermet-Gaudelus 2021 [34]	Prior infection by seasonal coronaviruses, as assessed by serology, does not prevent SARS-CoV-2 infection and disease in children, France, April to June 2020	EUROSURVEILLANCE	17
Toh 2022 [35]	Comparison of Seroconversion in Children and Adults With Mild COVID-19	JAMA NETWORK OPEN	16
Bloise 2021 [36]	Serum IgG levels in children 6 months after SARS-CoV-2 infection and comparison with adults	EUROPEAN JOURNAL OF PEDIATRICS	14
Seery 2021 [37]	Blood neutrophils from children with COVID-19 exhibit both inflammatory and anti-inflammatory markers	EBIOMEDICINE	13
Keuning 2021 [38]	Saliva SARS-CoV-2 Antibody Prevalence in Children	MICROBIOLOGY SPECTRUM	13
Vilibic-Cavlek 2021 [39]	SARS-CoV-2 Seroprevalence and Neutralizing Antibody Response after the First and Second COVID-19 Pandemic Wave in Croatia	PATHOGENS	12

In total, 57 journals published research articles in the field. The journals with the highest number of publications were Nature Communications (4 articles), Frontiers in Pediatrics (3), JAMA Network Open (3), Pathogens (3), Frontiers in Immunology (3), JCI Insight (3), eBioMedicine (3) and the Journal of Clinical Medicine (3); meanwhile, the journals that had the highest number of citations were the Journal of Pediatrics (1 article/192 citations), Science Translational Medicine (1/167), Nature Communications (4/140) and iScience (1/119).

Factorial analysis was used to identify the topics in the publications. Based on a keywords analysis, two clusters were identified (Figure 6). The red cluster includes the main terms related to the antibody responses and clinical characteristics exhibited in COVID-19 symptomatic and asymptomatic pediatric patients (included terms: IgG, IgM, IgA, spike, RBD, seropositive, seroprevalence, immunity, clinical, symptoms), while the blue cluster refers to SARS-CoV-2 antibody responses in the case of severe and MISC pediatric patients.

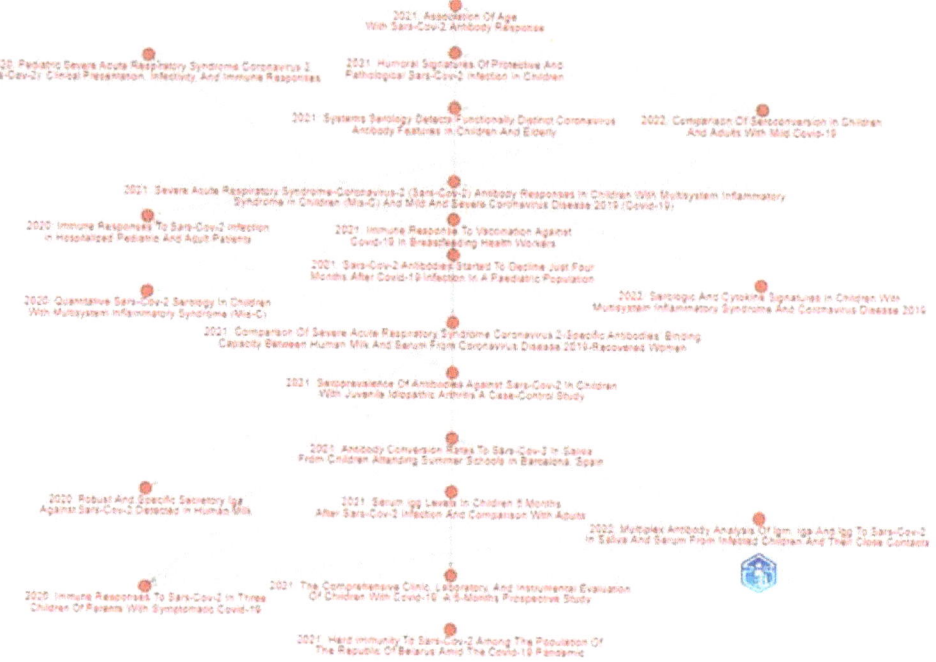

Figure 4. Bibliometrix historical analysis of direct citation of top-cited papers related to the researched topic. The nodes in the figure represent documents and the directional arrow represents the citation association between two documents.

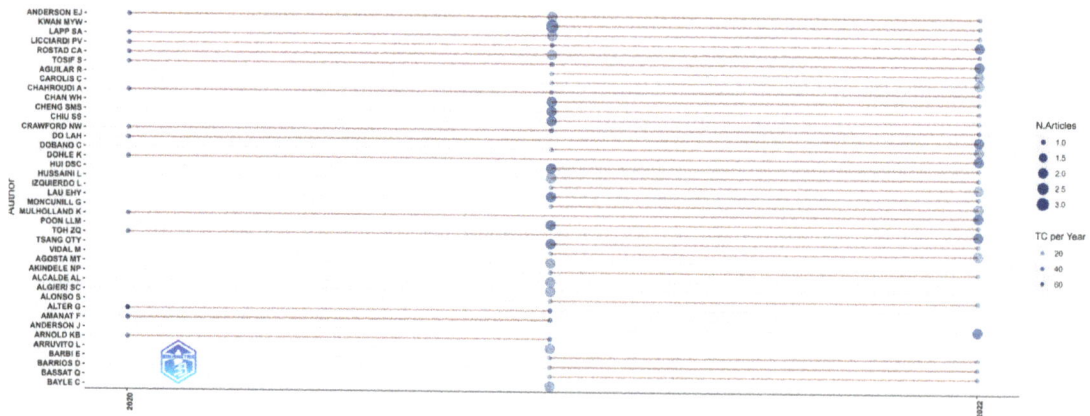

Figure 5. Top authors' production over time in the research field. The size of the circle is directly proportional to the number of documents, the shade of the color represents the number of citations; TC per Year—Total Citation per year.

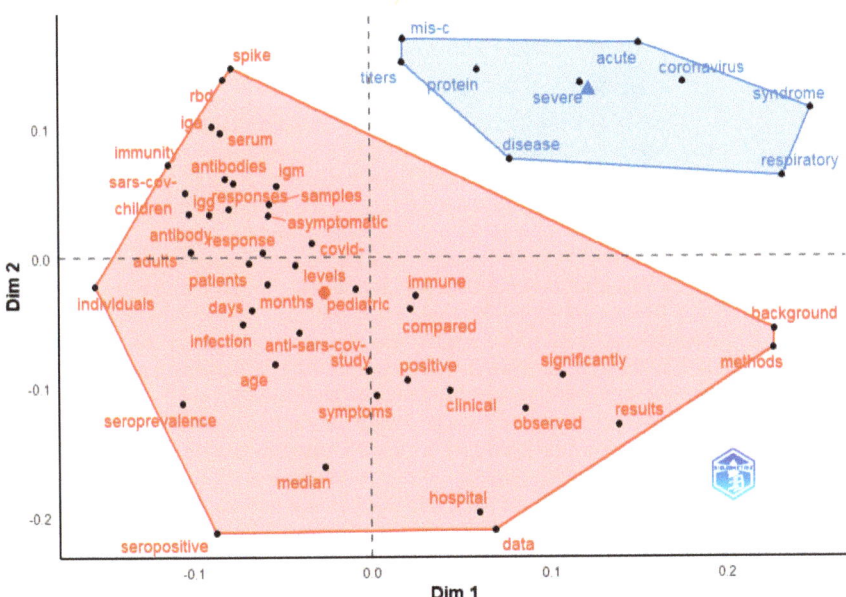

Figure 6. Bibliometrix conceptual structure map of terms from documents abstract. Factorial analysis method—multidimensional scaling.

4. Discussion

There have been a large number of articles published on COVID-19 since the beginning of the pandemic. Our bibliometric review focused on a specific portion of the scientific literature: those publications on the topic of SARS-CoV-2 antibody responses in the pediatric population. The analysis carried out using VOSviewer and Bibliometrix showed publication patterns, as well as country/organization/author collaborations. The country networks showed that the USA, Republic of China, and Italy were the most prolific countries in the field, while the most cited ones were the USA, Canada, and Australia. Moreover, collaboration patterns can be observed between the USA–Netherlands–Australia–Japan–France–China; UK–Italy–India–Israel; and Russia–Austria–Poland–Belarus. In Australia, the University of Melbourne, in the USA, Emory University, and in China, the University of Hong Kong and the Chinese University of Hong Kong, collaborated on research with other institutions; meanwhile, collaboration between the Harvard Medical School–Massachusetts General Hospital–Brigham and Women's Hospital, and the Albert Einstein College of Medicine–Children's Hospital at Montefiore–Montefiore Medical Center–Yale University, led to the publication of articles on the list of top ten most cited articles related to the analyzed topic. An analysis of the studies conducted by research centers/institutes revealed a focus on performing comparative analyses between the coronavirus antibody responses present in children and adults/elderly with COVID-19, and/or healthy patients (University of Melbourne, Australia), the inflammatory markers and SARS-CoV-2 antibody profiles of MIS-C patients (University of Melbourne, USA), humoral and cellular (T cell) responses, and the long-term persistence of SARS-CoV-2-neutralizing antibody responses in recovered children and adolescents (University of Hong Kong and the Chinese University of Hong Kong, China). Articles were published in journals concerning pediatrics, medicine in general and internal, research and experimental science, biochemistry and molecular biology, cell biology, microbiology, immunology and multidisciplinary sciences. The results of the keywords analysis identified two clusters, including terms related to the antibody responses and clinical characteristics exhibited in COVID-19 symptomatic and asymptomatic pediatric patients, and terms related to SARS-CoV-2 antibody responses in the case of severe and MISC pediatric patients.

4.1. Antibodies Levels and Disease Severity

In the analyzed studies, the SARS-CoV-2 antibodies were detected in serum/plasma, mucosa/nasal fluid, saliva, breast milk, and cerebrospinal fluid.

In the study of [40], the positive rates of anti-spike IgG, antiSARS-CoV-2 IgG, and of neutralizing antibodies in the case of symptomatic children gradually increased and reached 100% within 14–28 days after onset, and there was a plateau at two months after the onset of COVID-19 symptoms. In contrast, positive anti-S IgA were detected within 14–28 days after onset in both symptomatic (75%) and asymptomatic children (60%).

Disease severity is associated with a greater antibody response [37,41–43]. Akindele et al. [43] reported elevated levels of IgG titers in MISC patients (median 6.75, IQR 0.84–10.88) compared with acute COVID-19 patients (median 2.98, IQR 0.28–5.76), but the difference was not statistically significant ($p = 0.241$). A study from India [44] reported a median IgG antibody titer of 54.8 AU/mL (range 11.09–170.9), with significantly higher levels among children with MISC (median 60.3 AU/mL, range: 12.3–170.9 vs. children without MISC—median 54.8 AU/mL, range 11.0–144.3), and with significantly lower levels among children with MISC needing intensive care (PICU) (median 45.72, range: 18.92–156.37 vs. children who did not require PICU—median 81.28, range: 12.32–170.21). The study [45] reported high anti-spike IgG and IgA levels (in the sera and saliva of young infants compared with their parents) and low but detectable SARS-CoV-2-specific $CD4^+$ and $CD8^+$ T cell responses in young infants. In terms of IgM, the study from India [44] reported positive SARS-CoV-2 IgM antibodies in only 14% of children from the study. All children with positive IgM had no features suggestive of MISC and half of them also had a positive IgG test result. The median IgM antibody titer was 31.1 AU/mL (range 11.9–139.9). The study [24] reported that 100% of MIS-C and 80% of COVID-19 patients had detectable IgM antibodies against SARS-CoV-2 RBD (indicating a recent SARS-CoV-2 infection.)

The results of another study [36] showed that the IgM and IgG antibody levels were significantly lower at 180 days after infection in children (IgM median 0.74 (0.64–1.01) AU/mL, IgG median 16.53 (9.1–24.1) AU/mL) compared with levels at 30 days (IgM median 1.29 (1.02–1.47) AU/mL, IgG median 90.61 (71.5–101) AU/mL). Moreover, at 180 days after infection in children, these were at a lower level compared to their parents (parents IgM median 0.83 (0.53–1.19) AU/mL, IgG median 92.7 (44.1–163.3) AU/mL).

In study [22], both anti-SARS-CoV-2 IgA and IgG were quantified in nasal fluid and showed similar levels. In the study of [46], breast milk and serum anti-SARS-CoV-2 IgG and IgA, in the case of vaccinated breastfeeding women, were reported. The breast milk IgG and IgA levels were highly correlated ($r = 0.89$; $r = 0.83$, $p < 0.001$) to serum IgG and IgA levels.

Higher antibody levels were observed in symptomatic children in comparison with asymptomatic cases. In study [47], symptomatic children had significantly higher IgM levels (N CT, N FL, RBD, RBD Alpha, RBD Beta, RBD Gamma, RBD Delta, S, S1, S2) and IgG levels (N FL, RBD, RBD Alpha, RBD Beta, RBD Delta, RBD Gamma, S, and S2) in comparison with asymptomatic cases.

Children with MISC had higher antibody levels than non-MISC cases. In study [47], pediatric patients with MISC had significantly higher IgG levels (N FL, N CT, the S, S1, S2, RBD located in S1, from the Wuhan strain, RBD Alpha, RBD Beta, RBD Gamma, RBD Delta), higher IgA levels (for all tested antigens, except N-CT), and higher IgM levels (RBD, RBD Alpha, RBD Delta, S1) in comparison with non-MISC cases. In study [19], elevated IgM and IgG SARS-CoV-2 levels were observed in severe MISC cases in comparison with mild MISC cases. In a prospective study [24] analyzing children with MISC, symptomatic COVID-19, Kawasaki disease (KD), and hospitalized pediatric controls, higher levels of IgM, RBD IgG, full-length spike, and nucleocapsid protein antibody titers were encountered in the case of MISC in comparison to other groups. In addition, study [29] reported elevated levels of IgG antibody titers against SRBD and full-length S, and IgA antibody titers against full-length S (but not S-RBD) in patients with MISC compared to patients with severe COVID-19 (majority of whom had undetectable levels of the spike or nucleocapsid proteins of IgG antibodies). In the case of IgM antibody titers and anti-SARS-CoV-2 N antibodies, the differences were not statistically significant. The same study also reported no differences between the IgG antibody (directed to spike or nucleocapsid proteins) levels in children with or without immunodeficiency.

A correlation between saliva and plasma antibodies has been detected in COVID-19 pediatric patients [48]. The collection of SARS-CoV-2-specific saliva antibodies is a cost-effective, non-invasive and easy assay that may be used to determine levels of immunity after infection or immunization with COVID-19 vaccines, at an individual or population level [48,49].

Immunoglobulin A has an important role in fighting infectious pathogens from the point of entry (respiratory and digestive system), acting as an immune barrier; it has the ability to neutralize them before they enter the body and bind to epithelial cells [50]. A systematic review and meta-analysis of the role of IgA in COVID-19 diagnosis or severity, including 38 scientific articles from PubMed database, observed that IgA production correlates with disease severity (IgA is produced more effectively in patients after severe disease compared with mild or asymptomatic patients), and concluded that further studies should establish the roles of mucosal/systemic IgA responses in the protection/immunopathology of COVID-19 [51]. Mucosal vaccination therapy may be an effective treatment strategy by which to induce a local protective immunity within the mucosa.

4.2. Relationship between SARS-CoV-2 Antibodies and Inflammatory Markers

Several studies have analyzed the correlations between SARS-CoV-2 antibodies and cytokines, chemokines, neutrophils, C-reactive protein (CRP), ferritin (a marker of macrophage activation) and the erythrocyte sedimentation rate (ESR—systemic inflammation marker).

Some studies have analyzed antibody and cytokine responses in COVID-19 pediatric patients in order to investigate the relationship between the early responses of inflammatory cytokines, the late-stage responses of anti-SARS-CoV-2 IgG/IgM antibodies, and disease severity. The invasion of SARS-CoV-2 leads to the activation of innate immunity, and to determinate host cells initiating the inflammatory response and the release of large amount of cytokines and chemokines [52–55]. The results of a study analyzing anti–SARS-CoV-2 IgG/IgA, cytokines, and total protein using nasal mucosal secretions [22] indicated that there was not a strong correlation between antibodies and cytokines (IL-1, IFN-α2, IFN-γ, IP-10, IL-8, IL-1α, IL-1β, IL1-RA, MCP1), except for IL-18. There was a strong inverse correlation between IL-18 and anti–SARS-CoV-2 IgG (anti-S1, anti-S2, anti-RBD and anti-NC) and IgA (anti-S1, anti-S2, anti-RBD, anti-NC). In a study [56] analyzing SARS-CoV-2 antibody profiles in a case series of five children with neuropsychiatric symptoms associated with COVID-19, the antibodies of four SARS-CoV-2 antigens (S1 N-terminal domain (NTD), the S1 receptor binding domain (RBD), full-length spike (S), nucleocapsid (N)) correlated with pro-inflammatory cytokines and chemokines (in this study, the SARS-CoV-2 antibodies, cytokines, and chemokines were collected from cerebrospinal fluid). In particular, the antibodies to the N protein correlated most strongly with pro-inflammatory cytokines (GM-CSF, IL-2, IL-8, IL-13, IP-10, MCP-1, MIP-1 β, and TNF-α). Another study [43] reported higher levels of 14 of 37 cytokines/chemokines (IL-1RA, IL-2RA, IL-6, IL-8, tumor necrosis factor-α, IL-10, IL-15, IL-18, MCP-1, IP-10, MIP-1α, MCP-2, MIP-1β, eotaxin, regardless of age or sex, duration of symptoms, length of hospital stay, nasopharyngeal viral RNA levels) and high IgG titers in children with MIS-C compared to those with acute COVID-19. The study of [37] suggests a differentiation (that might be used at hospital admission) between symptomatic (mild/moderate) and asymptomatic patients based on the neutrophil expression of CD64 and serum levels of IgG antibodies (spike protein of SARS-CoV-2); there were higher levels in symptomatic patients compared with asymptomatic patients. A study from India [44] also reported increased neutrophil counts and higher levels of IgG antibodies in children with MISC compared with COVID-19 patients without MISC. Pierce and colaborators [22] reported that SARS-CoV-2-specific IgA and IgG concentrations were detected in nasopharyngeal samples, being negatively correlated with mucosal IL-18 levels. IL-18, a cytokine predominantly produced by macrophages, under the action of the NLRP3 inflammasome is cleaved to its active form and then the production of IFN-γ takes place. The early release of IL-18 is thought to moderate the adaptive response, with elevated serum levels of IL-18 being associated with disease severity. IFN-β1 was used for the early treatment of COVID-19 according to the study [57]. The results showed an association between disease severity and the joint action of various cytokines and chemokines. These findings of cytokine/chemokine dysregulation are consistent with results from studies on adults [55,58–61].

In study [19], in the case of MIS-C patients, NT-proBNP significantly positively correlated with IgG SARS-CoV-2 RBD ($p = 0.008$), but not with IgM SARS-CoV-2 BRD ($p = 0.73$). Correlation between SARS-CoV-2 IgG and NT-proBNP could indicate mechanism/disease severity. In the same study, no correlation between CRP and IgM/IgG SARS-CoV-2 RBD was encountered, while ferritin positively correlated with IgM/IgG SARS-CoV-2 BRD ($p = 0.03/0.10$). Ferritin (high) levels and their correlation with SARS-CoV-2 serology suggest an interplay between SARS-CoV-2 antibodies and monocyte/macrophage activation in MIS-C patients. In study [24], also in the case of MIS-C patients, RBD IgG antibody levels correlated with the erythrocyte sedimentation rate ($p = 0.046$), but not with CRP.

Overall, this study provides insights into the research directions in the field of SARS-CoV-2 antibody responses in the pediatric population and may provide a starting point for the future research directions of practitioners/policymakers/researchers/patients/organizations, etc. The study was limited to documents published in English, from WOS, up to November 2022. Searches using other databases, such as Scopus, PubMed, EMBASE, Google Scholar, Dimension, etc., and using a different time range (taking into account the growing body of scientific literature) may give a different set of records.

Author Contributions: Conceptualization, M.T. and I.M.; methodology, I.M., M.T., G.C.M. and N.G.; software, I.M. and G.C.M.; validation, M.T., E.A., L.D. and N.G.; formal analysis, I.M. and M.T.; investigation, M.T., E.A., L.D., N.G., I.M. and G.C.M.; data curation, M.T., I.M. and G.C.M.; writing—original draft preparation, M.T. and I.M.; writing—review and editing, M.T., I.M. and G.C.M. All authors have read and agreed to the published version of the manuscript.

Funding: Project financed by Lucian Blaga University of Sibiu through the research grant LBUS-IRG-2022-08.

Institutional Review Board Statement: Not applicable.

Informed Consent Statement: Not applicable.

Data Availability Statement: The data are available on request from the correspondent author.

Conflicts of Interest: The authors declare no conflict of interest.

References

1. Zheng, J.; Deng, Y.; Zhao, Z.; Mao, B.; Lu, M.; Lin, Y.; Huang, A. Characterization of SARS-CoV-2-specific humoral immunity and its potential applications and therapeutic prospects. *Cell. Mol. Immunol.* **2021**, *19*, 150–157. [CrossRef] [PubMed]
2. Kudlay, D.; Kofiadi, I.; Khaitov, M. Peculiarities of the T Cell Immune Response in COVID-19. *Vaccines* **2022**, *10*, 242. [CrossRef] [PubMed]
3. Deeks, J.J.; Dinnes, J.; Takwoingi, Y.; Davenport, C.; Spijker, R.; Taylor-Phillips, S.; Adriano, A.; Beese, S.; Dretzke, J.; Di Ruffano, L.F.; et al. Antibody tests for identification of current and past infection with SARS-CoV-2. *Cochrane Database Syst. Rev.* **2020**, *6*, CD013652. [PubMed]
4. VanEck, N.; Waltman, L. Software survey: VOSviewer, a computer program for bibliometric mapping. *Scientometrics* **2010**, *84*, 523–538. [CrossRef]
5. VanEck, N.J.; Waltman, L. *VOSviewer Manual*; Univeristeit Leiden: Leiden, The Netherlands, 2013.
6. Hosseini, M.R.; Martek, I.; Zavadskas, E.K.; Aibinu, A.A.; Arashpour, M.; Chileshe, N. Critical evaluation of off-site construction research: A Scientometric analysis. *Autom. Constr.* **2018**, *87*, 235–247. [CrossRef]

7. Grosseck, G.; Țîru, L.G.; Bran, R.A. Education for sustainable development: Evolution and perspectives: A bibliometric review of research, 1992–2018. *Sustainability* **2019**, *11*, 6136. [CrossRef]
8. Maniu, I.; Costea, R.; Maniu, G.; Neamtu, B.M. Inflammatory Biomarkers in Febrile Seizure: A Comprehensive Bibliometric, Review and Visualization Analysis. *Brain Sci.* **2021**, *11*, 1077. [CrossRef]
9. Fiore, U.; Florea, A.; Kifor, C.V.; Zanetti, P. Digitization, Epistemic Proximity, and the Education System: Insights from a Bibliometric Analysis. *J. Risk Financ. Manag.* **2021**, *14*, 267. [CrossRef]
10. Gajdosikova, D.; Valaskova, K. A Systematic Review of Literature and Comprehensive Bibliometric Analysis of Capital Structure Issue. *Manag. Dyn. Knowl. Econ.* **2022**, *10*, 210–224.
11. Cretu, D.M.; Morandau, F. Initial Teacher Education for Inclusive Education: A Bibliometric Analysis of Educational Research. *Sustainability* **2020**, *12*, 4923. [CrossRef]
12. Tomaszewska, E.J.; Florea, A. Urban smart mobility in the scientific literature—Bibliometric analysis. *Eng. Manag. Prod. Serv.* **2018**, *10*, 41–56. [CrossRef]
13. Maniu, I.; Maniu, G.; Totan, M. Clinical and Laboratory Characteristics of Pediatric COVID-19 Population—A Bibliometric Analysis. *J. Clin. Med.* **2022**, *11*, 5987. [CrossRef] [PubMed]
14. Morante-Carballo, F.; Montalván-Burbano, N.; Arias-Hidalgo, M.; Domínguez-Granda, L.; Apolo-Masache, B.; Carrión-Mero, P. Flood Models: An Exploratory Analysis and Research Trends. *Water* **2022**, *14*, 2488. [CrossRef]
15. Fiore, U.; Florea, A.; Pérez Lechuga, G. An Interdisciplinary Review of Smart Vehicular Traffic and Its Applications and Challenges. *J. Sens. Actuator Netw.* **2019**, *8*, 13. [CrossRef]
16. Florea, A. Digital design skills for factories of the future. In Proceedings of the 9th International Conference on Manufacturing Science and Education—MSE 2019 "Trends in New Industrial Revolution", Sibiu, Romania, 5–7 June 2019; Volume 290, p. 14002.
17. Ratiu, A.; Maniu, I.; Pop, E.-L. EntreComp Framework: A Bibliometric Review and Research Trends. *Sustainability* **2023**, *15*, 1285. [CrossRef]
18. Aria, M.; Cuccurullo, C. Bibliometrix: An R-tool for comprehensive science mapping analysis. *J. Informetr.* **2017**, *11*, 959–975. [CrossRef]
19. Yonker, L.M.; Neilan, A.M.; Bartsch, Y.; Patel, A.B.; Regan, J.; Arya, P.; Gootkind, E.; Park, G.; Hardcastle, M.; St. John, A.; et al. Pediatric severe acute respiratory syndrome coronavirus 2 (SARS-CoV-2): Clinical presentation, infectivity, and immune responses. *J. Pediatr.* **2020**, *227*, 45–52. [CrossRef]
20. Bartsch, Y.C.; Wang, C.; Zohar, T.; Fischinger, S.; Atyeo, C.; Burke, J.S.; Kang, J.; Edlow, A.G.; Fasano, A.; Baden, L.R.; et al. Humoral signatures of protective and pathological SARS-CoV-2 infection in children. *Nat. Med.* **2021**, *27*, 454–462. [CrossRef]
21. Pierce, C.A.; Preston-Hurlburt, P.; Dai, Y.; Aschner, C.B.; Cheshenko, N.; Galen, B.; Garforth, S.J.; Herrera, N.G.; Jangra, R.K.; Morano, N.C.; et al. Immune responses to SARS-CoV-2 infection in hospitalized pediatric and adult patients. *Sci. Transl. Med.* **2020**, *12*, eabd5487. [CrossRef]
22. Pierce, C.A.; Sy, S.; Galen, B.; Goldstein, D.Y.; Orner, E.; Keller, M.J.; Herold, K.C.; Herold, B.C. Natural mucosal barriers and COVID-19 in children. *JCI Insight* **2021**, *6*, e148694. [CrossRef]
23. Fox, A.; Marino, J.; Amanat, F.; Krammer, F.; Hahn-Holbrook, J.; Zolla-Pazner, S.; Powell, R.L. Robust and specific secretory IgAagainst SARS-CoV-2 detected in human milk. *iScience* **2020**, *23*, 101735. [CrossRef] [PubMed]
24. Rostad, C.A.; Chahroudi, A.; Mantus, G.; Lapp, S.A.; Teherani, M.; Macoy, L.; Tarquinio, K.M.; Basu, K.R.; Kao, C.; Linam, W.M.; et al. Quantitative SARS-CoV-2 serology in children with multisystem inflammatory syndrome (MIS-C). *Pediatrics* **2020**, *146*, e2020018242. [CrossRef] [PubMed]
25. Yang, H.S.; Costa, V.; Racine-Brzostek, S.E.; Acker, K.P.; Yee, J.; Chen, Z.; Karbaschi, M.; Zuk, R.; Rand, S.; Sukhu, A.; et al. Association of age with SARS-CoV-2 antibody response. *JAMA Netw. Open* **2021**, *4*, e214302. [CrossRef]
26. Tosif, S.; Neeland, M.R.; Sutton, P.; Licciardi, P.V.; Sarkar, S.; Selva, K.J.; Do, L.A.H.; Donato, C.; Quan Toh, Z.; Higgins, R.; et al. Immune Responses to SARS-CoV-2 in Three Children of Parents with Symptomatic COVID-19. *Nat. Commun.* **2020**, *11*, 5703. [CrossRef] [PubMed]
27. Selva, K.J.; van de Sandt, C.E.; Lemke, M.M.; Lee, C.Y.; Shoffner, S.K.; Chua, B.Y.; Davis, S.K.; Nguyen, T.H.O.; Rowntree, L.C.; Hensen, L.; et al. Systems Serology Detects Functionally Distinct Coronavirus Antibody Features in Children and Elderly. *Nat. Commun.* **2021**, *12*, 2037. [CrossRef]
28. Cohen, C.A.; Li, A.P.Y.; Hachim, A.; Hui, D.S.C.; Kwan, M.Y.W.; Tsang, O.T.Y.; Chiu, S.S.; Chan, W.H.; Yau, Y.S.; Kavian, N.; et al. SARS-CoV-2 Specific T Cell Responses Are Lower in Children and Increase with Age and Time after Infection. *Nat. Commun.* **2021**, *12*, 4678. [CrossRef]
29. Anderson, E.M.; Diorio, C.; Goodwin, E.C.; McNerney, K.O.; Weirick, M.E.; Gouma, S.; Bolton, M.J.; Arevalo, C.P.; Chase, J.; Hicks, P. Severe acute respiratory syndrome-coronavirus-2 (SARS-CoV-2) antibody responses in children with multisystem inflammatory syndrome in children (MIS-C) and mild and severe coronavirus disease 2019 (COVID-19). *J. Pediatr. Infect. Dis. Soc.* **2021**, *10*, 669–673. [CrossRef]
30. Isoldi, S.; Mallardo, S.; Marcellino, A.; Bloise, S.; Dilillo, A.; Iorfida, D.; Testa, A.; Del Giudice, E.; Martucci, V.; Sanseviero, M.; et al. The comprehensive clinic, laboratory, and instrumental evaluation of children with COVID-19: A 6-months prospective study. *J. Med. Virol.* **2021**, *93*, 3122–3132. [CrossRef]

31. Lau, E.H.; Hui, D.S.; Tsang, O.T.; Chan, W.H.; Kwan, M.Y.; Chiu, S.S.; Cheng, S.M.; Ko, R.W.; Li, J.K.; Chaothai, S.; et al. Long-term persistence of SARS-CoV-2 neutralizing antibody responses after infection and estimates of the duration of protection. *EClinicalMedicine* **2021**, *41*, 101174. [CrossRef]
32. Woudenberg, T.; Pelleau, S.; Anna, F.; Attia, M.; Donnadieu, F.; Gravet, A.; Lohmann, C.; Seraphin, H.; Guiheneuf, R.; Delamare, C.; et al. Humoral immunity to SARS-CoV-2 and seasonal coronaviruses in children and adults in north-eastern France. *EBioMedicine* **2021**, *70*, 103495. [CrossRef]
33. Shrwani, K.; Sharma, R.; Krishnan, M.; Jones, T.; Mayora-Neto, M.; Cantoni, D.; Temperton, N.J.; Dobson, S.L.; Subramaniam, K.; McNamara, P.S.; et al. Detection of Serum Cross-Reactive Antibodies and Memory Response to SARS-CoV-2 in Prepandemic and Post–COVID-19 Convalescent Samples. *J. Infect. Dis.* **2021**, *224*, 1305–1315. [CrossRef] [PubMed]
34. Sermet-Gaudelus, I.; Temmam, S.; Huon, C.; Behillil, S.; Gajdos, V.; Bigot, T.; Lurier, T.; Chrétien, D.; Backovic, M.; Delaunay-Moisan, A.; et al. Prior Infection by Seasonal Coronaviruses, as Assessed by Serology, Does Not Prevent SARS-CoV-2 Infection and Disease in Children, France, April to June 2020. *Eurosurveillance* **2021**, *26*, 2001782. [CrossRef] [PubMed]
35. Toh, Z.Q.; Anderson, J.; Mazarakis, N.; Neeland, M.; Higgins, R.A.; Rautenbacher, K.; Dohle, K.; Nguyen, J.; Overmars, I.; Donato, C.; et al. Comparison of Seroconversion in Children and Adults with Mild COVID-19. *JAMA Netw. Open.* **2022**, *5*, e221313. [CrossRef]
36. Bloise, S.; Marcellino, A.; Testa, A.; Dilillo, A.; Mallardo, S.; Isoldi, S.; Martucci, V.; Sanseviero, M.T.; Giudice, E.D.; Iorfida, D.; et al. Serum IgG Levels in Children 6 Months after SARS-CoV-2 Infection and Comparison with Adults. *Eur. J. Pediatr.* **2021**, *1850*, 3335–3342. [CrossRef]
37. Seery, V.; Raiden, S.C.; Algieri, S.C.; Grisolía, N.A.; Filippo, D.; De Carli, N.; Di Lalla, S.; Cairoli, H.; Chiolo, M.J.; Meregalli, C.N.; et al. Blood neutrophils from children with COVID-19 exhibit both inflammatory and anti-inflammatory markers. *EBioMedicine* **2021**, *67*, 103357. [CrossRef] [PubMed]
38. Keuning, M.W.; Grobben, M.; de Groen, A.-E.C.; Berman-de Jong, E.P.; Bijlsma, M.W.; Cohen, S.; Felderhof, M.; Pajkrt, D. Saliva SARS-CoV-2 Antibody Prevalence in Children. *Microbiol. Spectr.* **2021**, *9*, e0073121. [CrossRef]
39. Vilibic-Cavlek, T.; Stevanovic, V.; Ilic, M.; Barbic, L.; Capak, K.; Tabain, I.; Krleza, J.L.; Ferenc, T.; Hruskar, Z.; Topic, R.Z.; et al. SARS-CoV-2 Seroprevalence and Neutralizing Antibody Response after the First and Second COVID-19 Pandemic Wave in Croatia. *Pathogens* **2021**, *10*, 774. [CrossRef]
40. Han, M.S.; Um, J.; Lee, E.J.; Kim, K.M.; Chang, S.H.; Lee, H.; Kim, Y.K.; Choi, Y.Y.; Cho, E.Y.; Kim, D.H.; et al. Antibody Responses to SARS-CoV-2 in Children With COVID-19. *J. Pediatr. Infect. Dis Soc.* **2022**, *11*, 267–273. [CrossRef]
41. Gong, F.; Dai, Y.; Zheng, T.; Cheng, L.; Zhao, D.; Wang, H.; Liu, M.; Pei, H.; Jin, T.; Yu, D.; et al. Peripheral CD4+ T cell subsets and antibody response in COVID-19 convalescent individuals. *J. Clin. Investig.* **2020**, *130*, 6588–6599. [CrossRef]
42. Lucas, C.; Klein, J.; Sundaram, M.; Liu, F.; Wong, P.; Silva, J.; Mao, T.; Oh, J.E.; Tokuyama, M.; Lu, P.; et al. Kinetics of antibody responses dictate COVID-19 outcome. *medRxiv* **2020**.
43. Peart Akindele, N.; Kouo, T.; Karaba, A.H.; Gordon, O.; Fenstermacher, K.Z.J.; Beaudry, J.; Rubens, J.H.; Atik, C.C.; Zhou, W.; Ji, H.; et al. Distinct cytokine and chemokine dysregulation in hospitalized children with acute Coronavirus Disease 2019 and Multisystem Inflammatory Syndrome with similar levels of nasopharyngeal severe acute respiratory syndrome Coronavirus 2 shedding. *J. Infect. Dis.* **2021**, *224*, 606–615. [CrossRef] [PubMed]
44. Venkataraman, A.; Balasubramanian, S.; Putilibai, S.; Lakshan Raj, S.; Amperayani, S.; Senthilnathan, S.; Manoharan, A.; Sophi, A.; Amutha, R.; Sadasivam, K.; et al. Correlation of SARS-CoV-2 Serology and Clinical Phenotype Amongst Hospitalised Children in a Tertiary Children's Hospital in India. *J. Trop. Pediatr.* **2021**, *67*, fmab015. [CrossRef] [PubMed]
45. Goenka, A.; Halliday, A.; Gregorova, M.; Milodowski, E.; Thomas, A.; Williamson, M.K.; Baum, H.; Oliver, E.; Long, A.E.; Knezevic, L.; et al. Young Infants Exhibit Robust Functional Antibody Responses and Restrained IFN-γ Production to SARS-CoV-2. *Cell Rep. Med.* **2021**, *2*, 100327. [CrossRef] [PubMed]
46. Jakuszko, K.; Kościelska-Kasprzak, K.; Żabińska, M.; Bartoszek, D.; Poznański, P.; Rukasz, D.; Kłak, R.; Królak-Olejnik, B.; Krajewska, M. Immune Response to Vaccination against COVID-19 in Breastfeeding Health Workers. *Vaccines* **2021**, *9*, 663. [CrossRef] [PubMed]
47. De la Torre, E.P.; Obando, I.; Vidal, M.; de Felipe, B.; Aguilar, R.; Izquierdo, L.; Carolis, C.; Olbrich, P.; Capilla-Miranda, A.; Serra, P.; et al. SARS-CoV-2 Seroprevalence Study in Pediatric Patients and Health Care Workers Using Multiplex Antibody Immunoassays. *Viruses* **2022**, *14*, 2039. [CrossRef]
48. Dobaño, C.; Alonso, S.; Vidal, M.; Jiménez, A.; Rubio, R.; Santano, R.; Barrios, D.; Tomas, G.P.; Casas, M.M.; García, M.H.; et al. Multiplex antibody analysis of IgM, IgA and IgG to SARS-CoV-2 in saliva and serum from infected children and their close contacts. *Front. Immunol.* **2022**, *13*, 85. [CrossRef]
49. Li, D.; Calderone, R.; Nsouli, T.M.; Reznikov, E.; Bellanti, J.A. Salivary and serum IgA and IgG responses to SARS-CoV-2-spike protein following SARS-CoV-2 infection and after immunization with COVID-19 vaccines. *Allergy Asthma Proc.* **2022**, *43*, 419–430. [CrossRef]
50. Chao, Y.X.; Rötzschke, O.; Tan, E.K. The role of IgA in COVID-19. *Brain Behav. Immun.* **2020**, *87*, 182. [CrossRef]
51. Rangel-Ramírez, V.V.; Macías-Piña, K.A.; Garrido, R.R.S.; de Alba-Aguayo, D.R.; Moreno-Fierros, L.; Rubio-Infante, N. A systematic review and meta-analysis of the IgA seroprevalence in COVID-19 patients; Is there a role for IgA in COVID-19 diagnosis or severity? *Microbiol. Res.* **2022**, *263*, 127105. [CrossRef]
52. Schultze, J.L.; Aschenbrenner, A.C. COVID-19 and the human innate immune system. *Cell* **2021**, *184*, 1671–1692. [CrossRef]

53. Tay, M.Z.; Poh, C.M.; Rénia, L.; MacAry, P.A.; Ng, L.F. The trinity of COVID-19: Immunity, inflammation and intervention. *Nat. Rev. Immunol.* **2020**, *20*, 363–374. [CrossRef] [PubMed]
54. Lucas, C.; Wong, P.; Klein, J.; Castro, T.B.; Silva, J.; Sundaram, M.; Ellingson, F.K.; Mao, T.; Oh, J.E.; Israelow, B.; et al. Longitudinal analyses reveal immunological misfiring in severe COVID-19. *Nature* **2020**, *584*, 463–469. [CrossRef] [PubMed]
55. Jing, X.; Xu, M.; Song, D.; Yue, T.; Wang, Y.; Zhang, P.; Zhang, Y.; Zhang, M.; Lam, T.T.-K.; Faria, N.R.; et al. Association between inflammatory cytokines and anti-SARS-CoV-2 antibodies in hospitalized patients with COVID-19. *Immun. Ageing* **2022**, *19*, 12. [CrossRef] [PubMed]
56. Ngo, B.; Lapp, S.A.; Siegel, B.; Patel, V.; Hussaini, L.; Bora, S.; Philbrook, B.; Weinschenk, K.; Wright, L.; Anderson, E.J.; et al. Cerebrospinal fluid cytokine, chemokine, and SARS-CoV-2 antibody profiles in children with neuropsychiatric symptoms associated with COVID-19. *Mult. Scler. Relat. Disord.* **2021**, *55*, 103169. [CrossRef]
57. Monk, P.D.; Marsden, R.J.; Tear, V.J.; Brookes, J.; Batten, T.N.; Mankowski, M.; Gabbay, F.J.; Davies, D.E.; Holgate, S.T.; Ho, L.-P.; et al. Safety and efficacy of inhaled nebulised interferon beta-1a (SNG001) for treatment of SARS-CoV-2 infection: A randomised, double-blind, placebo-controlled, phase 2 trial. *Lancet Respir. Med.* **2021**, *9*, 196–206. [CrossRef]
58. Guo, Y.; Li, T.; Xia, X.; Su, B.; Li, H.; Feng, Y.; Han, J.; Wang, X.; Jia, L.; Bao, Z.; et al. Different profiles of antibodies and cytokines were found between severe and moderate COVID-19 patients. *Front. Immunol.* **2021**, *12*, 3344. [CrossRef]
59. Coomes, E.A.; Haghbayan, H. Interleukin-6 in COVID-19: A systematic review and meta-analysis. *Rev. Med. Virol.* **2020**, *30*, 1–9. [CrossRef]
60. Schultheiß, C.; Willscher, E.; Paschold, L.; Gottschick, C.; Klee, B.; Henkes, S.S.; Bosurgi, L.; Dutzmann, J.; Sedding, D.; Frese, T.; et al. The IL-1β, IL-6, and TNF cytokine triad is associated with post-acute sequelae of COVID-19. *Cell Rep. Med.* **2022**, *3*, 100663. [CrossRef]
61. Okba, N.M.; Müller, M.A.; Li, W.; Wang, C.; GeurtsvanKessel, C.H.; Corman, V.M.; Lamers, M.M.; Sikkema, R.S.; De Bruin, E.; Chandler, F.D.; et al. Severe acute respiratory syndrome coronavirus 2− specific antibody responses in coronavirus disease patients. *Emerg. Infect. Dis.* **2020**, *26*, 1478. [CrossRef]

Disclaimer/Publisher's Note: The statements, opinions and data contained in all publications are solely those of the individual author(s) and contributor(s) and not of MDPI and/or the editor(s). MDPI and/or the editor(s) disclaim responsibility for any injury to people or property resulting from any ideas, methods, instructions or products referred to in the content.

MDPI
St. Alban-Anlage 66
4052 Basel
Switzerland
www.mdpi.com

Biomedicines Editorial Office
E-mail: biomedicines@mdpi.com
www.mdpi.com/journal/biomedicines

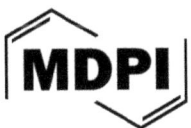

Disclaimer/Publisher's Note: The statements, opinions and data contained in all publications are solely those of the individual author(s) and contributor(s) and not of MDPI and/or the editor(s). MDPI and/or the editor(s) disclaim responsibility for any injury to people or property resulting from any ideas, methods, instructions or products referred to in the content.

www.ingramcontent.com/pod-product-compliance
Lightning Source LLC
LaVergne TN
LVHW070651100526
838202LV00013B/936